Medical Nutrition Therapy for Dietary Managers

By Sue Grossbauer, RD

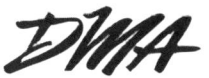

Copyright © 2004 Dietary Managers Association
406 Surrey Woods Dr
St. Charles, IL 60174

www.dmaonline.org

ISBN 0-9753476-0-8

Printed in the United States of America

ACKNOWLEDGEMENTS

We would like to express our appreciation to many individuals who have contributed to the development of this textbook, including Karen Eich Drummond, EdD, RD, FADA and Linda S. Eck, MBA, RD, FADA, as an enormous amount of their content developed for the DMA book, *Diet Therapy for the Dietary Manager, Third Edition*, has been adapted for this textbook.

In addition, we would like to recognize the enormous contributions of the review team who generously invested their professional expertise and valuable time to offer many recommendations for achieving the educational objectives of this textbook:

Charalee Allen, RD, LD
Cincinnati, OH

Yvette M. LeBlanc, PhD, LDN, RD
Lake Charles, LA

Bonnie Bakos, MS, RD
Johnstown, PA

Helenka Livingston, MS, RD
Oakland, CA

Marian Benz, RD, MS, CDE
Wauwatosa, WI

Grace Mitchell, RD, LDN
Tega Cay, SC

Jodie Ferrari, MS, RD, CDN
White Plains, NY

Cynthia Piland, MS, RD, LD
LaGrange, TX

Nancy Norwell Gasser, MS, RD, LD
Madison, WI

Becky Rude, MS, RD
Grand Forks, ND

Juanita Gunnell, MS, RD, LDN
Lincolnton, NC

Nancy Satterwhite, RD, LD
Hickory, NC

Beth Harrell, MS, RD, LD
Lee's Summit, MD

Linda Wozniak, RD, LDN
Hendersonville, NC

Christina Hasemann, MS, RD, CDN
Binghamton, NY

Furthermore, the ongoing efforts of the developers of the Dietary Manager Training Curriculum, Susan Davis Allen, MS, RD, Marian Benz, MS, RD, and The Certifying Board for Dietary Managers have done much to focus the development of this textbook.

We also wish to express gratitude for the intensive efforts of the editorial and production team of The Grossbauer Group in Chesterton, IN:

Sarah Holden and Susie Burnett

Finally, we express heartfelt thanks to

Pam Himrod, RD, CDM, CFPP, DMA Director of Education

and the entire staff of DMA for their support and direction, their ongoing commitment to enhancing the profession of dietary management, and their dedication to the members of Dietary Managers Association.

A PERSONAL INVITATION

We at Dietary Managers Association would like to extend a personal invitation to every student enrolled in a dietary manager training program to join DMA. We recognize the value of your career choice, and would like to offer you the many benefits of DMA membership. As a student, you are welcome to join today and establish your professional footing through your participation in this professional association.

Dietary Managers Association (DMA) is a national not-for-profit association established in 1960 that today has over 15,000 professionals dedicated to the mission: "to provide optimum nutritional care through foodservice management."

DMA is the premier resource for foodservice managers, directors, and those aspiring to careers in food service management. DMA achieves its mission through:

Education

Advocacy

Networking

Research

DMA members work in hospitals, longterm care, schools, correctional facilities, and other non-commercial settings. The association provides foodservice reference, publications and resources, employment services for members, continuing education and professional development, and certification programs. DMA monitors industry trends and legislative issues, and publishes one of the industry's most respected magazines, *DIETARY MANAGER*.

The DMA Annual Meeting & Expo also offers a unique opportunity to enjoy timely educational sessions and network with colleagues. DMA also provides industry leadership in the area of food protection, and offers online resources about food safety and sanitation.

For more information about DMA, please contact Dietary Managers Association by telephone at 800.323.1908 or 630.587.6336, or visit the DMA website at www.dmaonline.org to join online.

TABLE OF CONTENTS

CHAPTER 1 FOOD PREFERENCES AND CUSTOMS

To provide nutritional care, dietary managers need to understand what motivates people to eat, and how clients choose their foods. Dietary managers also need to recognize cultural, religious, and regional influences on food choices.

After completing this chapter, you should be able to:

- ▶ Explain that food is not only nutrition, but that it also has cultural, religious, social, and psychological meanings.
- ▶ List factors that influence food choices.
- ▶ List food preferences associated with religious beliefs and cultural traditions.
- ▶ Identify factors that may affect food intake.

Food is essential for life. In this book, you will learn a great deal about nutrition science. As you will learn in later chapters, food provides many nutrients. Without these nutrients, we could not survive. However, food means more than survival. People do not eat based on science alone. In fact, most of us have complex reasons for choosing the foods we do. In addition, the choices we make each time we eat are quite individual.

Food has many meanings, even though we may not think about these meanings from day to day. To provide effective dietary care, it is important to recognize what food means to individuals, and how dietary choices come about.

First, consider food as part of our culture. To understand this aspect of food, try asking yourself some questions. What does *turkey and dressing with cranberry sauce* mean to you? Many people will answer: *Thanksgiving*. This food has become part of a cultural tradition. Now, think about a wedding celebration. What food will always be served? Most people will answer: *a wedding cake*. Or, in China, the answer may be: *roasted pig*. Now, try another question. What food has become a symbol of American heritage and pride? Many people will answer: *apple pie*. From these examples, you can see that we regard food choices as cultural symbols. The meaning of these foods is much deeper than a sum of protein, carbohydrate, fat, vitamins, and minerals—the sheer nutritional values. When we want to reinforce a cultural event, we often choose food accordingly.

Clearly, food choices have some depth, and reflect who we are as a group—and as individuals. Let's take a closer look at some of the factors that influence what foods we choose, and how we feel about dietary choices. These factors include: cultural heritage, regional trends, religious practices, social and emotional meanings, availability of food, personal taste, aesthetic influences, attitudes and values, lifestyle, and personal health.

CULTURAL HERITAGE

No one is born craving beans and rice, or lamb chops, or pot roast with potatoes and pearl onions, or fast food French fries. Many food choices arise from what we learn through our own cultural experiences. Holidays, festivals, and important events each have associated foods. In addition, daily food choices vary by culture. Traditional German cuisine, for example, is likely to include sausage, schnitzel, spaetzel, beer, and other specialties. Japanese cuisine includes sushi, tempura, and rice. Swedish cuisine may include pancakes, even at meals other than breakfast. Mexican cuisine includes staples such as tortillas, rice, and refried beans. Creole cuisine, popular in New Orleans, represents a synthesis of French cooking with locally available foods, and the influences of Caribbean and Spanish cultures.

As a land of immigrants, the US enjoys multi-faceted cultural diversity. Our food choices are as rich and complex as our population itself. Here are more examples of cultural and ethnic food influences:

Latinos. Latinos are individuals of Latin American or Spanish background. Their diet contains a variety of vegetables. The major meats used are hamburger and chicken. These meats are often mixed with vegetables. Legumes are a good source of protein. Milk is not widely used, but cheese is a frequent ingredient. Corn is an important grain and is often used to make tortillas. Foods are often highly seasoned with chili peppers, onion, or garlic. Coffee with hot milk is a common beverage.

Indian Americans (from India). Staples of the Indian diet include rice, beans, lentils, and bread. Rice is usually served steamed and mixed with flavorings. Indian breads include chapatis, round flatbread made of whole wheat flour, and naan, a bread that uses yeast. Many Indians are Hindus and believe that cows are sacred, so they do not eat beef. Chicken or lamb is sometimes used. Dried beans, lentils, and split peas are popular in vegetarian dishes. Vegetables are often fried in vegetable oil with spices. Vegetables may also be mashed and shaped into balls and fried. Onions, garlic, and ginger are used for flavoring. Popular vegetables include cauliflower, okra, potatoes, and spinach. Most Indian main dishes are accompanied by chutneys or raitas. Chutney is a relish made from fruits, vegetables, and herbs. Raita is yogurt mixed with grated vegetables. Indian cooking also uses many strong spices. The heart of Indian cooking is the combination of spices that gives each dish its unique flavor.

Chinese Americans. Vegetables, rice and noodles, fruits, and foods made from soybeans (such as tofu and soy milk) are very important foods in the Chinese-American diet. Plain rice is served at all meals. Sometimes fried rice is served. Fried rice is made by adding egg to plain rice and stir-frying it. Pork, poultry, and fish are popular. Foods are often seasoned with soy sauce, which is high in sodium. (Low-sodium versions can be purchased). Corn oil, sesame oil, and peanut oil are used. Tea is the main beverage and it is always enjoyed black—without sugar, cream, or milk. Cow's milk and dairy products are not used often. Fruits are important and few sweets are eaten.

Japanese Americans. Some people are surprised to learn that Japanese food is quite different in appearance and taste from Chinese food. While Chinese food is often stir-fried, Japanese food is often simmered, boiled, steamed, or broiled. Also, Japanese foods are not as highly seasoned as Chinese dishes. Rice is the staple of many Japanese American diets, along with a variety of noodles. As in Chinese cooking, soybean products, such as soy sauce, are important. Seafood is generally more popular than meat and poultry. Vegetables, such as watercress and carrots, are an important part of most meals. Tea is the most popular beverage.

Middle Eastern Americans. Foods of choice in a traditional Middle Eastern diet include yogurt, cheeses (such as feta and goat cheese), lamb, poultry, chick peas, lentils, lemons, eggplant, pine nuts, olives, and olive oil. A Greek specialty is baklava, a baked dessert made with nuts and filo dough. Common cooking styles are grilling, frying, and stewing.

Cultural contributions to cuisine include the choices of ingredients, the style of preparation, the equipment used to cook food, the seasonings, and styles for displaying and serving. Dining itself is also cultural. Washing hands at the table with a warm, moist cloth is a common practice in some cultures. Choices for dining room décor, table settings, eating utensils, ambiance, music, lighting, accepted dress, and even the timing of meals all reflect cultural patterns.

While many of us carry on food-related practices passed on by parents, grandparents, and our individual cultural backdrops, the US has also become a fusion culture in many respects. Foods with cultural identity are popular everywhere. Think of enchiladas, or curries, or pasta with pesto, or pad thai. All are popular and easy to find in today's restaurants, cookbooks, and magazines. Most of us enjoy food choices stemming from a variety of cultures. Today, a key culinary trend goes one step further. Leading-edge chefs seek to mix flavors, ingredients, and cooking styles to create **fusion cuisine**, like pizza with pineapple and sweet-and-sour meats, or spicy Thai chicken wrapped in green tortillas.

REGIONAL TRENDS

Part of the cultural heritage unique to the US is the development of regional culinary trends. Often, these trends reflect a mix of native cultures, foods that are grown and harvested in the area, and ethnic traditions contributed by settlers and immigrants over time. For example, New England is known for maple syrup, Boston beans, brown bread, and cranberry muffins. Maine is recognized for lobster. Blueberries are important in New Jersey and in the Midwest, where many are grown. In Pennsylvania and parts of Ohio, the Pennsylvania Dutch heritage gives rise to scrapple (a loaf made from meat scraps, broth, and flour), homemade noodles, and shoofly (molasses) pie.

Vidalia onions are a hallmark of Georgia's cuisine and are the official state vegetable. Peanuts and peaches are also key crops in Georgia. Florida is known for key limes and key lime pie, coquina soup, and other specialties. Kuchen is the official state dessert in South Dakota. Most people associate Idaho with potatoes, and New Orleans with Creole cuisine, such as jambalaya, "dirty" rice, and gumbo. Barbecued meats and pickled okra have special significance in Texas. In the Southwest (Arizona, New Mexico, Oklahoma, Texas), Mexican-style foods such as burritos and tacos are popular. Garlic is so important in California that the town of Gilroy celebrates an annual garlic festival. In fact, food celebrations, such as strawberry harvest festivals, maple syrup festivals, and many others are key events in all parts of the country.

RELIGIOUS PRACTICES

Religious beliefs, along with religious custom and ritual, can exert strong influence on eating habits. Here are some examples.

Jewish Dietary Laws. The Jewish dietary laws are called *kashrut* or keeping **kosher**. Some Jews follow all the Jewish dietary laws all the time; others follow the laws not at all or to varying degrees, perhaps only on special holidays. The word *kosher* means fit, proper or in agreement with religious law. Basic concepts of Jewish dietary law include the following:

> Pig and pork products are not kosher so they are not eaten. Also, birds of prey are not kosher (this includes wild chickens and turkey). Domestic chicken, turkey, goose, pheasant, and duck are fine.

> All kosher animals must be slaughtered in such a way that the animal is killed instantly and painlessly. If the animal is killed in any other way, it is not kosher. Because Jewish dietary laws forbid eating blood from animals, the meat is put through another step called *koshering* after slaughtering. During koshering the meat or poultry is either soaked and salted or broiled to remove all traces of blood.

> According to Jewish dietary laws, only fish with both fins and scales are considered kosher. All finfish are acceptable, but shellfish, crustaceans, and fish-like mammals are not allowed. This includes shrimp, lobster, oysters, clams, scallops, crab, catfish, shark, and frog. Fish do not have to be koshered like meats and poultry.

> Meat and meat products may not be cooked or served with any dairy products. For example, chicken a la king and creamed chipped beef are forbidden unless made with nondairy products. Pots and pans in which meat is cooked and dishes on which it is served may not be used for dairy products. Separate sets of utensils and dishes are

necessary. Dairy products may be eaten from one to six hours after meat is eaten (the amount of time depends upon an individual's traditions).

All fruits, vegetables, and starches are considered kosher as well as *pareve* (meaning neutral) so they can be served with meat or dairy meals. A foodservice operation offering kosher food must be sure that all aspects of the operation are in accordance with kosher dietary laws.

Other Religions. Muslims abstain from eating pork and using alcohol. All meat must be slaughtered in a prescribed manner. Some Muslims choose to eat kosher meat or fish.

Buddhists may be vegetarians, avoiding animal products (sometimes fish as well). All Hindus regard the cow as sacred and do not eat beef or beef products. Some Hindus will not eat fish; some will not eat eggs, and some are vegetarian. Seventh Day Adventists are usually vegetarians who will eat no animal products except eggs and dairy. They also usually do not drink caffeine-containing beverages such as coffee, tea, or colas. Latter-Day Saints (Mormons) also do not consume caffeine-containing beverages, or alcohol.

SOCIAL AND EMOTIONAL MEANINGS

Eating has many social and emotional meanings to us. In the heritage of every human culture, a meal is enjoyed with family and friends and is often an event unto itself. Even the food preparation can be a social event complete with rituals and traditions. With today's fast-paced lifestyles, however, more people eat while doing something else—such as while working, driving, or walking. Companionship, though, makes a meal more satisfying. We can see how important this is by thinking about food and social events. Food is always part of a celebration. Food is part of courtship and dating. People go to restaurants to have fun together. When a visitor comes to your home or place of work, the custom is to offer food or drink. Food is fundamental to hospitality.

Emotionally, foods can represent comfort. Many adults associate particular foods with happy childhood memories, or talk about the favorites that "Mom (or Dad or another family member) used to make". Food that is very familiar and part of longstanding habits can also be comforting. Any food that imparts a unique sense of emotional well-being is a **comfort food**. Which foods provide comfort vary from one person to the next, but some foods have built a reputation for comfort. For some people, mashed potatoes and fried chicken are comfort foods. Other comfort foods may include things like chocolate cake, or grilled cheese sandwiches and cream of tomato soup. Whatever a person associates with good feelings and family routines can become a comfort food.

When someone is not feeling well, the value of comfort foods increases. Often, a food that is well tolerated has emotional meaning, too. Chicken soup, for example, not only has some medicinal value for someone suffering from a cold. It may also feel emotionally soothing. Sometimes, food as comfort plays a strong role in an individual's nutrition. Food has such powerful emotional overtones that it can take on its own meaning. Some people eat when they feel lonely, or nervous, or stressed.

Social and emotional meanings of food can exert strong influence on the foods each of us chooses to eat. Meanings such as these play an important role in dietary care. Because food is not just "chow," we all need a comfortable social environment, companionship, and a certain amount of familiar fare to feel satisfied from a meal. In fact, research shows that in a longterm care environment, residents eat better when they are with others, and in a relaxed environment.

AVAILABILITY OF FOOD
Another factor that influences food choices is simply what is available. This relates to cash on hand, and what food a person can afford to buy. It relates to ability to go shopping. Someone who cannot go to a grocery store on a regular basis is more likely to rely on canned and dried foods that store well in a cupboard. Someone who has access to a garden during the growing season may eat a great deal of fresh vegetables.

Availability also relates to local crops. Certain foods are more available in some areas than others. In coastal areas, fresh seafood may be key to the cuisine because it is caught close by. Pineapple is used extensively in Hawaii, because it is fresh and readily available. This distinction is blurring somewhat with the globalization of the US food supply. Today, American consumers can enjoy food from anywhere in the world. However, price factors affect choices, and some imported foods may not be as fresh or as economical as local specialties.

Another aspect of availability comes into play when an individual is eating away from home, or when home is an institution. If someone else is providing meals, the menu dictates what foods are available. Preferred foods may not be options. An individual will then choose something else. Over time, this can vastly alter a person's dietary habits and nutritional state. In particular, if preferred foods are not available, some individuals simply will not eat adequately.

PERSONAL TASTE
Personal taste is really a combination of biology and preferences we develop. The biological sense of taste arises from contact of food with the tongue and soft palate, where taste buds sense four types of tastes—bitter, sweet, sour and salty. Scientists say there may be a fifth taste, named *unami* by the Japanese scientists who identified it. Unami is the taste sensation from glutamate (an ingredient in MSG, a common flavor-enhancing ingredient). Unami can be described as "savory" or "meaty".

From the tongue and soft palate, taste sensations transfer to the brain, where we process them. One misconception is that certain parts of the tongue sense certain tastes—such as the tip of the tongue for sweetness, or the sides of the tongue for saltiness. Actually, this is not true. Experts say that tastes buds can sense all flavors on all areas of the tongue. How the brain interprets these signals and puts them together may vary from one person to another. Taste has its basis in taste genes, which were recently identified.

Along with what the taste buds sense, other factors contribute to our sense of taste. Smell is very important. The aroma of good food enhances taste tremendously. Conversely, someone suffering from a cold virus and stuffy nose may notice that food doesn't have much "flavor". This is because sense of smell is reduced. An unpleasant smell can ruin a meal. Another component of taste is called **mouthfeel**. This describes how food feels in the mouth as we eat it. Mouthfeel can be crunchy or smooth, creamy or lumpy. This has a strong impact on what we describe as the taste of food.

In general, we all tend to select foods that taste good to us. Preferences vary considerably. Many develop from habit, as well as from individual variations in how we sense the flavors of foods. While cultural influences and food habits are part of the picture, biology is another part.

AESTHETIC INFLUENCES

Sometimes, for holiday fun, people change the color of food. Think of St. Patrick's Day and green food. Green milkshakes are commonly available at this time. Many people enjoy green shakes because they taste like mint. We think of "green" and "mint" as belonging together. But what happens when we color mashed potatoes or cheese sauce green? These foods may not be appealing. Why? Because they just don't look right. Some people may even associate green in these foods with mold. Clearly, we have expectations about how food should look. Most of the time, we don't even think about these expectations.

The visual impact of food and the way it is presented are quite powerful. Think about this example: Maybe you really enjoy beef stew. The colorful assortment of shapes and flavors can be very attractive—brown chunks of meat, creamy-white potatoes, orange carrot slices, and light-green celery bits. Now, what happens if you blenderize the stew and put it in a cup? Will you enjoy the food in the same way? It may now look like a medium brown-colored sludge. The flavors, though, haven't changed. Most of us will say this doesn't sound appealing.

Again, this example demonstrates our need for visual appeal when we eat. As it turns out, this example represents a key challenge in providing dietary care. Sometimes, clients are unable to chew or swallow well, and need to receive blenderized food. A dietary manager may be called upon to overcome this aesthetic disadvantage when serving pureed food.

In addition, some people will respond strongly to whether foods are mixed together or presented separately. This can be personal choice, but can also have cultural influences. For example, a person raised in traditional Appalachian culture may never have seen a casserole. A person influenced by traditional Japanese culinary practices will expect to see each food separate from others, and may feel uncomfortable with mixed dishes.

Color of food is just one factor in the aesthetic impression food conveys. Presentation is also significant. How food looks on a plate—or in a bowl—influences how we believe it will taste. How is meat sliced? How are fruit pieces cut? Does the food have appealing shapes? What sauces and garnishes appear? What kind of dishware, trays, and table settings provide the backdrop for the meal? The finest chefs give tremendous attention to these details. Much like the first impressions we form of people we meet, the visual first impressions of meals affect how much we enjoy them.

ATTITUDES AND VALUES

What do you think of when you hear words like: Broccoli? Tomatoes? Fresh blueberries? These are among the foods believed to impart special health benefits, as part of a new understanding of functional foods. **Functional foods** are foods that convey health benefits beyond the nutrients (e.g. vitamins or minerals) they contain, through the presence of natural compounds. An example is tomatoes, which contain *lycopene*, a naturally-occurring chemical. Lycopene is touted as a preventative for cancer and heart disease. Today, many people choose foods such as tomatoes, soybean products, garlic, blueberries, or many others specifically to achieve health benefits. See *Nutrition in the News* (ADA Diet Survey) at the end of this chapter for more details about how a desire for health affects eating patterns.

Some individuals choose foods with the idea of losing weight, or gaining weight and building muscle. Some are motivated by physical performance. Sometimes, a desire to avoid diseases in the future affects food choices. For example, one person may avoid eggs and butter and eat fish to reduce a risk of heart disease.

In addition, we tend to assign value judgments to food. Some reflect a sense of status. It's easy to picture this idea when we think of caviar or high-priced champagne. These are perceived as "high-status" foods because of their price tags. Some people may perceive a meal made from dried beans as "low-status" because it is inexpensive. Value assignments and attitudes also affect the range of foods a person will try. Ask yourself: How do you feel about eating crawdads, or escargot (snails), or frogs' legs, or turtle soup, or rabbit meat, or dog meat, or venison? Some people may consider some of these delicacies, while others may reject them, often based on attitudes towards foods or what they represent. Political convictions may play a role in food choices, too. For example, some consumers may boycott particular products based on company practices.

The choice to follow a **vegetarian diet** can also stem from attitudes and values. A vegetarian diet is one that eliminates meats—usually red meat and poultry at a minimum. Some vegetarians avoid fish and seafood. Some avoid all animal products, including milk, cheese, and eggs. A diet with no animal products is called a **vegan diet**. Some people choose to avoid animal foods out of values and convictions regarding animal rights and humane treatment, while others choose vegetarian diets for health or religious reasons.

Value judgments also come into play as consumers evaluate special food categories, like genetically engineered foods and organic foods. To make **genetically engineered foods**, scientists take a selected gene from one plant (or animal) and place it into the genetic structure of another to change its characteristics. In food crops, a gene may be changed to improve resistance to pests and improve crop yields, or to improve shelf life after harvest, or to produce yeast that makes bread rise better, or to enhance nutritional components of a food. Most genetically engineered foods do not require special marketing approval from the FDA or any other government agency to reach the market.

Proponents of the process say that genetically engineered foods can have a tremendous economic impact and allow more of the world's hungry to be fed. They say that genetic engineering can reduce the need for pesticides or make more nutritious food. Meanwhile, some consumers feel that these foods should be identified. Some cite safety concerns, environmental concerns, and fears that genetic engineering could result in mistakes. Some restaurants have enacted policies for avoiding genetically engineered foods. Consumers who have reservations about genetically engineered foods may choose to avoid them.

The burgeoning organic foods trend is another current food issue that affects many consumers' food choices. **Organic foods** are grown without genetic engineering, without use of inorganic (chemically synthesized) growth hormones, antibiotics, pesticides, herbicides, or fertilizers. Part of the idea of growing food organically is conservation of soil, water, and other natural resources. Some consumers embrace this concept out of concern for environmental protection. Organic farmers may use organic fertilizers and natural pest control (insect traps, predator insects to eliminate harmful insects, etc.). They may practice crop rotation. Organic foods, according to their legal definition enacted with the National Organic Standards Program in 2002, contain at least 95% organic ingredients. Foods that meet this requirement can bear a USDA organic seal.

Yet another food term that elicits value judgments from many consumers is natural foods. **Natural foods**, as defined by the US Food Safety and Inspection Service, contain no artificial ingredients or added color and are only minimally processed. For some, the natural foods trend has become part of consumer backlash to today's advanced field of food technology. In a related vein, some consumers choose foods based on distance of transport—wanting locally grown foods. Or, they choose based on packaging—preferring minimal packaging to protect the environment.

Note that knowledge and education can be critical factors shaping dietary choices, too. While the US population devotes a great deal of attention to nutrition and food issues, reported facts can seem confusing. Nutrition advice can even seem contradictory. Knowledge may be incomplete, and not everyone is a nutrition scientist. Thus, some attitudes and values can evolve out of ignorance or uncertainty.

LIFESTYLE

A critical factor driving food choices today is lifestyle. According to the National Restaurant Association (NRA), eating out is big business—estimated at over $426 billion for the year 2003. This includes fast food dining, and eating on-the-run. In fact, a report from the NRA in 2000 indicates that 41% of all cellular phone users use their phones to make restaurant takeout or delivery orders. This is a powerful reflection of the lifestyle issues that have molded dietary habits in America.

On college campuses and in business environments, foodservice operators are scrambling to provide more and more "grab-and-go" food solutions. In the retail arena, operators are increasing shelf space for home meal replacements, convenience foods, and takeout items. In all, the average American consumer cooks from scratch much less than in the past. Families often do not eat together. Some of the traditional ritual and social venue of meals is giving way to hectic routines and busy schedules. The result in essence becomes an "availability of foods" concern. Dietary choices can be limited by what foods are available within lifestyle constraints, or what will be fast, easy, and convenient.

PERSONAL HEALTH

Aside from health beliefs, many personal diets are affected by health status. As an example, one person may be diagnosed with diabetes and face prescribed dietary changes. Another may be diagnosed with high blood cholesterol levels and be advised to follow a low fat diet. In this book, you will become familiar with many dietary changes dictated by health conditions. As a group, these are called **therapeutic diets**. Some individuals follow therapeutic diets more meticulously than others. In general, though, dietary advice offered by a physician, dietitian, or other health professional is likely to influence food choices.

At the same time, a person who is not feeling well may suffer a loss of appetite. A person taking one of many common medications may experience changes in how foods taste. One person may avoid what used to be favorite foods, or even develop a new list of food preferences based on medical changes. Yet another medication may increase a person's sense of hunger or thirst, bringing on a round of unplanned dietary changes. One person may have experienced loss of teeth or other dental conditions that affect ability to chew. Yet another may suffer a neurological disorder and find an ordinary diet difficult to swallow. Many women experiencing premenstrual syndrome (PMS) may face food cravings late in the menstrual cycle. Most likely, there is a biological basis for these cravings. Similar findings relate to food cravings during pregnancy. These are all examples of ways in which personal health status may result in dietary changes.

Finally, a dietary practice that sometimes occurs among low-income groups is called pica. **Pica** is the practice of eating items that are not actually food—such as laundry starch, clay, or paste. Some researchers believe that pica occurs most often among women or children who lack iron in their bodies. Ironically, though, eating these items does not improve nutritional state.

NUTRITION VERSUS DIET

In all, it's clear there is a big difference between nutrition and diet. **Nutrition** is the science of how components in food nourish the body. As you will discover in Chapter 2, these components include carbohydrates, fats, proteins, vitamins, and minerals. A **diet** is the foods and beverages a person consumes. Any person's diet reflects individual choices stemming from cultural heritage, regional trends, religious practices, social and emotional meanings, availability of food, personal taste, aesthetic influences, attitudes and beliefs, lifestyle, and personal health. In addition, dietary choices tend to become habit for most people. Dietary choices include not only what a person chooses to eat, but also what foods a person chooses to *avoid*.

Nutrition alone can, in theory, be provided by chemical formulations. However, we do not generally choose to obtain nutrition in this way, due to the powerful meaning of food to us as humans. Instead, we enjoy a rich, personal experience related to food. Thus, to provide nutritional care, a dietary manager must consider both nutrition and diet to develop plans that will help clients maintain or improve health. An effective dietary plan weaves comfortably into personal dietary choices. It respects heritage and preferences. It supports habits that have become meaningful for each of us as individuals. A critical factor driving food choices today is lifestyle.

AMERICAN DIETETIC ASSOCIATION DIET SURVEY FINDINGS
PEOPLE ARE TAKING MORE CARE TO ACHIEVE BALANCED NUTRITION AND HEALTHY DIET

CHICAGO – The percentage of Americans who carefully select what they eat to maximize their nutrition and health is higher than at any time in eight years, according to the American Dietetic Association's new national public opinion survey, *Nutrition and You: Trends 2000.*

And the number who say they're doing all they can to attain balanced nutrition and a healthy diet is on a slow upward trend.

According to the survey, 40 percent are either "very careful" or "somewhat careful" in selecting foods to achieve balanced nutrition and a healthy diet. That is up 6 percent since ADA's 1997 survey and the highest since ADA's first survey in 1991.

"It's great to see the trend heading upward, but there is definitely still room for improvement in Americans' eating habits," says Chicago registered dietitian and ADA spokesperson Diane Quagliani.

The *Nutrition and You: Trends 2000* survey found 41 percent of Americans are doing "all they can" to achieve balanced nutrition and a healthy diet—up slightly from 39 percent in 1997 and 35 percent in 1995.

Asked if they are doing more, the same or less than two years ago, 47 percent said more, 43 percent said the same and just 9 percent said less.

Those who said they were doing "the same" or "less" than two years ago were asked why they were not doing more. Their primary reasons were "I don't want to give up the foods I like" and "I am satisfied with the way I currently eat" (respondents could give more than one answer):

- *I don't want to give up the foods I like* was given as a "major reason" by 44 percent and a "minor reason" by 31 percent
- *I am satisfied with the way I currently eat* was a major reason for 39 percent, a minor reason for 36 percent
- *It takes too much time to keep track of my diet* was a major reason for 38 percent and a minor reason for 19 percent
- *I don't know or understand nutrition guidelines* was a major reason for 29 percent, a minor reason for 7 percent
- *I need more practical tips to help me eat right* was a major reason for 34 percent, a minor reason for 11 percent

"Not wanting to give up favorite foods is a popular reason for not doing more," Quagliani says. "But there's no reason you have to give up hot fudge sundaes or French fries. All foods can be a part of a healthful eating plan—it's all a matter of minding how often and how much you eat of some foods."

"Lack of time to eat well is another popular misconception," Quagliani says. "There are plenty of quick options—washed and cut fruits and vegetables, quick-cooking whole grain pasta. It doesn't take any extra time to choose non-fat milk or lean meats.

▶ Food has many meanings. To provide effective dietary care, it is important to recognize what food means to individuals, and how dietary choices come about.

▶ Factors that influence dietary choices include cultural heritage, regional trends, religious practices, social and emotional meanings, availability of food, personal taste, aesthetic influences, attitudes and values, lifestyle, and personal health.

▶ Cultural contributions to cuisine include the choices of ingredients, the style of preparation, the equipment used to cook food, the seasonings, and styles for displaying and serving.

▶ Personal taste is really a combination of biology and preferences we develop. Preferences vary considerably. Many develop from habit, as well as from individual variations in how we sense the flavors of foods.

▶ The visual impact of food and the way it is presented are quite powerful.

▶ A dietary manager can apply an understanding of why we choose the foods we do to support nutrition.

Comfort food: any food that imparts a unique sense of emotional well-being

Diet: the foods and beverages a person consumes

Functional foods: foods that convey health benefits beyond the nutrients (e.g. vitamins or minerals) they contain, through the presence of natural compounds

Fusion cuisine: a culinary trend that mixes flavors, ingredients, and cooking styles from various cultures

Genetically engineered food: a food whose genetic structure has been modified by the addition of a selected gene from another plant or an animal to change its characteristics

Kosher: a Hebrew word meaning fit, proper or in agreement with religious law, used to describe a particular diet followed by many Jewish people

Mouthfeel: how food feels in the mouth as we eat it

Natural food: a food that contains no artificial ingredients or added color and is only minimally processed

Nutrition: the science of how components in food nourish the body

Organic food: a food grown without genetic engineering, without use of inorganic (chemically synthesized) growth hormones, antibiotics, pesticides, herbicides, and fertilizers

Pica: the practice of eating items that are not actually food—such as laundry starch, clay, or paste

Therapeutic diet: a diet dictated by a health condition

Vegetarian diet: a diet that eliminates meats

Vegan diet: a diet with no animal products at all

1. Apple pie is meaningful to many Americans as:
   A. The best source of lycopene
   B. A symbol of patriotic pride
   C. An economic gold standard
   D. A traditional food for wedding celebrations

2. Tortillas are common in:
   A. Mexican cuisine
   B. Greek cuisine
   C. Lebanese cuisine
   D. French cuisine

3. Scrapple is a meat characteristic of:
   A. Latin American cuisine
   B. Italian cuisine
   C. Pennsylvania Dutch cuisine
   D. Japanese American cuisine

4. A comfort food is one that:
   A. Minimizes the side effects of medications
   B. Provides extra vitamins
   C. Soothes emotions
   D. Is easy to swallow

5. Which of the following is a component of Kosher dietary laws?
   A. Beef is prohibited.
   B. Fresh fruits are prohibited.
   C. Meat and meat products may be cooked or served only with dairy products.
   D. Meat and meat products may not be cooked or served with any dairy products.

6. Which of the following is characteristic of Hindu practices?
   A. Beef is prohibited.
   B. Fresh fruits are prohibited.
   C. Meat and meat products may be cooked or served only with dairy products.
   D. Meat and meat products may not be cooked or served with any dairy products.

7. Seventh-Day Adventists usually:

   A. Are under-nourished
   B. Favor eating poultry
   C. Follow vegetarian diets
   D. Eat tempura

8. Organic foods are grown:

   A. Without any form of fertilizer
   B. On the same land year after year
   C. With genetically engineered seeds
   D. Without antibiotics, growth hormones, synthetic pesticides, herbicides, or fertilizers

9. Basic taste sensations are:

   A. Curry, peppery, and salty
   B. Oniony, peppery, and salty
   C. Sweet and salty
   D. Sweet, sour, salty, bitter, and possibly unami

10. A therapeutic diet is:

    A. A set of dietary changes dictated by health conditions
    B. A dietary fad designed to promote weight loss
    C. A drug therapy
    D. A set of religious dietary laws

In order to plan and implement menus, a dietary manager needs to master nutrition concepts. An understanding of basic nutrients is also essential for planning therapeutic diets.

After completing this chapter, you should be able to:

- Explain what a nutrient is.
- List six nutrient groups and provide examples.
- Name key functions of each of the six nutrient groups.
- List some food sources for nutrients.
- List the energy content of nutrients.
- Provide examples of *nutrient-dense* foods.

As explained in Chapter 1, nutrition is the science of how components in food nourish the body. Nutrition also explores how substances in food relate to health and disease. Almost daily, we are bombarded with news reports that something in the food we eat is not good for us—or is very good for us. We hear that food-related factors may cause, complicate, prevent or even combat conditions such as heart disease, hypertension, cancer, arthritis, attention deficit disorder, or Alzheimer's disease…to name a few. While not all health claims in popular media are valid, substantial scientific research indicates that diet is indeed relevant to health.

The science of nutrition addresses the processes by which we choose kinds and amounts of foods, and the balance of foods and nutrients in our diets. Lastly, nutrition looks at how the body digests, absorbs, transports, utilizes, and excretes the foods we eat. These topics will be further discussed in Chapter 4.

Now let's go back to the concept of nutrients. **Nutrients** are substances in food that provide energy and/or promote the growth and maintenance of the body. Nutrients also help regulate many body processes—such as pumping blood through the heart, or thinking, or even breathing from minute to minute. Sound nutrition supports the optimum health of the body. Nutrients fall into six groups as follows:

- Carbohydrates
- Lipids (includes fats and oils)
- Proteins
- Vitamins
- Minerals
- Water

Figure 2.1

FUNCTIONS OF NUTRIENTS

Carbohydrates: Provide energy

Lipids and proteins: Provide energy, promote growth and maintenance, regulate body processes

Vitamins: Regulate body processes

Minerals: Promote growth and maintenance, regulate body processes

Water: Promotes growth and maintenance, regulates body processes

The functions of each group of nutrients are shown in Figure 2.1.

Most foods are a mixture of carbohydrates, proteins, and lipids, and contain smaller quantities of other nutrients, such as vitamins and minerals. It's been said many times: "You are what you eat." Indeed, the nutrients you eat are in your body. Water accounts for about 50-70% of body weight. Lipids (fats) account for about 4-27% of body weight, and protein accounts for about 14-23% of body weight. Carbohydrates comprise only 0.5%. (Even though carbohydrates are important nutrients, most do not remain as carbohydrates in the body.) The remainder of body weight includes minerals, such as calcium in bones, and traces of vitamins.

NUTRIENTS: TERMINOLOGY

Most, but not all, nutrients are considered essential nutrients. **Essential nutrients** either cannot be made in the body or cannot be made in the quantities needed by the body; therefore, we must obtain them through food. Thus, "essential" in this term means it is *essential* that we consume these nutrients; they are *essential* components of our diets. Carbohydrates, vitamins, minerals, water, and some parts of lipids and proteins are considered essential. Note that we do not usually eat nutrients by themselves. Nutrients are components of foods. For example, a glass of milk contains carbohydrates, lipids, protein, vitamins, minerals, and water.

Some nutrients provide energy, as discussed later in this chapter. These are called **energy-yielding nutrients**—carbohydrates, lipids (fats), and protein. A **calorie** is a unit of measurement of heat or energy. Although we use the term calorie in our speech, and will use it in this book, calorie is actually a shortened form of the term "kilocalorie" (which means 1,000 calories). Of the nutrients, only carbohydrates, lipids, and protein provide energy as follows.

Carbohydrates: 4 calories per gram

Lipids: 9 calories per gram

Protein: 4 calories per gram

A gram is a unit of weight; there are 28 grams in one ounce. Vitamins, minerals, and water do not have any calories. Alcohol, although not a nutrient, provides seven calories per gram.

Energy-yielding nutrients also commonly serve as building blocks for body tissues. This is particularly true of proteins and lipids (fats). Because these nutrients give our bodies energy, we tend to consume these in large amounts. Thus, they are sometimes called **macronutrients**. Nutrients we use in smaller quantities, such as vitamins and minerals, may be called **micronutrients**. *Macro* means great or large; *micro* means small. Now, let's take a close look at the six nutrient categories, starting with the macronutrients—carbohydrates, lipids, and protein.

CARBOHYDRATES

Carbo means carbon, and *hydrate* means water. **Carbohydrates** do indeed contain carbon and the two chemical elements that make up water: hydrogen and oxygen. The main function of carbohydrates is to provide energy to the body. In fact, the central nervous system, including the brain and nerve cells, relies almost exclusively on a form of carbohydrate called glucose for energy.

Carbohydrates fall into two categories: simple carbohydrates (commonly called sugars), and complex carbohydrates (commonly called starch and fiber). Carbohydrate-rich foods include nutritious foods such as breads and cereals, fruits and vegetables, dried beans and peas, as well as not-so-nutritious foods such as cupcakes and soft drinks. To better understand carbohydrates, let's take a closer look at simple and complex carbohydrates.

Simple Carbohydrates (Sugars)

Simple carbohydrates are so named because their chemical structure is fairly simple. In fact, the simple carbohydrates are building blocks for the complex carbohydrates. A familiar name for simple carbohydrates is sugar. There are six forms of simple carbohydrates or sugars that are nutritionally important:

- Glucose
- Sucrose
- Fructose
- Lactose
- Galactose
- Maltose

As you can see, all of these names end in *ose*, which means sugar.

Glucose, also called dextrose or blood sugar, is found in sweet fruits such as grapes and berries, and in trace amounts in most plant foods. In the body, glucose is called **blood sugar** because it circulates in the blood at a relatively

Figure 2.2

RELATIVE SWEETNESS OF SWEETENERS

SWEETENER	APPROXIMATE SWEETNESS (as compared to sucrose)
Saccharin	300
Aspartame	200
Fructose	1.5
Glucose	0.7
Lactose	0.15

constant level. Blood sugar is extremely important because it provides most of the energy that will be burned by the millions of cells in the body. Although glucose appears in certain foods, it is not the major source of glucose in the body. Instead, starch and most other sugars become glucose in the body. Fructose, also called fruit sugar, is found in ripe fruits and honey. Fructose is a very sweet sugar, as shown in Figure 2.2. Some chemicals that provide a sweet taste are not sugars at all. Instead, they are artificial sweeteners. Saccharin and aspartame, for example, are not sugars. However, they can substitute for sugar in the diet by providing a sweet taste. For more information on artificial sweeteners, see *Nutrition in the News* (More Choices for the Sweet Life) at the end of this chapter.

Galactose does not appear in foods by itself; it is only present bound to glucose in a sugar called *lactose*. Glucose, fructose, and galactose are single sugars, also referred to as monosaccharides. (*Mono* means one; *saccharide* means sugar unit and refers to a molecule of sugar.) The remaining three sugars, sucrose, lactose, and maltose, have two sugars units and are called disaccharides. (*Di* means two.) Sucrose is the chemical name for what we know as table sugar or refined sugar. It is composed of two single sugars: glucose and fructose. Table sugar is made from sugar cane or sugar beets and is used to sweeten many foods such as soft drinks, many baked goods, jams, and jellies. Sucrose appears naturally in some foods. For example, there are small amounts of sucrose in many fruits and vegetables. Lactose is the sugar found naturally only in milk and certain other dairy products. Although lactose is considered a sugar, it is not a very sweet sugar. Lactose is made of two single sugars linked together: glucose and galactose. Maltose is made of two glucose units. It is present in germinating seeds, beer, malted breakfast cereals, and other malt products.

Sugar in Food

Besides sweetening foods, sugars prevent spoilage in jams and jellies and perform several functions in baking, such as browning the crust and retaining moisture in baked goods. Sugar also acts as a food for yeast in breads. When yeast "eats" sugar, carbon dioxide (a gas) is produced. Carbon dioxide makes bread rise and gives it an airy texture.

In addition to occurring naturally in some foods, sugar is often added to foods to sweeten them. Added sugars are often table sugar, high fructose corn syrup, or corn syrup. Although a natural sugar, honey is primarily fructose and glucose, the same two components as table sugar. They both contribute only energy and no other nutrients in significant amounts, and because honey is more concentrated, it has twice as many calories as the same amount of table sugar. Fruits are an excellent source of natural sugar. Canned fruits are packed in four different ways: in water, fruit juice, light syrup, and heavy syrup. Both light syrup and heavy syrup have sugar added, with heavy syrup containing more added sugar. Dried fruits are much more concentrated sources of sugar than fresh fruits because they contain much less water. Lactose, or milk sugar, is present in large amounts in milk, ice cream, ice milk, sherbet, cottage cheese, cheese spreads and other soft cheeses, eggnog, and cream. Hard cheeses contain only traces of lactose.

Figure 2.3 lists added sugars (also called refined sugars) commonly found in foods. Sucrose and corn sweeteners are the most frequently used sugars. Added sugars are used to sweeten soft drinks, breakfast cereals, candy, baked goods such as cakes and pies, syrups, jams and jellies. One-quarter of the sugar

COMMON FORMS OF ADDED SUGARS

FORM OF SUGAR	DESCRIPTION
Table sugar (granulated sugar, sucrose)	Obtained in crystalline form from cane and beets. Is about 99.9% pure and is sold in granulated or powdered form.
Corn sweeteners	Corn syrup and other sugars made from corn.
Corn syrup	Made from cornstarch. Mostly glucose. Only 75% as sweet as sucrose. Less expensive than sucrose. Used extensively in baked goods. Also used in canned goods.
High fructose corn syrup	Corn syrup treated with an enzyme that converts glucose to fructose, which results in a sweeter product. Used in soft drinks, baked goods, jelly, syrups, fruits, and desserts.
Brown sugar	Sugar crystals contained in a molasses syrup with natural flavor and color; 91 to 96% sucrose.
Molasses	Thick syrup left over after making sugar from sugar cane. Brown in color with a high sugar concentration.
Turbinado sugar	Sometimes viewed incorrectly as raw sugar. Produced by separating raw sugar crystals and washing them with steam to remove impurities.

Figure 2.3

Figure 2.4

SUGAR CONTENT OF FOODS

FOOD/PORTION . . . . .TEASPOONS OF SUGAR

Dairy

Skim milk, 1 cup 3

Swiss cheese, 1 ounce . . . . .Less than 1

Vanilla ice cream, ½ cup .4

Meat, Poultry, & Fish

Meat, poultry, or fish, 3 ounces 0

Eggs

Egg, 1 0

Grains

White bread, 1 slice . . . . .Less than 1

English muffin, 1 . . . . .Less than 1

White rice, cooked, ½ cup . . . . .Less than 1

Cheerios cereal, 1 cup . . . . .Less than 1

Honey Nut Cheerios, 1 cup 3

Quaker Oatmeal Squares, 1 cup 2

Fruits

Apple, 1 medium 4.5

Banana, 1 medium 7

Orange, 1 medium 3

Raisins, 14 grams 2.5

FOOD/PORTION . . . . .TEASPOONS OF SUGAR

Vegetables

Broccoli, ½ cup raw chopped . . . . . . .Less than 1 gram

Mixed vegetables, ⅓ cup . . . . .Less than 1 gram

Beverages

Cola soft drink, 12 fluid ounces 10

Cakes, Cookies, Candies, & Pudding

Brownie, 1 average 6

Chocolate graham crackers, 8 2

Chocolate chip cookies, 3 3

Lemon drops, 4 piece 2.5

M&M's™ candy, 70 pieces 7

Vanilla pudding, ½ cup 6

Sweeteners

White sugar, 1 Tablespoon 4

Honey, 1 Tablespoon 4

High fructose corn syrup, 1 Tablespoon 4

Source: USDA

consumed in the United States is in soft drinks. While table sugar consumption has dropped over the past 15 years, consumption of high fructose corn syrup has increased almost 250%, according to figures from the U.S. Department of Agriculture. Figure 2.4 lists the sugar content of some foods.

Sugarless gums use sweeteners such as sorbitol or mannitol. These substances are called sugar alcohols. Sorbitol is 60% as sweet as sucrose, with about the same number of calories per gram. Sorbitol is used in such products as sugarless hard and soft candies, chewing gums, jams, and jellies. Xylitol, another sugar alcohol, is about as sweet as table sugar and is absorbed very slowly. A third sugar alcohol, mannitol, is poorly digested, so it does not contribute a full four calories per gram. It occurs naturally in pineapple, olives, sweet potatoes, and carrots, and is added to sugarless gums. Both mannitol and sorbitol, when taken in large amounts, can cause diarrhea. Products whose reasonably foreseeable consumption may result in a daily ingestion of 50 grams of sorbitol or 20 grams mannitol must bear the labeling statement, "Excess consumption may have a laxative effect."

Complex Carbohydrates: Starches

Whereas sugars are chemically made up of one or two units of sugar molecules, **starch** is more complex. Chemically, starches and fiber—both forms of complex carbohydrates—consist of many sugar molecules strung together. This is why we refer to them as *complex*. Another term for complex carbohydrates is polysaccharides. *Poly* means many, so a polysaccharide is made up of many glucose units. A single starch molecule (or chain) may contain 300 to 1,000 or more sugar units. The giant molecules are packed side by side in a plant root or seed, providing energy for the plant. All starches are plant materials.

Cereal grains, which are the fruits or seeds of cultivated grasses, are rich sources of starch. Examples include wheat, corn, rice, rye, barley, and oats. Wheat and other grains consist of three parts: the starchy endosperm, the vitamin-rich germ, and the bran, the protective outer coat that contains fiber. Figure 2.5 is a diagram of a grain of rice. Cereal grains are used to make breads, breakfast cereals, and pastas. Starches are also found in potatoes, vegetables, and dried beans and peas. Figure 2.6 identifies common sources of starch in the diet.

Starches are a key component of a healthful diet. As you might guess from the chemical structure, a starch molecule is a terrific way for the body to store sugar for future use. In fact, this is one way the body uses starch. Some starch breaks down immediately after a meal and is used as sugar to fuel body functions. But blood sugar sometimes goes the other way. Extra sugar in the body may be built back into starch and stored for energy in the future. The body's form of stored starch is called **glycogen**. Glycogen is stored in muscles and in the liver. Glycogen is not really a food component; it is a special form of carbohydrate the body makes.

Figure 2.5

FIGURE 2.5. A GRAIN OF RICE

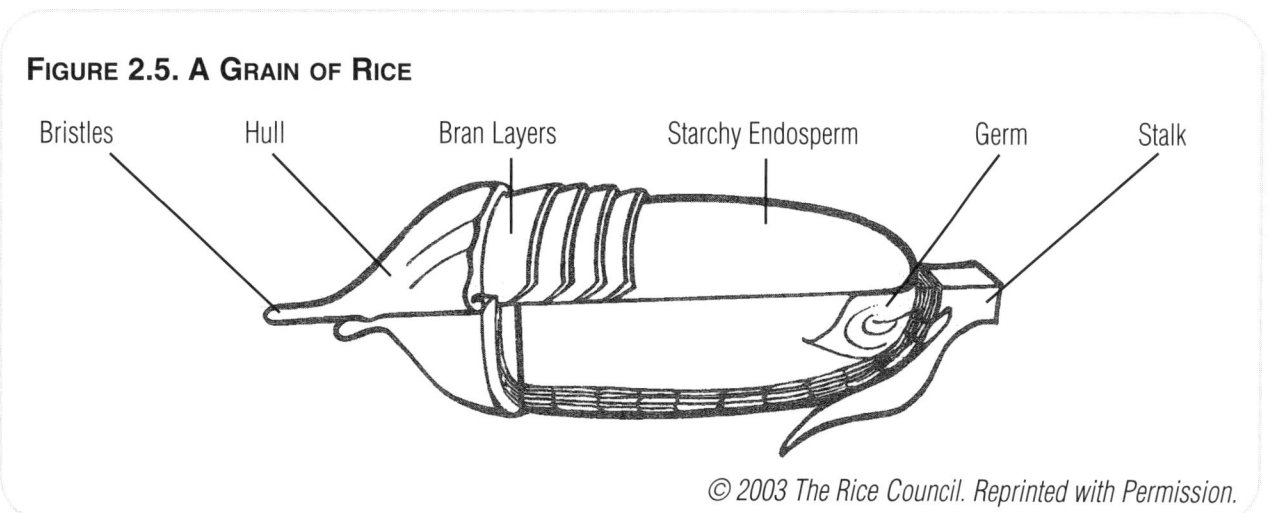

Bristles Hull Bran Layers Starchy Endosperm Germ Stalk

Figure 2.6

GOOD SOURCES OF STARCH

Breads, both whole grain and white

Breakfast cereals, cooked and ready-to-eat

Flours, whole grain and white

Pastas, such as macaroni and spaghetti

Grains, such as barley and rice

Legumes, such as dried peas, beans, and lentils

Starchy vegetables, such as potatoes, corn, sweet peas, and lima beans

Complex Carbohydrates: Dietary Fiber

The term **dietary fiber** describes a variety of carbohydrate compounds from plants that are not digestible. Like starch, most fibers are chains of glucose units bonded together, but what's different is that the chains can't be broken down or digested. In other words, most fiber passes through the stomach and intestines unchanged and is excreted in the feces. Unlike sugars or starches, fiber does not give rise to sugar in the body. Fiber was called *roughage* a few generations ago. Fiber is found only in plant foods where it supports the plant's stems, leaves, and seeds.

There are two major types of fiber—insoluble and soluble. **Soluble fiber** simply means fiber that dissolves in water, forming a gel. **Insoluble fiber** also dissolves in water, but not nearly to the extent as soluble fiber.

Soluble fibers include gums, mucilages, pectin, and some hemicelluloses. These are components of foods such as apples, oats, and dried beans (see Figure 2.7). In the body, they slow down the movement of food through the lower digestive tract. They slow down the release of glucose from other foods into the body, which may be beneficial to someone with diabetes who needs to control blood sugar. They also help control blood cholesterol levels.

Insoluble fibers include cellulose, lignin, and some hemicelluloses. These fibers occur in bran (wheat bran, corn bran, whole grain breads), and vegetables. Insoluble fibers form the structures of plants, such as skins, and the bran of the wheat kernel. You have seen insoluble fiber in the skin of whole kernel corn and the strings of celery. Insoluble fibers speed up the movement of food through the lower digestive tract and can help prevent constipation. Like soluble fibers, they also slow down the release of glucose from other foods into the body.

The amount of fiber in a plant varies from one kind of plant to another and may vary within a species or variety, depending on growing conditions and

Figure 2.7

SOLUBLE AND INSOLUBLE FIBER IN FOODS

FOODS CONTAINING SOLUBLE FIBERS
Beans and peas, such as:
　　kidney beans
　　pinto beans
　　chick peas
　　split peas
　　and lentils

Some cereal grains, such as:
　　oats
　　barley

Some fruits and vegetables, such as:
　　apples
　　grapes
　　citrus fruits
　　carrots

FOODS CONTAINING INSOLUBLE FIBERS
Wheat bran

Whole grains such as:
　　whole wheat
　　brown rice

Products made with whole grains such as:
　　whole wheat bread
　　rye bread

Many vegetables, such as:
　　potatoes
　　green beans
　　cabbage
　　celery
　　corn

maturity of the plant at the time of harvest. Like starch, fiber is found abundantly in plants, especially in the outer layers of cereal grains and the fibrous parts of legumes (dried beans and peas), fruits, vegetables, nuts, and seeds. Fiber is not found in animal products such as meat, poultry, fish, dairy products, and eggs. Most foods contain both soluble and insoluble fibers.

Whenever the fiber-rich bran and the vitamin-rich germ are left on the endosperm of a grain, the grain is called whole grain. Examples of whole grains include whole wheat, whole rye, bulgur (whole wheat grains that have been steamed and dried), oatmeal, whole cornmeal, whole hulled barley, popcorn, and brown rice. The milling of whole wheat in the United States to produce white flour removes the bran and germ and leaves behind mostly starch.

By law, white flour and other refined grain products must be **enriched**, meaning that certain nutrients (thiamin, riboflavin, niacin, and iron) are added in amounts approximately equivalent to those originally present in the whole grain but lost through milling. Unfortunately, enrichment does not replace the fiber removed by milling, and it only replaces some of the nutrients lost. Whole wheat flour (particularly if stone-ground) retains most of the original nutrients and has more fiber, vitamin B6, magnesium, and zinc than enriched white flour.

As a general rule, unrefined foods contain more fiber than refined foods because fiber is usually removed in processing. For example, raw apples contain much fiber in the skin, but the skin is removed to make applesauce or canned sliced apples. Although fiber supplements are available, they are not generally recommended. Whole foods contain a greater variety of fibers, as well as many other nutrients. Purified fibers in large amounts can be harmful, and certain purified fibers may not have the same effect in the body as the actual fiber in food.

Since insoluble fiber holds water and speeds the movement of wastes through the intestines, stools produced by a high fiber diet tend to be bulkier and softer and pass more quickly and more easily through the intestines. A diet high in insoluble fiber helps prevent and treat hemorrhoids and diverticulosis, a disease of the large intestine in which the intestinal walls become weakened and bulge out into pockets. Insoluble fibers may also reduce the risk of colon cancer.

Studies indicate that soluble fibers play a role in reducing the level of cholesterol in the blood. Eating soluble fiber may help lower blood cholesterol when part of an overall health plan that includes eating less fat and cholesterol. Soluble fiber helps people with diabetes maintain control of their blood sugar levels. Lastly, fiber-rich foods usually require more chewing and provide an increased sense of fullness or satiety, so they are excellent choices for anyone trying to lose weight.

LIPIDS

Lipids is the scientific name for a diverse group that includes fats, oils, and cholesterol. These are important for providing energy and for helping the body absorb fat-soluble vitamins (discussed later in this chapter). Fats and oils are the most plentiful lipids in nature. It is customary to call a lipid a *fat* if it is a solid at room temperature and an *oil* if it is a liquid at the same temperature. Lipids from animal sources, such as butter, are usually solid, whereas oils are liquid and generally of plant origin (such as corn oil). A few exceptions to this rule of thumb include coconut oil and palm kernel oil. These are fats from plant sources that may be solid at room temperature. We commonly speak of "animal fats" and "vegetable oils". For the purposes of this book, we will use the word "fat" to refer to both fats and oils.

In recent years there has been much discussion about how much fat and cholesterol we eat, what kind of fat we eat, and the relationship between dietary fats and cholesterol and cardiovascular (heart and artery) disease. A high level of blood cholesterol has been identified as one of the major risk factors for having a heart attack or a stroke. This is important because diet, particularly fat intake, influences blood cholesterol levels. Chapter 3 addresses the relationship between fat intake and heart disease.

Triglycerides

The bulk of the body's fat tissue is in the form of **triglycerides**, and most of the fats in foods are also in the form of triglycerides. Figure 2.8 shows what a triglyceride looks like. It is composed of three fatty acids attached to glycerol. Each fatty acid is made up of carbon atoms joined like links on a chain. The carbon chains vary in length, with most fatty acids containing four to 20

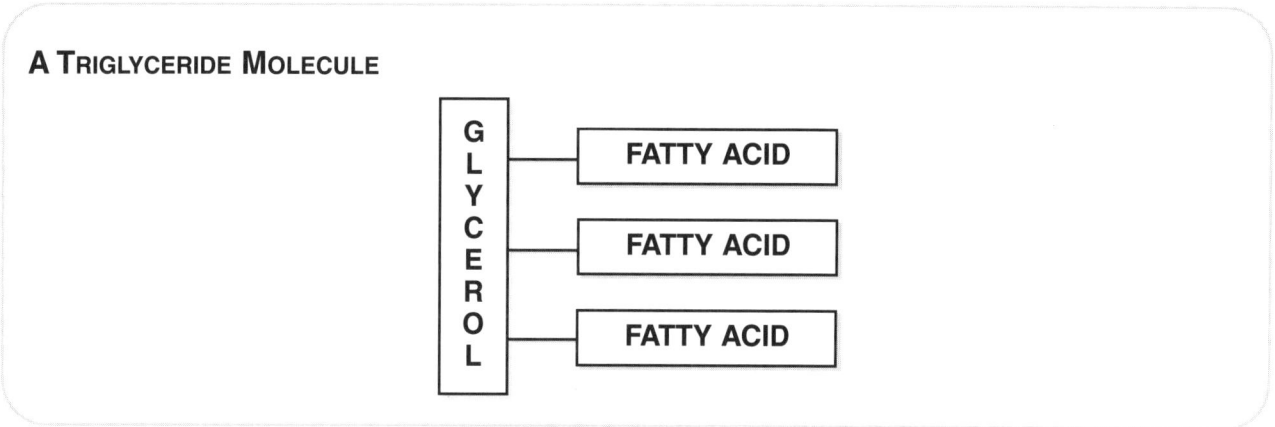

A TRIGLYCERIDE MOLECULE

carbon atoms. Each carbon has hydrogen attached, much like charms on a charm bracelet.

Types of Fatty Acids

Fatty acids may be one of three different types:

- Saturated
- Monounsaturated
- Polyunsaturated

These terms relate to chemistry. "Saturated" describes the chemical structure. When each carbon atom in the chain holds as many hydrogen atoms as it can (two), it is called a saturated fatty acid. A **saturated fatty acid** is therefore filled, or saturated, with hydrogens. When a double bond forms between two neighboring carbons, two hydrogens are missing, so the carbons are not saturated. This type of fatty acid is called an **unsaturated fatty acid**. A fatty acid that contains one double bond in the chain is a **monounsaturated fatty acid**. (*Mono* means one). A fatty acid containing more than one double bond is a **polyunsaturated fatty acid (PUFA)**. *Poly* means many, so this term means that the fatty acid is unsaturated in many places. Another fatty acid, **trans-fatty acid**, has its hydrogen atoms in an unusual location. Trans-fatty acids are made during the process in which vegetable oils are partially hydrogenated to make them more solid. Hydrogenated oils are used in margarines and shortening. This may sound like a great deal of technicality. But in fact, these chemical distinctions have a serious impact on how these fats affect the body, as you will learn later in this book.

Two of the fatty acids in food are considered to be **essential fatty acids (EFA)** because the body can't make them. They are essential in our diets. The names of the two essential fatty acids are *linoleic acid* and *linolenic acid*. Linoleic acid is polyunsaturated and is found in corn, cottonseed, soybean, and safflower oil. It is also found in nuts, seeds, and whole grain products. Linolenic acid is also polyunsaturated and appears in some vegetable oils such as canola, walnut, soybean oils, and in fatty fish. Another type of fatty acid receiving much attention today is called omega-3 fatty acid. "Omega-3" just refers to the location of the first double bond in the chain. Omega-3 is a type of polyunsaturated fatty acid.

Triglycerides in Foods

The fat in our diets is both visible and invisible. When we think about fats, most of us think about only the visible fats—butter, margarine, and cooking oils. But much of the fat in the diet comes from less visible sources—the fatty streaks in meat, the fat under the skin of poultry, the fat in milk and cheese, the fat in many baked goods, fried foods, nuts, and the fat contained in many processed foods such as candy, chips, crackers, canned soups, and convenience frozen dinners. Unprocessed cereal grains, fruits and vegetables (except avocados and olives), flour, pasta, breads, and most cereals have little or no fat.

All fats in foods are made up of mixtures of fatty acids. If a food contains mostly saturated fatty acids, it is considered a key source of saturated fat. If it contains mostly polyunsaturated fatty acids, it is a key source of polyunsaturated fat. Monounsaturated fats contain mostly monounsaturated fatty acids.

Animal fats are generally more saturated than liquid vegetable oils. Figure 2.9 shows the proportions of fatty acids in fats from various sources. Saturated fat raises blood cholesterol more than anything else in the diet, so let's take a look at the foods in which it is found. Animal products are a major source of saturated fat in the typical American diet. The fat in whole-milk dairy products (like butter, cheese, whole milk, ice cream, and cream) contains high amounts of saturated fat. Saturated fat is also concentrated in the fat that surrounds meat and in the white streaks of fat in the muscle of meat (marbling). Well-trimmed cuts from certain sections of the animal, such as the round, are lower in saturated fat than well-marbled, untrimmed meat. Poultry, when the skin is removed, and most fish are lower in saturated fat.

A few vegetable fats—coconut oil, cocoa butter, and palm oil—are high in saturated fat. These may be used for commercial deep fat frying and in foods such as cookies and crackers, whipped toppings, coffee creamers, cake mixes, and even frozen dinners. Chocolate products, such as chocolate candy bars and baking chips, contain cocoa butter and sometimes also palm kernel oil or palm oil. Like saturated fat intake, trans-fatty acid fat intake also raises blood cholesterol, specifically a form called LDLs. High LDL raises the risk for heart disease. As mentioned, trans-fatty acids are found in vegetable shortenings and some margarines. Trans-fatty acids are also found in foods that contain shortening or margarines, such as crackers, cookies, and foods fried in partially hydrogenated fats.

Polyunsaturated fats are found in greatest amounts in safflower, corn, soybean, cottonseed, sesame, and sunflower oils, which are commonly used in salad

Figure 2.9

FATTY ACIDS IN FATS & OILS

Fats & Oils	Saturated Fatty Acids	Monounsaturated Fatty Acids	Polyunsaturated Fatty Acids
High in Saturated			
Coconut oil	11.8 grams	0.8 grams	0.2 grams
Palm kernel oil	11.1	1.5	0.2
Cocoa butter	8.1	4.5	0.4
Butter	7.1	3.3	0.4
Palm oil	6.7	5.0	1.3
Lard	5.0	5.8	1.4
High in Monounsaturated			
Olive oil	1.8	9.9	1.1
Canola oil	0.9	7.6	4.5
Peanut oil	2.3	6.2	4.3
High in Polyunsaturated			
Safflower oil	1.2	1.6	10.1
Corn oil	1.7	3.3	8.0
Soybean oil	2.0	3.2	7.9
Cottonseed oil	3.5	2.4	7.1
Sunflower oil	1.4	6.2	5.5
Margarine, liquid	1.8	3.9	5.1
Margarine, soft tub	1.8	4.8	3.9

Source: National Institutes of Health

dressings and for cooking oils. Nuts and seeds also contain some polyunsaturated fats. Examples of monounsaturated fats include olive oil, peanut oil, and canola oil. Like other vegetable oils, these are used in salad dressings and for cooking oils. Both monounsaturated and polyunsaturated fats tend to reduce blood cholesterol levels.

Cholesterol

Cholesterol is a type of sterol, which has most of its atoms arranged in a ring rather than a chain. All the cholesterol the body needs is made by the liver, so it is not technically an essential nutrient. The body uses cholesterol to build cell membranes and brain and nerve tissues. Cholesterol also helps the body produce steroid hormones needed for body regulation, bile acids needed for digestion, and a form of vitamin D.

Cholesterol is found only in foods of animal origin: egg yolks, meat, poultry, fish, milk, and milk products. Egg yolk and organ meats (liver, kidney, sweetbread, brain) are major sources of cholesterol. One egg yolk contains about 10 times as much cholesterol as one ounce of meat. Both the lean and fat of meat and the meat and skin of poultry contain cholesterol. In milk products, cholesterol is mostly in the fat, so lower fat products contain less cholesterol. Egg whites and foods that come from plants have no cholesterol. Figure 2.10 shows the cholesterol content of selected foods.

Functions of Lipids

Fat serves a variety of functions. Some fat is needed in the diet to provide the essential fatty acids. Fat in food also contains the fat-soluble vitamins (A, D, E, and K). Fat also provides a concentrated source of energy. About 15-20% of the

Figure 2.10

CHOLESTEROL IN FOODS

FOOD AND PORTION	CHOLESTEROL
Liver, braised, 3 ounces	333 milligrams
Egg, whole, 1	213
Beef, short ribs, braised, 3 ounces	80
Beef, ground, lean, broiled medium, 3 ounces	74
Beef, top round, broiled, 3 ounces	73
Chicken, roasted, without skin, light meat, 3$\frac{1}{2}$ ounces	75
Haddock, baked, 3 ounces	63
Mackerel, baked, 3 ounces	64
Swordfish, baked, 3 ounces	43
Shrimp, moist heat, 3 ounces	167
Milk, whole, 8 ounces	33
Milk, 2% fat, 8 ounces	18
Milk, 1% fat, 8 ounces	10
Skim milk, 8 ounces	4
Cheddar cheese, 1 ounce	30
American processed cheese, 1 ounce	27
Cottage cheese, low fat, $\frac{1}{2}$ cup	5

Source: National Institutes of Health

weight of healthy normal-weight men is fat (about 18-25% for women). At least half of fat deposits are located just beneath the skin, where they help to cushion body organs (acting like shock absorbers) and provide insulation (to help maintain a constant body temperature). Lipids are also an important component of cells, including the cell membrane (the outer layer of the cell). Because fats slow digestion and the emptying of the stomach, they delay the onset of hunger. In addition to creating a feeling of fullness, fats increase the palatability of foods by enhancing their aroma, taste, flavor, juiciness, and tenderness.

PROTEIN

To most Americans, the term "protein" means meat, and possibly poultry and fish, too. While these foods are all excellent sources of protein, there are other less well-known sources such as dried beans and peas, whole grains, and vegetables. Protein-rich meats, poultry, and fish rank high in the diets of Americans. In other parts of the world, plant-based protein sources are the foundation of the diet.

Like carbohydrates and fats, **proteins** contain carbon, hydrogen, and oxygen. But unlike these other nutrients, proteins contain the chemical element nitrogen. **Amino acids** are the nitrogen-containing building blocks of proteins. Proteins are strands of amino acids (Figure 2.11). This allows for an endless number of combinations and sequences in the amino acid chains and, therefore, a great variety of proteins in plants and animals.

THE AMINO ACIDS

ESSENTIAL AMINO ACIDS	NONESSENTIAL AMINO ACIDS*
Histidine	Alanine
Isoleucine	Arginine
Leucine	Aspartic acid
Lysine	Cysteine
Methionine	Cystine
Phenylalanine	Glutamic acid
Threonine	Glutamine
Tryptophan	Glycine
Valine	Proline
	Serine
	Tyrosine

*Under some circumstances, one or more of these may become essential.

Figure 2.11

When a new protein is made in a cell, the long string of amino acids (usually 35 to 300 amino acids long) quickly bends and coils into a three-dimensional form. Each protein has a unique sequence of amino acids and a unique way of bending and coiling that is necessary for the protein to function normally. Different tissues in the body, such as hair and skin, each have their own characteristic proteins. Because of the different shapes proteins take, they are able to perform many varied tasks in the body, yet each protein is designed to perform a specific function(s) and can't be replaced by another. When its unique three-dimensional structure becomes distorted and unfolds, the protein undergoes a process called *denaturation*. Once denatured, the protein can't function, and in most cases, the process can't be reversed. Denaturation can occur both with proteins in food and to proteins in the body. Causes for it include alcohol, high temperatures, very acidic substances (acids are solutions that usually have a sour taste, such as vinegar), agitation or whipping, or the salts of mercury, silver, and lead. Cooking an egg, for example, denatures protein. Some amino acids, called the essential amino acids, must be provided by food because the body can't make them. Without these amino acids, the body can't make the proteins it needs to rebuild tissue and do other tasks. Other amino acids are considered nonessential amino acids because they can be made by the human body.

Functions

Amino acids are required by the body for building and maintaining cells. For instance, proteins are found in the skin, bone, cartilage, and muscles. The greatest amounts of proteins are needed when the body is building new cells rapidly, such as during infancy, pregnancy, or when a mother is nursing a child. Proteins are also essential for maintenance of the body. Parts of the body are constantly being remodeled, that is to say they are being broken down and built again. For example, your skin today is not the same skin you had a few months ago. It has been rebuilt. Large amounts of protein are needed by individuals suffering from burns or infections, or recovering from surgery. The thousands of enzymes which speed up the numerous chemical reactions in the body are made of proteins. Many hormones (chemical messengers) that regulate metabolism are also made of protein.

Proteins also are needed for forming antibodies that fight infection. Antibodies travel in the blood, where it is their job to attack any foreign bodies that do not belong, such as a virus, bacteria, or a toxin. Antibodies actually combine with these foreign bodies, producing an immune response that helps ward off harmful infections. Proteins can be burned to supply energy. When the diet does not supply enough calories from carbohydrates or fats, proteins are used for energy, even at the expense of building body proteins. Some amino acids can even be converted to glucose, the sole fuel of the brain. Proteins are needed regularly in the diet because the body has little protein reserve. However, if more proteins and more calories are eaten than are needed by the body, the extra proteins are used for energy or are converted to body fat and stored in fat cells. Thus, a person can become overweight from eating excess calories in the form of proteins. Proteins also assist in maintaining water balance within the body and keeping the blood neutral, meaning neither too acidic nor too basic. Any solution can be measured on a scale, called the *pH scale*, to determine if it is acidic (pH is less than seven), neutral (pH is seven), or basic (pH is greater than seven). Normal processes of the body produce acids and bases that can cause major problems in the blood and in the body, such as coma and death, if not brought back to neutral. Proteins have the ability to neutralize both acids and bases.

During digestion, proteins are broken down into amino acids that are then absorbed into the blood. Amino acids travel through the blood into the body's cells. There is an amino acid pool in the body that provides the cells with a supply of amino acids for making protein. The *amino acid pool* refers to the overall amount of amino acids distributed in the blood, the organs (such as the liver), and the body's cells. Amino acids from foods, as well as amino acids from body proteins that have been dismantled, stock these pools. In this manner, the body recycles its own proteins. If there is a shortage of a nonessential amino acid during production of a protein, the cell will make it and add it to the protein strand. If there is a shortage of an essential amino acid, the protein can't be completed.

Protein deficiency in the US is usually due to illness, injury, or economic factors. In these cases, protein deficiency may cause wasting of muscles, weight loss, delayed wound healing, lowered immunity due to fewer antibodies being made, and edema. *Edema* is the abnormal pooling of fluid in the tissues, causing swelling of the part of the body where the pooling occurs. Edema is often seen in malnutrition. With appropriate nutritional intervention, extra protein can be given where there is a loss of body protein due to burns, surgery, stress, infections, skin breakdown, and similar situations. Protein deficiency commonly occurs in developing countries where children do not have enough to eat. It is rarely seen without a deficiency of calories and other nutrients as well. **Protein calorie malnutrition** is the name for a group of diseases characterized by both protein and energy deficiency. Protein-deficiency disease is called kwashiorkor, and energy-deficiency disease is called marasmus. *Kwashiorkor* is characterized by retarded growth and development, a protruding abdomen due to edema, peeling skin, a loss of normal hair color, irritability, and sadness. *Marasmus* is characterized by gross underweight, no fat stores, and wasting away of muscles. There is no edema, as seen in kwashiorkor, and individuals are apathetic. Whereas marasmus is usually associated with severe food shortage, prolonged semi-starvation, or early weaning, kwashiorkor is associated with poor protein intake.

Sources and Quality of Protein
Protein occurs in almost all foods of animal and plant origin. Animal sources of protein in the American diet include meat, poultry, seafood, eggs, milk, and

cheese. Plant sources include legumes, cereal grains, and products made with them, such as bread and ready-to-eat cereals, vegetables, nuts, and seeds. The legumes (beans, peas, and lentils) contain larger amounts and better quality proteins than other plant sources. Fruits contain very little protein. Animal sources of protein almost always have fat, especially saturated fat, while plant sources contain very little fat.

The quality of a particular protein depends on its content of essential amino acids. Food proteins providing all of the essential amino acids in the proportions needed by the body are called *complete* or high-quality proteins. Meat, poultry, fish, milk and milk products, and eggs are all sources of complete proteins. Animal proteins are much better absorbed than plant proteins; over 90% of the amino acids are absorbed into the body. Plant proteins are usually low in one or more of the essential amino acids and are called *incomplete* proteins. The amino acid that is in short supply is called the *limiting amino acid*. Plant proteins are not absorbed as well as animal proteins. About 80% of the protein in legumes is absorbed, while 60 to 90% of the protein in cereal grains and other plant foods is absorbed. Although plant proteins are incomplete proteins, they are the major source of protein for many people around the world. To *complement* proteins means to eat either some animal protein (such as milk or eggs) with vegetable protein, or to combine two plant sources, such as grains and legumes, so that the essential amino acids deficient in one are present in the other.

VITAMINS

Vitamins are essential in small quantities for growth and good health. Vitamins are similar to each other because they are made of the same elements—carbon, hydrogen, oxygen, and sometimes nitrogen or cobalt. They are different in that their elements are arranged differently, and each vitamin performs one or more specific functions in the body. In the early 1900s, scientists thought they had found the compounds needed to prevent two diseases caused by vitamin deficiencies: scurvy and pellagra. These compounds originally were believed to belong to a class of chemical compounds called amines. Their name comes from the Latin *vita*, or life, plus *amine*—vitamine. Later, the "e" was dropped when it was found that not all of the substances were amines. At first, no one knew what they were chemically, and they were identified by letters. Later, what was thought to be one vitamin turned out to be many, and numbers were added; the vitamin B complex is the best example (for example, vitamin B1 and vitamin B6). When they were found unnecessary for human needs, some vitamins were removed from the list, which accounts for some of the gaps in the numbers. For example, vitamin B8, adenylic acid, was later found not to be a vitamin. Others, originally designated differently from each other, were found to be one and the same. For example, vitamins H, M, S, W, and X were all shown to be biotin. Let's start with some basic facts about vitamins:

▶ Very small amounts of vitamins are needed by the human body, and very small amounts are present in foods. Some vitamins are measured in I.U.s (international units), a measure of biological activity; others are measured in weight in micrograms or milligrams. Some vitamins, such as Vitamin D, can be measured in I.U.s and micrograms. To illustrate how small these amounts are, remember that one ounce is 28.3 grams. A milligram is $\frac{1}{1000}$ of a gram, and a microgram is $\frac{1}{1000}$ of a milligram.

▶ Although vitamins are needed in small quantities, the roles they play in the body are enormously important.

▶ Vitamins must be obtained through foods because they are either not made in the body or not made in sufficient quantities.

▶ There is no perfect food that contains all the vitamins in just the right amounts. The best way to assure an adequate intake of vitamins is to eat a varied and balanced diet.

▶ Vitamins do not have any calories, so they do not directly provide energy to the body. However, they are involved in how the body uses energy and performs many of its necessary functions.

▶ Some substances considered to be vitamins in foods are not actually vitamins, but rather are precursors. In the body, the precursor is chemically changed to the active form of the vitamin, under proper conditions.

Vitamins are classified according to how soluble they are in either fat or water. Figure 2.12 lists the fat-soluble and water-soluble vitamins. The fat-soluble vitamins generally occur in foods containing fat and can be stored in the body, in

---

VITAMINS

FAT-SOLUBLE	WATER-SOLUBLE
Vitamin A	Vitamin C
Vitamin D	Thiamin
Vitamin E	Riboflavin
Vitamin K	Niacin
	Vitamin B6
	Folate
	Vitamin B12
	Pantothenic acid
	Biotin

Figure 2.12

fat tissue. The water-soluble vitamins are not stored appreciably in the body. Now let's take a closer look at 13 vitamins.

Vitamin A

Vitamin A is involved in many different functions. It plays a role in the formation and maintenance of healthy skin and hair, as well as in proper bone growth and tooth development in children. Vitamin A is also needed for the immune system to work properly (for fighting infections) and for maintenance of the protective linings of the lungs, intestines, urinary tract, and other organs. Vitamin A is essential for normal reproduction and, when eaten generously in the form of fruits and vegetables, may protect against certain forms of cancer. Vitamin A is well-known for its part in helping us see properly. Vitamin A is necessary for the health of the eye's cornea, the clear membrane that covers the eye. Without enough vitamin A, the cornea becomes cloudy and dry. Vitamin A is also necessary for night vision, the ability for eyes to adjust after seeing a flash of bright light at night. In night blindness, it take longer than normal to adjust to dim lights. This is an early sign of vitamin A deficiency. If the deficiency continues, it can eventually lead to blindness.

The form of vitamin A found in fruits and vegetables is actually a precursor of vitamin A called beta carotene. In the body, beta carotene is converted to

Figure 2.13

VITAMIN A IN FOODS

FOOD	RETINOL EQUIVALENTS
Liver, beef, 3 oz	9,011
Sweet potato, baked, 1 small	2,488
Carrots, raw, 1	2,025
Spinach, cooked, 1/2 cup	875
Squash, butternut, 1/2 cup	857
Cantaloupe, 1/4 melon	516
Milk, 2%, 1 cup	140
Apricots, dried, 4 large halves	127
Broccoli, cooked, 1/2 cup	110
Egg yolk, 1	97
Cheese, cheddar, 1 oz	86
Margarine, fortified, 1 tsp	47
Peach, 1 medium	47
Orange, 1 medium	27

Source: USDA

vitamin A. Beta carotene often gives foods an orange color. It occurs in dark green vegetables, such as spinach, and deep orange fruits and vegetables, such as apricots, carrots, and sweet potatoes (see Figure 2.13).

Other sources of vitamin A include animal products such as liver (a very rich source), egg yolk, butter, milk, fortified margarine, cream, cheese, and fortified cereals. Low fat and skim milks are often fortified with vitamin A because the vitamin is removed from the milk when the fat is removed. **Fortified** foods have one or more nutrients added. Most ready-to-eat and instant-prepared cereals are also fortified with vitamin A. *Retinol*, the active form of vitamin A found in animal foods, is used in fortification.

Nutrient needs for vitamin A are expressed in *retinol equivalents (REs)*. Retinol equivalents measure the amount of retinol the body will actually obtain from eating foods with various forms of vitamin A, e.g. retinol or beta carotene.

Because the body stores vitamin A, it is not absolutely necessary to eat a good source every day. Vitamin A deficiency is not seen often in the US and other developed countries. Unfortunately, it is of concern in third-world countries where a lack of vitamin A causes poor growth, infection, blindness, and death. Although there may not be agreement on exactly how much vitamin A can be considered a toxic dose, excessive use of vitamin A may cause dry, scaly skin, bone pain, soreness, stunted growth, liver damage, nausea, and diarrhea. *Megadoses* (more than 10 times the estimated nutrient need) are particularly dangerous for pregnant women and children.

Vitamin D

Vitamin D differs from the other fat-soluble vitamins in that it can be made in the body and it acts more like a hormone than like a vitamin. Acting like a hormone or chemical messenger, vitamin D maintains blood calcium and phosphorus levels so that there is enough calcium and phosphorus present for building bones and teeth. Vitamin D also helps the body absorb calcium and phosphorus from the digestive tract. Only small amounts of vitamin D are found in most foods. For this reason, milk is usually fortified with vitamin D. Other significant food sources of vitamin D include liver, egg yolks, and fish liver oils. Fortunately, many people make enough vitamin D to meet ongoing needs. When ultraviolet rays shine on the skin, a cholesterol-like compound is converted into a vitamin D precursor and absorbed into the blood. The precursor is then transformed into vitamin D. A light-skinned person needs only 10 to 15 minutes of sun each day to make enough vitamin D; a dark-skinned person needs several hours. Vitamin D deficiency, which is rare in the US, causes rickets in children and infants. In *rickets*, bones are soft and pliable because they lack enough calcium and phosphorus to become strong. When this happens, several problems develop: bowlegs, knock knees, chest deformities, and curving of the spine. Deficiency may also occur in adults who have little exposure to the sun and low intakes of vitamin D, calcium, and phosphorus. It is referred to as *osteomalacia* and is seen in the Middle East and the Orient. It is characterized by soft bones that break easily and bend easily as well, causing deformities of the spine, for example.

Vitamin D, when taken in excess, is the most toxic (poisonous) of all the vitamins. Toxicity symptoms include nausea, vomiting, diarrhea, fatigue, and thirst. It can lead to calcium deposits in the heart and kidneys that can cause severe health problems. Young children and infants are especially susceptible to the toxic effects of too much vitamin D; megadoses can cause growth failure.

Vitamin E

Vitamin E has an important function in the body as an antioxidant. **Antioxidants** combine with oxygen so oxygen is not available to oxidize, or destroy, important substances. Vitamin E prevents destruction of cells. Today, scientists suggest that antioxidants can slow down the normal aging process and provide important protection against cancer. Both vitamin E and vitamin C are considered antioxidant vitamins. Vitamin E is important for the health of the cell (especially the red blood cells), the proper functioning of the immune system, and the metabolism of vitamin A.

Vitamin E is widely distributed in plant foods. Rich sources include vegetable oils, margarine and shortening made from vegetable oils, and wheat germ. In oils, vitamin E acts like an antioxidant and thereby prevents the oil from going rancid or bad. Other good sources include whole grain cereals, green leafy vegetables, nuts, and seeds. Animal foods are poor sources, except for liver and egg yolk. Vitamin E deficiency is rare, as is toxicity due to large doses of vitamin E.

Vitamin K

Vitamin K has an essential role in the production of proteins involved in blood clotting. When the skin is broken, blood clotting is vital to prevent excessive blood loss. Vitamin K is also involved in calcium metabolism. Vitamin K appears in certain foods and is also made in the body. There are billions of bacteria which normally live in the intestines, and some of them produce vitamin K. It is thought that the amount of vitamin K produced by the bacteria is significant and may meet about half of body needs. Food sources of vitamin K provide the balance. Excellent sources of vitamin K include green leafy vegetables such as kale, spinach, cabbage, and liver. Other sources include milk and eggs. A deficiency of vitamin K is rare in adults. An infant is normally given this vitamin after birth to prevent bleeding, because the intestines do not yet have the bacteria to produce vitamin K.

Water-Soluble Vitamins

The water-soluble vitamins include vitamin C and the B-complex vitamins. The B vitamins work in every cell of the body where they function as coenzymes. A *coenzyme* works with an enzyme to make it active. An *enzyme* boosts chemical reactions in the body to support all kinds of body functions.

The body stores only limited amounts of water-soluble vitamins; excesses are excreted in the urine. Nevertheless, many water-soluble vitamins taken in excess (e.g. through massive supplementation) can cause toxic side effects.

Vitamin C

Vitamin C (also called ascorbic acid) is important in forming collagen, a protein that gives strength and support to bones, teeth, muscle, cartilage, blood vessels, and skin tissue. It has been said that vitamin C acts like cement, holding together our cells and tissues. Vitamin C also helps absorb iron into the body and strengthens resistance to infection. Like vitamin E, vitamin C is an important antioxidant, preventing the oxidation of vitamin A and polyunsaturated fatty acids in the intestine. Its antioxidant properties have made vitamin C widely used in foods as an additive. It may appear on the food label as sodium ascorbate, calcium ascorbate, or simply ascorbic acid.

Foods rich in vitamin C include citrus fruits (oranges, grapefruits, limes, and lemons) and tomatoes. Good sources include white potatoes, sweet potatoes, tomatoes, broccoli, and other green and yellow vegetables, as well as cantaloupe and strawberries (Figure 2.14). There is little or no vitamin C in meats

Figure 2.14

VITAMIN C IN FOODS

Food	Milligrams Vitamin C
FRUITS	
Orange, 1	.80
Kiwi, 1 medium	.75
Cranberry juice cocktail, ¾ cup	.67
Orange juice, from concentrate, ½ cup	.48
Papaya, ½ cup cubes	.43
Strawberries, ½ cup	.42
Grapefruit, ½	.41
Grapefruit juice, canned, ½ cup	.36
Cantaloupe, ½ cup cubes	.34
Tangerine, 1	.26
Mango, ½ cup, slices	.23
Honeydew melon, ½ cup cubes	.21
Banana, 1	.10
Apple, 1	.8
Nectarine, 1	.7

Food	Milligrams Vitamin C
VEGETABLES	
Broccoli, chopped, cooked, ½ cup	.49
Brussels sprouts, cooked, ½ cup	.48
Cauliflower, cooked, ½ cup	.34
Sweet potato, baked, 1	.28
Kale, cooked, chopped, ½ cup	.27
White potato, baked, 1	.26
Tomato, 1 fresh	.22
Tomato juice, ½ cup	.22
CEREALS	
Corn flakes, 1 cup	.15

Source: USDA

or dairy foods. Some juices are fortified with vitamin C, as are most ready-to-eat cereals. Certain situations raise the body's need for vitamin C. These include pregnancy and nursing, growth, fevers, infections, burns, fractures, surgery, cancer, heavy alcohol intake, and cigarette smoking. Megadoses of vitamin C often cause nausea, abdominal cramps, and diarrhea. Megadoses of vitamin C can also interfere with clotting medications (such as warfarin and dicoumarol) and cause incorrect urine test results for diabetes. A deficiency of vitamin C causes a disease called *scurvy*. Symptoms of scurvy include bleeding gums, weakness, growth failure, delayed wound healing, easy bruising, and iron-deficiency anemia. Many of these symptoms are due to the faulty formation of collagen. Vitamin C deficiency is of some concern in the US and is sometimes seen in elderly individuals, or among individuals who have inadequate diets. Of all the vitamins, vitamin C is the most fragile and the most easily destroyed during preparation, cooking, or storage.

Thiamin, Riboflavin, and Niacin

Thiamin, riboflavin, and niacin all play key roles as coenzymes in energy metabolism. Coenzymes are chemical compounds that help enzymes work. As mentioned earlier, enzymes are specialized proteins that speed up specific chemical reactions in the body. These vitamins are essential to release energy from glucose, fatty acids, and amino acids. Thiamin also plays a vital role in the normal functioning of the nervous system and appetite. Riboflavin is important for healthy skin and normal functioning of the eyes. Niacin is needed for the maintenance of healthy skin and the normal functioning of the nervous system and digestive tract. Because thiamin, riboflavin, and niacin all help release energy from food, the needs for these vitamins increase as calorie intake rises.

Thiamin is widely distributed in foods, but mostly in moderate amounts. Pork is an excellent source of thiamin. Other sources include liver, dry beans and peas, peanuts, peanut butter, seeds, and whole grain and enriched breads and cereals.

Milk is a major source of riboflavin; yogurt and cheese are also good sources. Other sources include organ meats like liver (very high in riboflavin), whole grain and enriched breads and cereals, and some meats.

The main sources of niacin are meat, poultry, and fish. Organ meats are quite high in niacin. All foods containing complete protein, such as those just mentioned and also milk and eggs, are good sources of the precursor of niacin, tryptophan. *Tryptophan* is an amino acid present in some of these foods that is converted to niacin (with the help of riboflavin and vitamin B6). Whole-grain and enriched breads and cereals supply niacin.

A thiamin deficiency causes a disease called *beriberi*, which is characterized by poor appetite, depression, confusion, weakness, wasting, heart problems, and deterioration of the nervous system. Thiamin deficiency is not common in developed countries, except in alcoholics, who get most of their calories from alcohol rather than from food. Most deficiencies of B vitamins include more than just one vitamin, so it is not surprising to find riboflavin lacking, along with thiamin. Because the symptoms of a thiamin deficiency are more severe, the signs of a riboflavin deficiency (cracks at the corner of the mouth, skin rash, poor healing, burning and itching eyes) may never be seen. Niacin deficiency still occurs in poor urban areas, possibly because there is poor intake of complete protein sources that contribute much of the niacin in the diet. The effects of *pellagra*, the niacin-deficiency disease, are easy to remember as the "4 Ds"— diarrhea, dermatitis (skin inflammation), dementia, and ultimately death. Niacin deficiency first appears as fatigue, poor appetite, indigestion, and a skin rash. Later, nervous system symptoms appear, including confusion and disorientation.

Toxicity is not a problem with these vitamins, except for niacin. Nicotinic acid, a form of niacin, has been prescribed by physicians to lower elevated blood cholesterol levels. Unfortunately, it has some undesirable side effects. Starting at doses of 100 milligrams, typical symptoms include flushing, rashes, tingling, itching, hives, nausea, diarrhea, and abdominal discomfort. Flushing of the face, neck, and chest lasts for about 20 minutes after taking a large dose. More serious side effects of large doses include liver malfunction, high blood sugar levels, and abnormal heart rhythm.

Vitamin B6

Vitamin B6 plays an important role as part of a coenzyme involved in carbohydrate, fat, and protein metabolism. It is particularly important in protein metabolism. Vitamin B6 is also used to make red blood cells, which transport oxygen around the body. It helps convert tryptophan, an amino acid, to niacin. The need for vitamin B6 is directly related to protein intake. As the intake of protein increases, the need for vitamin B6 increases.

Good sources of vitamin B6 include organ meats, meat, poultry, and fish. Vitamin B6 also appears in plant foods; however, it is not as well absorbed from these sources. Good plant sources include whole grains, potatoes, some fruits (such as bananas and cantaloupe), and some leafy green vegetables (such as broccoli and spinach). Fortified ready-to-eat cereals are also good sources of vitamin B6. Deficiency of vitamin B6 causes muscle twitching, rashes, greasy skin, and a type of anemia called *microcytic anemia*, a small cell anemia. Excessive use of vitamin B6 (more than two grams daily for two months or more) can cause irreversible nerve damage and symptoms such as numbness in hands and feet, and difficulty walking.

Folate

Folate is also called folic acid, its synthetic form used in fortified foods and supplements. Folate is part of a coenzyme used to make new cells, including red blood cells, white bloods cells, and digestive tract cells. A deficiency of folate can cause *megaloblastic anemia*, a condition in which the red blood cells are

Figure 2.15

VITAMINS: FUNCTIONS AND FOOD SOURCES

VITAMIN	FUNCTIONS	FOOD SOURCES
Vitamin E	Antioxidant; protects red and white blood cells	Vegetable oils, margarine, shortening, seeds, nuts, wheat germ, whole grain and fortified breads and cereals, soybeans
Vitamin K	Blood clotting; makes protein used in making bones	Dark green leafy vegetables, cabbage, intestinal bacteria
Vitamin C	Antioxidant; formation of collagen; wound healing; iron absorption; functioning of immune system	Citrus fruits, bell peppers, kiwifruit, broccoli, strawberries, tomatoes, potatoes, juices and cereals fortified with vitamin C
Thiamin	Coenzyme in energy metabolism; functioning of nervous system; normal growth	Pork, sunflower seeds, wheat germ, peanuts, dry beans, and whole grain and enriched/fortified breads and cereals
Riboflavin	Coenzyme in energy metabolism; healthy skin; normal vision	Milk and milk products, whole grain and enriched/fortified breads and cereals, some meats, eggs
Niacin	Coenzyme in energy metabolism; healthy skin; normal functioning of nervous system	Meat, poultry, fish, whole grain and enriched/fortified breads and cereals, milk, eggs
Vitamin B6	Coenzyme in carbohydrate, fat, and protein metabolism; synthesis of blood cells	Meat, poultry, fish, fortified cereals, some leafy green vegetables, potatoes, bananas, watermelon
Folate	Formation of new cells	Green leafy vegetables, legumes, orange juice, enriched/fortified breads and cereals
Vitamin B12	Activation of folate; normal functioning of the nervous system	Meat, poultry, seafood, eggs, dairy products, fortified breads and cereals
Pantothenic Acid	Energy metabolism	Widespread
Biotin	Energy metabolism; carbohydrate, fat, and protein metabolism	Widespread

oversized and function poorly. Other symptoms may include digestive tract problems, such as diarrhea, and mental depression. During pregnancy, the need for folate increases because of its vital role in producing new cells. Folate is needed both before and during pregnancy to help reduce the risk of certain serious and common birth defects called neural tube defects, which affect the brain and spinal cord. The tricky part is that neural tube defects can occur in an embryo before a woman realizes she's pregnant. Luckily, folate occurs naturally in a variety of foods, including liver; dark-green leafy vegetables such as collards, turnip greens, and Romaine lettuce; broccoli and asparagus; citrus fruits and juices; whole grain products; wheat germ; and dried beans and peas, such as pinto, navy, and lima beans, and chick-peas and black-eyed peas. By law, many grain products are fortified with folate. This gives women another way to get sufficient folate.

Vitamin B12

Vitamin B12, also called cobalamin and cyanocobalamin, is present in all body cells. Along with folate, vitamin B12 is involved in making new cells in the body and in the growth of healthy red blood cells. It also helps in the normal functioning of the nervous system by maintaining the protective cover around nerve fibers. Vitamin B12 is different from other vitamins in that it is found only in animal foods such as meat, poultry, fish, shellfish, eggs, milk, and milk products. Plant foods do not contain any vitamin B12. Vegetarians who do not eat any animal products will need to include fortified soy milk in their diet, or take supplements.

Vitamin B12 is also different from other vitamins in that it requires a compound called *intrinsic factor* (produced in the stomach) to be absorbed. A deficiency of vitamin B12 in the body is usually not due to poor intake, but rather due to a problem with absorption. When there is a problem with absorption of vitamin B12, *pernicious anemia* develops. Pernicious anemia results in macrocytic anemia, as seen when there is a folate deficiency. Therefore, folate supplementation may mask the symptoms of pernicious anemia. Pernicious anemia is also characterized by deterioration in the functioning of the nervous system that, if untreated, could cause significant and sometimes irreversible damage. Therapy includes vitamin B12 injections.

Pantothenic Acid and Biotin

Both pantothenic acid and biotin are involved in energy metabolism. Pantothenic acid is part of a coenzyme used in energy metabolism. Biotin is part of a coenzyme used in energy metabolism, fat synthesis, amino acid metabolism, and glycogen synthesis. Both pantothenic acid and biotin are widespread in foods, and deficiency is rare. Intestinal bacteria make considerable amounts of pantothenic acid. There is no known toxicity of either pantothenic acid or biotin.

Figure 2.15 summarizes the functions and food sources of vitamins.

MINERALS

If you were to weigh all the minerals in the body, they would only amount to four or five pounds. We need only small amounts of minerals in the diet, but they perform enormously important jobs—such as building bones and teeth, regulating heartbeat, and transporting oxygen from the lungs to tissues.

Some minerals are needed in relatively large amounts in the diet—over 100 milligrams daily. (A paper clip weighs about 1 gram. A milligram is $\frac{1}{1000}$ of a gram.) These minerals are called *major minerals* and include calcium, chloride, magnesium, phosphorus, potassium, sodium, and sulfur. Other minerals, called

Figure 2.16

ESSENTIAL MINERALS

MAJOR MINERALS	TRACE MINERALS
Calcium	Chromium
Chloride	Cobalt
Magnesium	Copper
Phosphorus	Fluoride
Potassium	Iodine
Sodium	Iron
Sulfur	Manganese
	Molybdenum
	Selenium
	Zinc

trace minerals or trace elements, are needed in smaller amounts—less than 100 milligrams daily. Iron, fluoride, and zinc are examples of trace minerals. Figure 2.16 lists major and trace minerals.

Minerals have some distinctive properties not shared by other nutrients. For example, whereas over 90% of the carbohydrate, fat, and protein in the diet is absorbed into the body, the percentage of minerals absorbed varies tremendously. As examples, only 5-10% of dietary iron is normally absorbed; about 30% of calcium is absorbed; yet almost all of dietary sodium is absorbed. Unlike some vitamins, minerals are not easily destroyed in storage or preparation. Like vitamins, minerals can be toxic when consumed in excessive amounts.

Calcium and Phosphorus

Calcium and phosphorus are used for building bones and teeth. They give rigidity to the structures. Bone is being constantly rebuilt, with new bone being formed, and old bone being taken apart, every day. Teeth are also rebuilt, but at a much slower rate.

Calcium also circulates in the blood and appears in other body tissues, where it helps blood clot, muscles contract (including the heart muscle), and nerves transmit impulses. Calcium helps maintain normal blood pressure and immune defenses.

Phosphorus is involved in the release of energy from fats, proteins, and carbohydrates during metabolism, and in the formation of genetic material and many enzymes. Phosphorus also helps in the absorption and transport of fats and assists in keeping blood chemistry neutral. Phosphorus has the ability to buffer or neutralize both acids and bases.

The major sources of calcium are milk and milk products. Not all milk products are as rich in calcium as milk (Figure 2.17). As a matter of fact, butter, cream, and cream cheese contain very little calcium. Other good sources of calcium include canned salmon and sardines (containing bones), oysters, calcium-fortified foods such as orange juice, and greens such as broccoli, collards, kale, mustard greens, and turnip greens. Other greens such as spinach, beet greens, Swiss chard, sorrel, and parsley are rich in calcium but also contain a binder (called *oxalic acid*) that prevents calcium from being absorbed. Dried beans and peas and certain shellfish contain moderate amounts of calcium but are usually not eaten in sufficient quantities to make a significant contribution. Meats and grains are poor sources.

Even though only about 30% of the calcium we eat is absorbed, the body absorbs more calcium (up to 60%) when it is needed—such as during growth and pregnancy, and also when there is inadequate calcium in the diet. Vitamin D aids in calcium absorption.

Phosphorus is widely distributed in foods and is not likely to be lacking in the diet. Milk and milk products are excellent sources. Good sources are meat, poultry, fish, eggs, legumes, and whole grain foods. Fruits and vegetables are generally low in this mineral. Compounds that include phosphorus are used in processed foods, especially soft drinks.

CALCIUM IN SELECTED FOODS

FOOD	CALCIUM CONTENT (MG)
Milk, skim, 8 ounces	302
Milk, 2%, 8 ounces	297
Milk, whole, 8 ounces	291
Yogurt, low fat, 1 cup	415
Yogurt, low fat with fruit, 1 cup	345
Yogurt, frozen, 1 cup	200
Ice cream, 1 cup	176
Cottage cheese, creamed, 1 cup	147
Swiss cheese, 1 ounce	272
Parmesan, 1 ounce	390
Cheddar, 1 ounce	204
Mozzarella, 1 ounce	183
American cheese, 1 ounce	174

FOOD	CALCIUM CONTENT (MG)
Cheese pizza, 1/4 of 14 " pie	332
Macaroni and cheese, 1/2 cup	181
Orange juice, calcium-fortified, 8 ounces	300
Sardines with bones, 3 ounces	372
Oysters, 1 cup	226
Shrimp, 3 ounces	98
Tofu, 3 1/2 ounces	128
Dried navy beans, cooked, 1 cup	95
Turnip greens, frozen and cooked, 1 cup	249
Kale, frozen and cooked, 1 cup	179
Mustard greens, 1 cup	104
Broccoli, frozen and cooked, 1 cup	94

Source: USDA

Figure 2.17

When there isn't enough calcium in the diet, calcium is removed from the bones, a problem that over time will weaken the bone structure and lead to a disease called *osteoporosis* or adult bone loss. Sometimes individuals who are aware of the problems of osteoporosis take calcium supplements. Many calcium supplements provide mixtures of calcium with other compounds, such as calcium carbonate, a good source of calcium. There are also powdered forms of calcium-rich sources, such as bone meal and dolomite (a rock mineral). These are dangerous, as they may contain lead and other elements in amounts that would constitute a risk. Calcium supplements should not be taken without guidance from a physician or Registered Dietitian.

Sodium

Sodium is a critical mineral that helps the body maintain water balance and acid-base balance. It also plays an important role in helping contract muscles and transmit nerve impulses. Meat, poultry, fish, eggs, and milk are high in natural sodium when compared to fruits and vegetables, but are still quite low compared to processed foods.

Deficiency of sodium is not a problem in the US. The estimated minimum requirement is 500 mg per day. The sodium intake of Americans is easily six times this amount—varying from three to eight grams daily.

Potassium

Potassium is an electrolyte found mainly inside the body's cells. In the cell, potassium is needed for making protein. Along with sodium, it helps maintain water balance and acid-base balance. Potassium is also needed to release energy from carbohydrates, fats, and proteins. In the blood, potassium assists in muscle contraction, helps maintain a normal heartbeat, and helps send nerve impulses.

Potassium is distributed widely in foods, both plant and animal. Unprocessed, whole foods are the best sources of potassium, such as fruits and vegetables (winter squash, potatoes, oranges, and grapefruits), milk, grains, meat, poultry, fish, and legumes.

A potassium deficiency is very uncommon in healthy people, but may result from dehydration or from using a certain class of blood pressure medications called *diuretics*. Diuretics cause increased urine output and some cause an increased excretion of potassium as well. Symptoms of a deficiency include weakness, nausea, and abnormal heart rhythms that can be very dangerous, even fatal.

Excessive potassium is equally dangerous and megadoses of it can cause numbness, abnormal heart rhythms, and cardiac failure, in which the heart stops beating. It is not recommended to take potassium supplements without the advice of a physician. Some salt substitutes contain potassium instead of sodium. Some healthcare facilities require a doctor's order to give salt substitutes to a client. A good alternative to using salt substitutes is a packet of herbs and spices that help flavor foods without sodium or potassium.

Chloride

Chloride is another important electrolyte in the body. It helps maintain water balance and acid-base balance. Chloride is also part of hydrochloric acid, found in quite high concentration in the juices of the stomach. Hydrochloric acid aids in protein digestion, as explained in Chapter 4. The most important source of chloride in the diet is sodium chloride or salt. If sodium intake is adequate, there will be ample chloride as well.

Magnesium

Magnesium is found in all body tissues, with about 60-70% being in the bones, and the remainder in the muscles and other soft tissues. It is an essential part of many enzyme systems responsible for energy conversions in the body. Magnesium is used in building bones and teeth and works with calcium, potassium, and sodium to contract muscles and transmit nerve impulses. Magnesium also has a role in making protein.

Magnesium is a part of the green pigment called chlorophyll that is found in plants. Good sources include green leafy vegetables, nuts (especially almonds and cashews), seeds, whole grain cereals, and legumes such as soybeans. Seafood is also a good source. Deficiency symptoms are rare.

Sulfur

Sulfur is found in three of the amino acids. The protein in hair, skin, and nails is particularly rich in sulfur. Sulfur is also a part of two vitamins, thiamin and biotin. High protein foods supply plentiful amounts of sulfur and a deficiency is not known to occur.

Trace Minerals

Most of the trace minerals do not occur in the body in their free form, but are bound to organic compounds on which they depend for transport, storage, and function. Our understanding of many trace minerals is just starting to emerge. All the trace minerals are toxic in excess.

Fluoride

Fluoride is the term used for the form of fluorine as it appears in drinking water and in the body. The terms fluoride and fluorine are used interchangeably. Fluoride contributes to solid tooth formation and results in a decrease of dental caries (cavities), especially in children. There is also evidence that fluoride helps retain calcium in the bones of older people.

The major source of fluoride is drinking water. Some supplies of drinking water are naturally fluoridated, and many supplies of water have fluoride added, usually at a concentration of one part fluoride to one million parts water. In nearly all areas where fluoridation of water has been introduced, the incidence of dental caries in children has been reduced by 50% or more. In areas where there is too much natural fluoride in the water, teeth become discolored, but there are no undesirable health effects.

Iodine

Iodine is required in extremely small amounts for the normal functioning of the thyroid gland. The thyroid gland is located in the neck and is responsible for producing two important hormones that maintain a normal level of metabolism in the body. These hormones are essential for normal growth and development.

With a deficiency of dietary iodine, thyroid enlargement (called *goiter*) occurs. Iodine-deficiency goiter was common in certain inland areas of the United States where the soil contains little iodine. (Foods grown along the seacoast are goods sources of iodine as well as saltwater fish and shellfish). Iodized salt was introduced in 1924 to combat iodine deficiencies. Iodine also finds its way accidentally into milk, because cows receive drugs containing iodine and feed containing iodine—and into baked goods through iodine-containing compounds used in processing.

Iron

Iron is an important part of compounds necessary for transporting oxygen to the cells and making use of the oxygen when it arrives. It is widely distributed in the body, where much of it is in the blood as the *heme* portion of hemoglobin. Hemoglobin is the oxygen carrier found in red blood cells. Iron is also part of the protein *myoglobin* in muscles, which makes oxygen available for muscle contraction. Iron works with many enzymes in energy metabolism.

Liver is an excellent source of iron. Other sources are meats, egg yolks, seafood, green leafy vegetables, legumes, dried fruits, and whole grain and enriched breads and cereals.

The ability of the body to absorb and utilize iron from different foods varies from 3% for some vegetables to up to 30% from red meat. The form of iron in animal foods such as meat, poultry, and fish is absorbed and utilized more readily than iron in plant foods. The presence of these animal products in a meal increases the availability of iron from other foods, as well. The presence of vitamin C in a meal also increases iron absorption. Some foods actually decrease iron consumption: coffee, tea, calcium supplements, wheat bran, and other forms of fiber. The body adjusts its own iron absorption according to need. The body absorbs iron more efficiently when iron stores are low and during growth spurts or pregnancy.

The most common indication of poor iron status is *iron-deficiency anemia*, a condition in which the size and number of red blood cells are reduced. This condition may result from inadequate intake of iron or from blood loss.

Symptoms of iron-deficiency anemia include fatigue, pallor, irritability, and lethargy. Iron-deficiency anemia is a real concern in the US, more so for women than men. Iron requirements are higher for women of childbearing age than for men, because women have to replace menstrual blood losses.

Selenium

It was not known that selenium was an essential mineral until 1979. Selenium is part of an enzyme that acts like an antioxidant and prevents oxidative damage to tissues, much like vitamin E. Excellent sources include seafood, meat, and liver. Because selenium is sometimes found in the soil, whole grains may be a good source of selenium as well. Deficiency in the US is rare, and selenium can be toxic in large amounts.

Zinc

Zinc is involved in enzymes that promote at least 50 metabolically important reactions in the body. Zinc assists in wound healing, bone formation, development of sexual organs, and general growth and maintenance of all tissues. Zinc is also important for taste perception and appetite.

Protein-containing foods are all good sources of zinc, particularly meat, shellfish, eggs, and milk. Whole grains and some legumes are good sources as well, but zinc is much more readily available in animal foods. In general, iron and zinc are both found in the same foods.

Children, pregnant and premenopausal women, and the elderly are most at risk for being deficient in zinc. Children who are deficient in zinc typically have poor growth and little appetite. Other symptoms of zinc deficiency include diarrhea, impaired immune response, slowed metabolism, loss of taste and smell, confusion, and poor wound healing. Too much zinc interferes with copper metabolism and can cause other serious problems.

Other Trace Minerals

Chromium participates in carbohydrate and fat metabolism. Chromium actually works with insulin to get glucose into the body's cells. A chromium deficiency results in a condition much like diabetes, in which the glucose level in the blood is abnormally high. Good sources of chromium are liver, meat, the dark meat of poultry, whole grains, and brewer's yeast.

Cobalt is a part of vitamin B12 and is therefore needed to form red blood cells. We take in the cobalt we need by eating vitamin B12-rich foods. (Remember that vitamin B12 is found only in animal foods).

Copper is necessary along with iron for the formation of hemoglobin. As a part of many enzymes, it also helps make the protein collagen, assists in wound healing, and keeps nerves healthy. Copper occurs in most unprocessed foods. Organ meats, meats, shellfish, whole grain cereals, nuts, and legumes are rich

Figure 2.18

MINERALS: FUNCTIONS AND FOOD SOURCES

Mineral	Functions	Food Sources
MAJOR MINERALS:		
Calcium	Mineralization of bones and teeth; blood clotting; muscle contraction; transmission of nerve impulses	Milk and milk products, calcium-set tofu, calcium-fortified foods, broccoli, collards, kale, mustard greens, turnip greens, legumes, whole wheat bread
Phosphorus	Mineralization of bones and teeth; energy metabolism; formation of DNA and many enzymes; buffer	Milk and milk products, meat, poultry, fish, eggs, legumes
Magnesium	Energy metabolism; formation of bones and maintenance of teeth; muscle contraction, nerve transmission; immune system	Green leafy vegetables, potatoes, nuts, legumes, whole grain cereals
Sodium	Water balance; acid-base balance; buffer; muscle contraction; transmission of nerve impulses	Salt, processed foods, MSG
Potassium	Water balance; acid-base balance; buffer; muscle contraction; transmission of nerve impulses	Many fruits and vegetables (potatoes, oranges, grapefruit), milk and yogurt, legumes, meats
Chloride	Water balance; acid-base balance; part of hydrochloric acid in stomach	Salt
Sulfur	Part of some amino acids; part of thiamin	Protein foods
TRACE MINERALS:		
Copper	Iron metabolism; formation of hemoglobin; collagen formation; energy release	Seafood, whole grain breads and cereals, legumes, nuts, seeds
Fluoride	Strengthening of developing teeth	Water (naturally or artificially fluoridated), tea, seafood
Iodine	Normal functioning of thyroid gland; normal metabolic rate; normal growth and development	Iodized salt, saltwater fish
Iron	Part of hemoglobin and myoglobin; part of some enzymes; energy metabolism; needed to make amino acids	Red meats, shellfish, legumes, whole grain and enriched breads and cereals, green leafy vegetables
Selenium	Activation of antioxidant	Seafood, meat, liver, eggs, whole grains and vegetables (if soil is rich in selenium)
Zinc	Cofactor of many enzymes; wound healing; DNA and protein synthesis; bone formation; development of sexual organs; general growth and maintenance; taste perception and appetite	Protein foods; legumes, dairy products, whole grain products, fortified cereals
Chromium	Works with insulin	Liver, meats, whole grains, nuts

sources. Copper deficiency is generally not a problem (except in cases of malnutrition), and excessive copper intake can be toxic.

Manganese is needed for blood formation and bone structure, and as part of many enzymes involved in energy metabolism. Manganese is found in many foods, especially whole grains, legumes, nuts and seeds, and leafy vegetables. A deficiency is unknown.

Molybdenum is a cofactor in a number of enzyme systems and is possibly involved in the metabolism of fats. Deficiency does not seem to be a problem.

As time goes on, more trace minerals will probably be recognized as essential to human health. There are currently several trace minerals that are essential to animals and are likely to be essential to humans as well. They include arsenic, nickel, silicon, and boron.

Figure 2.18 summarizes this section on minerals.

WATER

Nothing survives without water, and virtually nothing takes place in the body without water playing a vital role. While variations may be great, the average adult's body weight is generally 50 to 60% water—enough, if it were bottled, to fill 40 to 50 quarts. For example, in a 150-pound man, water accounts for about 90 pounds, fat about 30 pounds, with proteins, carbohydrates, vitamins and minerals making up the balance. Men generally have more water than women. Some parts of the body have more water than others. Human blood is about 92% water; muscle and the brain are about 75%; and bone is about 22%.

The body uses water for virtually all its functions—digestion, absorption, circulation, excretion, transporting nutrients, building tissue, and maintaining temperature. Almost all of the body's cells depend on water to perform their functions. Water carries nutrients to the cells and carries away waste materials to the kidney. Water is needed in each step of the process of converting food into energy and tissue. Digestive secretions are mostly water, acting as a solvent for nutrients. Water in the digestive secretions softens, dilutes, and liquefies the food to facilitate digestion. It also helps move food along the gastrointestinal tract.

Water serves as an important part of lubricants, helping to cushion the joints and internal organs, keeping body tissues such as the eyes, lungs and air passages moist, and surrounding and protecting the fetus during pregnancy.

Many adults take in and excrete between eight and 10 cups of fluid daily. Nearly all foods have some water, too. Milk, for example, is about 87% water, eggs about 75%, meat between 40 and 75%, vegetables from 70 to 95%, cereals from eight to 20%, and bread around 35%.

The body gets rid of the water it doesn't need through the kidneys and skin and, to a lesser degree, from the lungs and gastrointestinal tract. The largest amount is excreted as urine by the kidneys. About a pint to more than two quarts a day are excreted as urine. The amount of urine reflects, to some extent, the amount of fluid intake of the individual, although no matter how little water one consumes, the kidneys will always excrete a certain amount each day to eliminate waste products generated by the body's metabolic actions. In addition to the urine, air released from the lungs contains some water. Evaporation that occurs from the skin (when sweating or not sweating) contains water as well.

If normal and healthy, the body maintains water at a constant level. A number of mechanisms, including the sensation of thirst, operate to keep body water content within narrow limits. We feel thirsty when the blood starts to become too concentrated. It is therefore very important not to ignore feelings of thirst. Most of the elderly cannot rely on the thirst mechanism to maintain adequate hydration status. For healthy individuals, it is not possible to drink too much water. It will simply be excreted.

There are, of course, conditions in which the various body mechanisms for regulating water balance do not work, such as severe vomiting, diarrhea, excessive bleeding, high fever, burns, and excessive perspiration. In these situations, large amounts of fluids and electrolytes (minerals) are lost. The management and treatment of these conditions are medical problems to be managed by a physician.

Figure 2.19

EXAMPLE OF EMPTY CALORIES

Homemade Cupcake with Icing

INFORMATION PER SERVING:
Serving Size = 1 Cupcake

Calories .170

Fat . . . . .5 grams

Sodium . . . . .110 milligrams

Carbohydrates . . . . .30 grams

Protein .2 grams

Vitamin A . . . .*

Vitamin C . . . .*

Calcium . . . .*

Iron . . . .*

*Less than 2% of recommended intakes

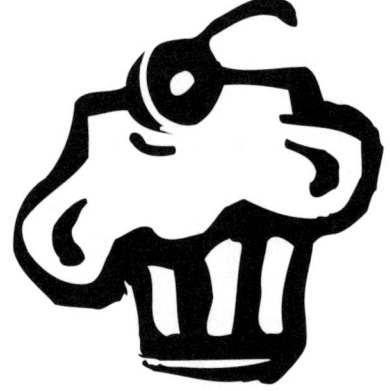

NUTRIENT DENSITY

Foods vary in how rich they are in nutrients. Foods that are nutrient-rich relative to their calorie (energy) content are said to be of high **nutrient density**. For example, one cup of broccoli has 25 calories and proportionally high levels of vitamins and minerals. It has a high nutrient density. In contrast, one cup of cola has 100 calories and no vitamins. You can think of calories as a "price" paid for vitamins, minerals, and other essential nutrients. If you pay a high price for a small amount of nutrients when you eat a particular food, that food is not nutrient dense. Sometimes people use the term **empty calories** to describe a food that has low nutrient density. See the sample in Figure 2.19. In the "price" analogy, if you pay a low price (caloric intake) and receive many nutrients, the food you are consuming is nutrient-dense. Sound dietary habits rely on nutrient-dense foods for many of the daily food choices.

MORE CHOICES FOR THE SWEET LIFE ● FOOD INSIGHT, SEPT./OCT. 2002

With an increasing focus on the rising rate of obesity in the United States and the associated health concerns, many consumers are seeking ways to manage their consumption of calories. Yet few find it easy to abandon their desire for even the occasional sweet food or beverage. For many, low-calorie or reduced-calorie sweeteners offer a means to manage caloric intake, allowing the substitution of lower-calorie foods and beverages for their higher-calorie counterparts. These foods can provide them with the sweet foods and beverages that they desire while allowing them to manage their caloric intake as well.

Low-calorie or high-intensity sweeteners are many times sweeter than sucrose (sugar) but add a taste to foods that is similar to that provided by regular sweeteners like sugar or corn syrup. The use of low-calorie sweeteners can substantially reduce the amount of calories in products such as soft drinks, candies, chewing gum, and desserts like pudding, gelatin, and ice cream. In addition, several low-calorie sweeteners are available for use as "tabletop sweeteners," which consumers add directly to foods like coffee, tea, fruits, or breakfast cereal.

The five intense, low-calorie sweeteners approved for use in the United States include acesulfame potassium, aspartame, neotame, saccharin, and sucralose. These sweeteners do not affect insulin or glucose levels and have long played a role in the food choices of people with diabetes and others who must manage their intake of carbohydrates.

LOW-CALORIE SWEETENERS CURRENTLY USED IN THE UNITED STATES

Acesulfame potassium

Acesulfame potassium—or acesulfame K as it is abbreviated on food labels—is calorie-free and is about 200 times sweeter than sugar. Acesulfame K is highly stable and has been approved for use in a wide variety of foods, beverages, and baked products. Acesulfame potassium is not broken down by the body and is eliminated without providing any calories.

Aspartame

Aspartame is a very low-calorie sweetener and is about 200 times sweeter than sugar. It is made by joining two amino acids; aspartic acid and the methyl ester of phenylalanine. The components of aspartame are also found naturally in common foods, including meat, dairy products, fruits, and vegetables. After ingestion, aspartame is broken down to its components and is utilized by the body in the same way that it is utilized when it is derived in much larger amounts from common foods. Persons with a rare hereditary disease known as phenylketonuria (PKU) must control their intake of phenylalanine from all sources, including aspartame. Although aspartame contains only a small amount of phenylalanine, the labels of foods and beverages containing aspartame must include a statement advising individuals with PKU of the presence of phenylalanine.

Neotame

Neotame received FDA approval for use in foods and beverages in the United States in July 2002. Neotame is a derivative of the dipeptide composed of the amino acids aspartic acid and phenylalanine. It is 7,000 to 13,000 times as sweet as sugar depending on its food application. It can be used alone or blended with other high-intensity or carbohydrate sweeteners. In addition, because the product is not metabolized to phenylalanine, no special labeling for individuals with phenylketonuria is required. Extensive research has been conducted on neotame to establish its safety as a sweetening ingredient. The FDA reviewed the findings from more than 100 scientific studies before approving neotame.

Saccharin

Saccharin is calorie-free and is about 300 times sweeter than sugar. Because saccharin is stable when heated, it is suitable for use in foods and beverages, and cooking and baking. It is not broken down by the body and is eliminated without providing any calories. Decades ago there were questions about whether saccharin could cause bladder cancer, based on animal studies. Numerous follow-up studies with animals and humans have shown no overall association between saccharin consumption and cancer incidence. Recently, after extensive review of the scientific data on the topic, the federal government removed saccharin from a list of potential cancer-causing agents.

Sucralose

Sucralose is calorie-free and is approximately 600 times sweeter than sugar. It is made from sugar through a patented, multistep process. Sucralose is highly stable and can be used in foods and beverages, and cooking and baking. The body does not recognize sucralose as a sugar or a carbohydrate. It is not broken down by the body and is eliminated without providing any calories.

The variety of sweeteners available to food manufacturers and consumers provides more options to sweeten different foods in different ways. Each sweetener has a slightly different intensity or character to its sweet taste. Some sweeteners may work well in applications like sugar-free soft drinks, and others may work best in baked goods or hard candy. Combinations of some sweeteners have been found to have a synergistic effect—that is, the taste of one sweetener is enhanced when it is combined with another one. The end result is that less sweetener blend is required to provide the same amount of sweetness.

A recent national consumer survey shows that more than 163 million Americans consume reduced-calorie or sugar-free foods and beverages.

(*Calorie Control Council, 2002.*) Consumers are fortunate to have so many choices today, for without low-calorie or reduced-calorie sweeteners, life for these consumers would simply not be as sweet.

HOW SWEETENERS ARE APPROVED

All low-calorie sweeteners have undergone extensive safety testing and have been carefully reviewed by the U.S. Food and Drug Administration (FDA). Before a low-calorie sweetener is approved for commercial use, it must undergo extensive testing and significant regulatory scrutiny. U.S. food safety laws prohibit FDA from approving a low-calorie sweetener (or any food ingredient) that has not been shown to have "a reasonable certainty in the minds of competent scientists that the substance is not harmful under the intended conditions of use." Manufacturers requesting approval are required to provide FDA with extensive data, including the name, chemical identity, and composition of the sweetener; the physical or other technical effects that the sweetener is intended to produce; and comprehensive reports of research concerning safety. FDA also considers projected consumption levels, as well as specific use levels. Information on projected consumption and specific levels is requested in the petition that the manufacturer submits to FDA for approval of a new product. All FDA-approved low-calorie sweeteners meet the same standard of safety and are safe for consumption by pregnant women and children.

Reduced-Calorie Sweeteners

Food manufacturers may use another group of ingredients to reduce the number of calories in food products. These reduced-calorie sweeteners are metabolized more slowly or incompletely by the body and thus provide fewer calories. They vary in sweetness, being from about half as sweet as the same amount of sugar to being equally as sweet as sugar.

These sweeteners are frequently combined with intense, low-calorie sweeteners, such as acesulfame potassium, aspartame, saccharin, and sucralose. These combinations are used in sugar-free chewing gums, candies, frozen desserts, and baked goods. Reduced-calorie sweeteners give these foods mild sweetness as well as the bulk and texture of sugar; the intense, low-calorie sweeteners bring the sweetness up to the level consumers expect.

Polyols—Polyols (or sugar alcohols) are a group of reduced-calorie sweeteners that contain some calories. Polyols are found naturally in berries, apples, plums, and other foods, and are manufactured from carbohydrates for use in sugar-free candies, cookies, chewing gums, and other reduced-calorie foods. Familiar names of polyols include sorbitol, mannitol, and isomalt.

Tagatose—Tagatose is a naturally occurring reduced-calorie bulk sweetener that can be found in some dairy products. Tagatose has a physical bulk similar to that of sucrose or table sugar and is almost as sweet. Tagatose has 1.5 calories per gram whereas sucrose has 4 calories per gram. Tagatose can therefore provide the bulk of sugar with significantly fewer calories.

HOW DID THEY DO THAT? ● FOOD INSIGHT, JANUARY/FEBRUARY 2001

Chances are that your kitchen cabinets or refrigerator contains at least one food product that has been changed in order to improve its nutritional profile. Fat-free cheeses, reduced-fat baked goods, fortified cereals and juices, and sugar-free beverages are all examples of products that showcase the nutritional benefits of food technology. Most food product development is complicated, and these types of products listed above are no exception. In fact, more times than not it's a long, drawn-out process of research and development, testing and re-testing, and heading back to the "drawing board" for another try at development of the food product being sought. Here, in the second part of Food Insight's two-part series on food ingredients, we provide the answers to some of your technical food development questions. Consider it "food for thought."

Q Why do some sugar-free foods use more than one type of sugar substitute?

A Sugar substitutes, also known as "very low-calorie sweeteners" or "intense sweeteners," are often combined in order to produce a taste that most closely mimics that of real sugar and because together they produce an improved simulation of a sugar-like taste than either one could achieve alone. "By combining sweeteners, a very precise taste can be achieved, aftertastes can be controlled, and costs can be optimized," says Mark Kantor, Ph.D., associate professor in the department of nutrition and food science at the University of Maryland. Combining sweeteners can result in a synergistic effect that also allows the food manufacturer to use less total sweetener overall— up to 40 percent less—without compromising taste. Sometimes

sweeteners are blended to obtain the best qualities of each, such as heat stability and the ability to retain sweetness over time. "It is possible that no one sweetener alone would result in the same desirable attributes that are achieved by using a combination," adds Kantor.

Q Why are some reduced-fat products not much lower in calories than their regular-fat versions?

A "When replacing fat in a food with something else, there is a net decrease in caloric value—after all, fat packs 9 calories per gram—more than proteins or carbohydrates" says Manfred Kroger, Ph.D., professor emeritus of food science at The Pennsylvania State University. However, there are a few reasons why reduced-fat foods aren't necessarily much lower in calories than their full-fat counterparts. First, reduced-fat products are not the same as fat-free products—some may have only a slight reduction in fat compared to a reference food. Second, although some ingredients used to reduce the amount of fat in foods are truly fat- and calorie-free (such as olestra, which is not absorbed by the body and which therefore contributes no calories), most of these ingredients contain from 1 to 5 calories per gram. Finally, in order to make a reduced-fat food have the same weight per serving as the regular-fat version (as required by the Food and Drug Administration), other ingredients must be added to the product, or a larger portion of the product must be considered as a serving. The additional ingredients contribute calories, and naturally, a larger portion of food per serving would also increase the number of calories per serving. Here's a simple example: removing 1 gram of fat from a typical cracker would lower the number of calories by 9. However, in reality, the inclusion of a fatreplacer ingredient would add calories back, resulting in a net reduction of perhaps 4 calories per gram of fat removed.

Q Do reduced-fat baked goods have extra sugar added to them?

A Sugar does make up a larger percentage of reduced-fat and fat-free foods. Why? One reason is that when an ingredient is removed from a product, the remaining ingredients in the product become, in effect, more "concentrated." In other words, even though the total amount of sugar is the same in both the regular and reduced- fat or fat-free version of a food, the proportion of sugar in the lower-fat version is greater. In some cases, when fat is removed from a food, a carbohydrate-based fat-replacer ingredient is added, which may also contribute to a higher "sugars" value on the product's nutrition label.

Q What are fat substitutes made of?

A Fat-reduction ingredients may be classified into three categories: carbohydrate-based, proteinbased, or fat- based. Polydextrose, modified food starch, maltodextrins, xanthan gum, and cellulose gel are examples of carbohydrate-based fat replacers, which provide 0 to 4 calories per gram. They contribute bulk, creaminess, thickening, and stabilization to reduced-fat and fatfree foods such as frozen desserts, baked goods, salad dressings, and dairy products. Protein-based fat replacers, such as those from whey or egg white, are produced by simultaneously heating and blending them to make protein emulsions that mimic the creamy mouth feel of fat. Soy and corn are also sources of protein for the production of these ingredients. Protein-based fat-reduction ingredients provide 1 to 4 calories per gram, and are used in such foods as mayonnaise, salad dressings, baked goods, and a variety of dairy products. The fat-based substitutes simulate real fat in taste, texture, and mouth feel. Some of these products can be used just like regular oils, such as for frying, while others are more suitable as food ingredients. Depending on the degree to which fat-based fat-reduction ingredients are absorbed by the body, they can provide between 0 and 5 calories per gram. Olestra, salatrim, and mono- and diglycerides are examples of fat-based fat-reduction ingredients.

Q How is reduced-fat peanut butter made?

A Regular peanut butters contain a minimum of 90 percent peanuts, whereas the reduced-fat varieties contain approximately 60 percent peanuts. The peanuts that are taken out in reduced-fat products are replaced by corn syrup solids, which give "body" to the product. Unlike the peanuts that they are replacing, the corn syrup solids have no fat, thereby reducing the overall fat content of the peanut butter. (The numbers of calories in reduced-fat peanut butters are not necessarily lower than the numbers of calories in regular versions of peanut butter, however.) Soy protein, vitamins, and minerals are also added to reduced-fat peanut butters in order to make them nutritionally equivalent to regular peanut butter.

Q What's in those new cholesterol-lowering spreads that makes them work?

A Today you can find two new types of products on the market—cholesterol-lowering spreads—and plant compounds are the keys to these products. One type of product contains a soybean extract called a plant sterol, whereas the other type contains a plant stanol ester found in small amounts in corn, wheat, and wood oils. Both types of the two new cholesterol-lowering table spreads function similarly to inhibit cholesterol absorption, decrease low-density lipoprotein (LDL) cholesterol (or "bad" cholesterol) levels, and maintain high-density lipoprotein (HDL), cholesterol (or "good" cholesterol) levels and thereby promote healthy blood cholesterol levels.

Q How do they get all those vitamins and minerals into fortified cereals?

A Adding nutrients to a cereal can cause taste and color changes in the product. This is especially true with added minerals. Since no one wants cereal that tastes like a vitamin supplement, a variety of techniques are employed in the fortification process. In general, those nutrients that are heat stable (such as vitamins A, and E and various minerals) are incorporated into the cereal itself: they're baked right in. Nonheat- stable nutrients (such as B-vitamins) are applied directly to the cereal after all heating steps are completed. Each cereal is unique—some can handle more nutrients than others can, which is one reason why fortification levels are different across all cereals.

© International Food Information Council (IFIC) Foundation. Reprinted with permission.

Key Points

- Nutrients are substances in food that provide energy and/or promote the growth and maintenance of the body. They help regulate many body processes—such as pumping blood through the heart, thinking, or breathing.

- There are six nutrient groups: carbohydrate, lipids (fats), protein, vitamins, minerals, and water.

- Carbohydrates fall into two categories: simple carbohydrates (commonly called sugars), and complex carbohydrates (commonly called starch and fiber).

- Sugars occur naturally in some foods, such as fruits and milk, and are often added to foods to sweeten them. Added sugars are often table sugar, high fructose corn syrup, or corn syrup.

- Starches and fiber consist of many sugar molecules strung together. This is why we refer to them as complex carbohydrates.

- The term dietary fiber describes a variety of carbohydrate compounds from plants that are not digestible.

- Lipids is the scientific name for a diverse group that includes fats, oils, and cholesterol. These are important for providing energy and for helping the body absorb fat-soluble vitamins.

- Fatty acids may be saturated, monounsaturated, or polyunsaturated. Animal products are a major source of saturated fat.

▶ Protein is found in meat, poultry, fish, dried beans and peas, whole grains, and some vegetables.

▶ The amino acids that make up protein are required by the body for building and maintaining the body's cells.

▶ Vitamins help regulate many body functions.

▶ Although vitamins are needed in small quantities, the roles they play in the body are enormously important.

▶ Vitamins must be obtained through foods because they are not made in the body or are not made in sufficient quantities.

▶ Some substances considered to be vitamins in foods are actually precursors. In the body, a precursor is chemically changed to the active form of the vitamin, under proper conditions.

▶ The fat-soluble vitamins are: A, D, E, and K. The body generally can store these.

▶ The water-soluble vitamins include B vitamins and vitamin C. The body generally cannot store these.

▶ Excessive doses of some vitamins or minerals can cause toxicity.

▶ Essential minerals include calcium and phosphorus, used for building bones and teeth, and iron, which helps the red blood cells deliver oxygen.

▶ Water itself is a nutrient. It is used for nearly all body functions.

▶ Foods that are nutrient-rich relative to their calorie (energy) content are of high nutrient density, and play an important role in good nutrition.

Amino acids: the nitrogen-containing building blocks of proteins

Antioxidants: substances that combine with oxygen so the oxygen cannot oxidize, or destroy, important substances

Blood sugar: glucose; circulates in our blood at a relatively constant level

Calorie: a unit of measurement of heat or energy. Technically, what we call a "calorie" is actually 1,000 calories—a kilocalorie.

Carbohydrates: key nutrients containing carbon, hydrogen, and oxygen and used primarily for energy; include simple carbohydrates (commonly called sugars), and complex carbohydrates (commonly called starch and fiber)

Key Terms

Cholesterol: a type of sterol, which has most of its atoms arranged in a ring rather than a chain; a risk factor for heart disease

Dietary fiber: a variety of carbohydrate compounds from plants that are not digestible

Empty calories: calories that provide little or no nutrient density

Energy-yielding nutrients: carbohydrates, lipids (fats), and protein, which provide energy

Enriched: containing certain nutrients (thiamin, riboflavin, niacin, and iron) added in amounts approximately equivalent to those originally present in the whole grain but lost through milling

Essential fatty acid (EFA): fatty acids that the body cannot make and that are essential in our diets

Essential nutrients: nutrients that either cannot be made in the body or cannot be made in the quantities needed by the body, and must be obtained through food

Fortified: containing one or more added nutrients

Glucose: a common form of sugar; the form of sugar the body uses

Glycogen: the body's form of stored starch, stored in muscles and in the liver

Insoluble fiber: fiber that does not dissolve well in water

Lipids: a diverse group that includes fats, oils, and cholesterol; important for providing energy and for helping the body absorb fat-soluble vitamins.

Macronutrients: energy-yielding nutrients present in large quantities in the diet; carbohydrate, lipids, and protein

Micronutrients: nutrients required in small quantities, such as vitamins and minerals

Monounsaturated fatty acid: a fatty acid in which a double bond forms between two neighboring carbons; two hydrogens are missing, so the carbons are not saturated

Nutrients: substances in food that provide energy and/or promote the growth and maintenance of the body

Nutrient density: the amount of nutrients a food contains relative to its calorie (energy) content

Polyunsaturated fatty acid (PUFA): a fatty acid containing more than one double bond between two neighboring carbons

Protein calorie malnutrition: a group of diseases characterized by both protein and energy deficiency

Proteins: food components that consist of strands of amino acids; used for building and maintaining the body's cells

Saturated fatty acid: a fatty acid that is filled, or saturated, with hydrogens

Soluble fiber: fiber that dissolves in water, forming a gel

Starch: a complex carbohydrate consisting of many sugar molecules strung together; also called polysaccharide.

Trans-fatty acids: fatty acids that have their hydrogen atoms in an unusual location; made during the process in which vegetable oils are partially hydrogenated to make them more solid

Triglyceride: a form of fat; composed of three fatty acids attached to glycerol

1. Which of the following is an example of an energy-yielding nutrient?
   A. Water
   B. Fat
   C. Vitamin C
   D. Magnesium

2. An essential fatty acid is one that:
   A. The body cannot make
   B. Raises blood cholesterol
   C. Lowers blood cholesterol
   D. Is found only in leafy green vegetables

3. Which of the following is a major food source for saturated fats?
   A. Canola oil
   B. Olive oil
   C. Butter
   D. Fresh apple

4. The building blocks for proteins are called:
   A. Dietary fiber
   B. Precursors
   C. Enzymes
   D. Amino acids

5. Which of the following is the most concentrated food source for protein?
   A. Whole grain bread
   B. Skim milk
   C. Potatoes
   D. Bananas

6. Beta carotene is:

   A. A form of vitamin A found in yellow vegetables
   B. A form of vitamin E found in oils
   C. A nonessential amino acid
   D. A trace mineral

7. Which of the following is the most concentrated food source for vitamin C?

   A. Rice
   B. Beef
   C. Tomato
   D. Celery

8. What two minerals are very important for building bones and teeth?

   A. Molybdenum and calcium
   B. Potassium and phosphorous
   C. Zinc and iron
   D. Calcium and phosphorous

9. Which mineral plays a strong role in wound healing?

   A. Calcium
   B. Chromium
   C. Selenium
   D. Zinc

10. Which of the following is the most nutrient-dense food?

   A. Cola drink
   B. Broccoli
   C. Shortening
   D. Chocolate chip cookie

A dietary manger needs to select and recommend foods according to established nutrition principles. In addition, a dietary manager needs to be able to apply guides and tools to assess nutritional adequacy.

After completing this chapter, you should be able to:

- Identify criteria for a healthful diet.
- List key health concerns related to dietary intake.
- Explain why food guides may be used.
- Describe the Food Guide Pyramid.
- Suggest meat alternatives.
- List the Dietary Guidelines for Americans.
- Describe the Five-a-Day concept.
- Recommend ways to adjust a diet for sugar, starch, and fiber.
- Recommend ways to adjust a diet for various types of fats.
- Recommend ways to adjust a diet for protein.
- Explain how Dietary Reference Intakes (DRIs) are used.
- Recommend ways to minimize nutrient loss during food preparation and service.
- Describe the concept of functional foods. (See *Nutrition in the News* at the end of this chapter).
- Explain the advantages of eating food, as compared with taking nutritional supplements.

With so many foods from which to choose, how do you know if a diet is nutritious and healthful? There are several approaches to answering this question. As you'll see later in this chapter, both government and private agencies have answered the question. Many guidelines and standards exist. Generally, sound nutrition advice hinges on a few key ideas:

- Adequacy
- Balance
- Moderation
- Variety

An *adequate* diet supplies enough energy and essential nutrients to maintain health. A *balanced* diet is one with a variety of foods that does not emphasize certain foods at the expense of others. For example, someone who drinks a lot of soda and little or no milk will get plenty of sugar. But the soda will crowd out nutrients, such as calcium and vitamin D, found in milk. A *moderate* diet is one that provides adequate amounts of fat, sugar, calories, and so on—but not too much. Lastly, a *varied* diet uses many different food choices to provide nutrients. Each food has its own nutrient profile. For example, three fruits may all offer vitamin C, but one also offers more fiber, while another offers more folacin or vitamin A. Thus, it is best not to rely on just one food to provide a key nutrient over and over. Varying selection of foods increases the likelihood of getting all needed nutrients and other food components over time.

HEALTH CONCERNS

Early nutrition scientists focused on identifying essential nutrients. A few decades ago, nutrition advice centered on encouraging intake of certain foods to prevent deficiencies and enhance growth. Today, however, nutrition scientists devote a great deal of research to an opposite problem: nutritional excess and imbalance. The Surgeon General's Report on Nutrition and Health in 1988 became a kind of turning point for nutritional planning. The report concluded that over-consumption of certain nutrients—not deficiency—should be our chief nutritional concern. Generally, the over-consumed nutrients are macronutrients. Some studies of over-consumption focus on fats and types of fats, as well as overall caloric intake.

Nutrition can play a role in the development or prevention of many common health problems. Some of these problems rank among the leading causes of illness and death in the United States, touch the lives of most Americans, and generate substantial healthcare costs.

As an example, the World Health Organization cites obesity as one of the top five health problems in the developed world (including in the US). Being overweight is measured through *body mass index (BMI)*. As you will learn in Chapter 8, BMI is simply a ratio of weight to height. The higher the weight (in

Figure 3.1

FIGURE 3.1. OBESITY: FAST FACTS

- In the past 30 years, the prevalence of obesity in the US has increased by more than 25%.
- Among young adults in the 1990s, obesity increased by 49%.
- Almost two-thirds of American adults are overweight or obese.
- Overweight and obesity are associated with heart disease, certain types of cancer, Type 2 diabetes, stroke, arthritis, breathing problems, and psychological disorders, such as depression.
- 300,000 deaths each year in the United States are associated with obesity.
- Obesity is responsible for about 5.5-7.8% of healthcare expenditures.
- The economic cost of obesity in the United States was about $117 billion in 2000.

Compiled from CDC, FDA, the Surgeon General, and other sources. Please see later chapters for more information about health conditions.

Figure 3.2

PHYSICAL ACTIVITY AND INACTIVITY

▶ It is recommended that Americans accumulate at least 30 minutes (adults) or 60 minutes (children) of moderate physical activity most days of the week. More may be needed to prevent weight gain, to lose weight, or to maintain weight loss.

▶ Less than ⅓ of adults engage in the recommended amounts of physical activity.

▶ Many people live sedentary lives; in fact, 40% of adults in the United States do not participate in any leisure time physical activity.

▶ 43% of adolescents watch more than 2 hours of television each day.

▶ Physical activity is extremely helpful in maintaining weight loss, especially when combined with healthy eating.

Source: US Surgeon General, American Cancer Society

relation to height), the higher the BMI. **Overweight** is defined as being at a BMI of 25-29.9. **Obesity** is defined as being at a BMI of 30 or greater. Figure 3.1 lists more facts about obesity.

What causes overweight and obesity? According to the US Surgeon General:

▶ Overweight and obesity result from an imbalance involving excessive calorie consumption and/or inadequate physical activity.

▶ For each individual, body weight is the result of a combination of genetic, metabolic, behavioral, environmental, cultural, and socioeconomic influences.

While food alone does not cause, cure, or control obesity, weight control is a nutritional issue. It is an issue of balance—the energy consumed versus the energy expended. When we consume more than we use, we gain weight. It is also often an issue of moderation. We can enjoy calorie-dense foods, but excesses may contribute to overweight.

Note that exercise is very important in managing weight and preventing disease. Exercising regularly helps a person achieve a healthy balance of energy consumed and energy used. But it also has a direct and positive effect on wellness. For example, exercise helps prevent heart disease by strengthening the heart and cardiovascular system. It also reduces the risk of developing breast cancer, colon cancer, and other forms of cancer. Some key facts about physical activity appear in Figure 3.2.

A complex of health issues hinges on this fundamental factor. In addition, many nutrition concerns have evolved specific to disease. For example, the American Heart Association lists risk factors for developing coronary heart disease (see Figure 3.3). A **risk factor** is a habit, trait, or condition of any individual that is

Figure 3.3

RISK FACTORS FOR CORONARY HEART DISEASE

MAJOR RISK FACTORS FOR CORONARY HEART DISEASE THAT CANNOT BE CHANGED:

Increasing age. About 85% of people who die of coronary heart disease are age 65 or older. At older ages, women who have heart attacks are twice as likely as men are to die from them within a few weeks.

Male gender. Men have a greater risk of heart attack than women, and they have attacks earlier in life. Even after menopause, when women's death rate from heart disease increases, it's not as great as men's.

Heredity (including race). Children of parents with heart disease are more likely to develop it themselves. African Americans have more severe high blood pressure than whites. Consequently, their risk of heart disease is greater.

MAJOR RISK FACTORS FOR CORONARY HEART DISEASE THAT CAN BE MODIFIED OR TREATED:
You can change or treat these factors to lower your risk by focusing on your lifestyle habits or, if needed, taking medicine.

Tobacco smoke. Smokers' risk of heart attack is more than twice that of nonsmokers. Cigarette smoking is the biggest risk factor for sudden cardiac death: smokers have two to four times the risk of nonsmokers. Smokers who have a heart attack are more likely to die and die suddenly (within an hour) than are nonsmokers. Available evidence also indicates that chronic exposure to environmental tobacco smoke (secondhand smoke, passive smoking) may increase the risk of heart disease.

High blood cholesterol levels. The risk of coronary heart disease and stroke rises as blood cholesterol levels increase. When other risk factors (such as high blood pressure and tobacco smoke) are present, this risk increases even more. A person's cholesterol level is also affected by age, gender, heredity and diet.

High blood pressure. High blood pressure increases the heart's workload, causing the heart to enlarge and weaken over time. It also increases the risk of stroke, heart attack, kidney failure and congestive heart failure. When high blood pressure exists with obesity, smoking, high blood cholesterol levels or diabetes, the risk of heart attack or stroke increases several times.

Physical inactivity. Lack of physical activity is a risk factor for coronary heart disease. Regular, moderate-to-vigorous exercise plays a significant role in preventing heart and blood vessel disease. Even moderate-intensity physical activities are beneficial if done regularly and long term. More vigorous activities are associated with more benefits. Exercise can help control blood cholesterol, diabetes and obesity as well as help to lower blood pressure in some people.

Obesity and overweight. People who have excess body fat are more likely to develop heart disease and stroke even if they have no other risk factors. Obesity is unhealthy because excess weight increases the strain on the heart. It's directly linked with coronary heart disease because it influences blood pressure, blood cholesterol and triglyceride levels, and makes diabetes more likely to develop. If you can lose as little as 10 to 20 pounds, you can help lower your heart disease risk.

Diabetes mellitus. Diabetes seriously increases the risk of developing cardiovascular disease. Even when glucose levels are under control, diabetes increases the risk of heart disease and stroke. Two-thirds of people with diabetes die of some form of heart or blood vessel disease. If you have diabetes, it's critically important for you to monitor and control any other risk factors you can.

Reproduced with permission. American Heart Association World Wide Web Site URL address www.americanheart.org/presenter.jhtml?identifier=235 © 2003, Copyright American Heart Association associated with an increased chance of developing a disease. Blood cholesterol levels and overall body weight are two of the factors that may be influenced by diet. Being overweight also increases the risk for developing Type 2 diabetes, and for having hypertension. Thus, many of these factors work in tandem to create health risks. Conversely, an individual who devotes special attention to sound nutrition and weight management may reduce risks for heart disease, hypertension, diabetes, cancer, joint problems, and more—all in one fell swoop.

Because nutrition can play a very strong role in preventing long-term and degenerative diseases such as heart disease, dietary guidelines center on limiting certain foods. Meanwhile, it is still important to consume adequate amounts of essential nutrients.

WHY USE FOOD GUIDES?

With so many nutrients—and so many foods from which to choose—eating a healthy diet sounds intimidating. Based on advice, it may be tempting to find out what amounts of each macronutrient and micronutrient occur in each food we eat, and then count and total nutrients each day. However, this is rarely practical. So how can we evaluate a diet? How can we plan an adequate menu? How can we advise a person to choose health-promoting foods?

The answer is through dietary guidelines and food guides. These are forms of food guidance. They provide shortcuts or easy-to-use tools that consumers can use to direct their own food choices. One such tool is the Food Guide Pyramid, explained in the next section. Dietary guidance also comes in the form of Dietary Guidelines for Americans, addressed later in this chapter as well. Other forms of guidance include the Five A Day concept, and the DRIs, also discussed later in this chapter.

Food Guide Pyramid

The **Food Guide Pyramid**, developed by the US Department of Agriculture (USDA) and the Department of Health and Human Services, provides practical guidance about how to eat. It offers a pattern for making dietary choices, based on sound nutrition. The Pyramid classifies foods into five groups for recommending eating, and one group to limit (see Figure 3.4.)

The food groups shown in the main sections of the Pyramid are:

- Bread, cereal, rice, and pasta group (6-11 servings per day)
- Fruit group (2-4 servings per day)
- Vegetable group (3-5 servings per day)
- Milk, yogurt, and cheese group (2-3 servings per day)
- Meat, poultry, fish, dry beans, eggs and nuts group (2-3 servings per day).

Figure 3.4

FOOD GUIDE PYRAMID

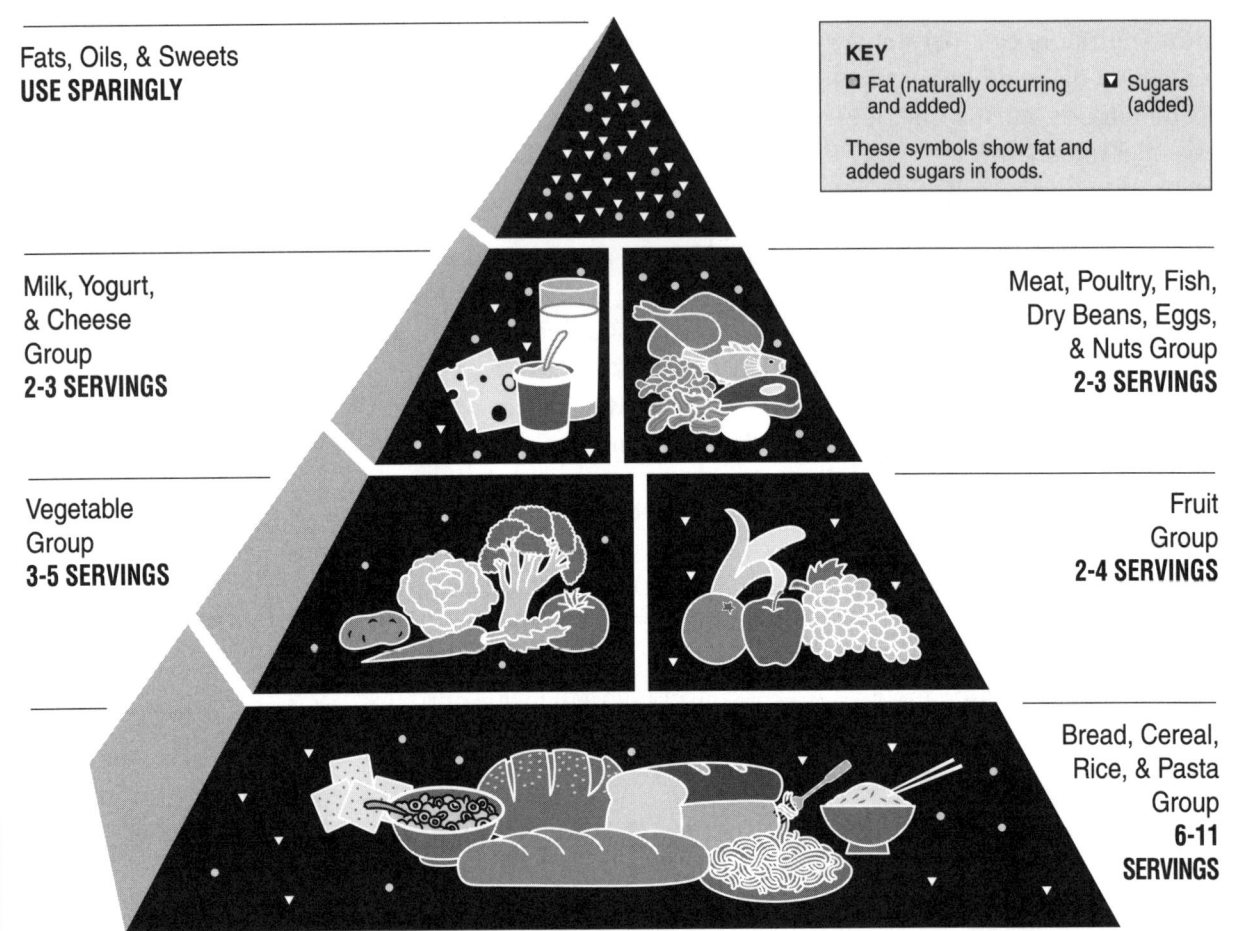

Food Guide Pyramid
A Guide to Daily Food Choices

Fats, Oils, & Sweets
USE SPARINGLY

KEY
□ Fat (naturally occurring and added)   ▼ Sugars (added)

These symbols show fat and added sugars in foods.

Milk, Yogurt, & Cheese Group
2-3 SERVINGS

Meat, Poultry, Fish, Dry Beans, Eggs, & Nuts Group
2-3 SERVINGS

Vegetable Group
3-5 SERVINGS

Fruit Group
2-4 SERVINGS

Bread, Cereal, Rice, & Pasta Group
6-11 SERVINGS

Source: U.S. Department of Agriculture/U.S. Department of Health and Human Services

The pyramid shape reflects the idea that foods at the base should be plentiful in a healthy diet. Foods at the tip should be used sparingly.

At the base of the Food Pyramid are breads, cereals, rice, and pasta—all foods from grains. These foods provide complex carbohydrates (starches), which are an important source of energy, fiber, vitamins, and minerals. Just above the base of the pyramid are vegetables and fruits—plant foods. Most people need to eat more of these foods for the vitamins, minerals, and fiber they supply.

Above vegetables and fruits are two groups of foods that come mostly from animals: milk, yogurt, and cheese; and meat, poultry, fish, dry beans, eggs, and nuts. These foods are important for protein, calcium, iron, and zinc.

The small tip of the Pyramid shows fats, oils, and sweets. These are foods such as salad dressings and oils, cream, butter, margarine, sugars, soft drinks, candies, and sweet desserts. These foods provide calories, and are generally not very nutrient-dense.

The Pyramid shows a range of servings for each major food group. The optimum number of servings depends on how many calories a person needs. In turn, calorie requirements depend on a person's age, sex, size, and level of physical activity. The following daily calorie level suggestions are based on recommendations of the National Academy of Sciences and on calorie intakes reported by people in national food consumption surveys:

- ▶ 1,600 calories is about right for many sedentary women and some older adults.
- ▶ 2,200 calories is about right for most children, teenage girls, active women, and many sedentary men. Women who are pregnant or breastfeeding may need somewhat more.
- ▶ 2,800 calories is about right for teenage boys, many active men, and some very active women.

Now take a look at Figure 3.5, which shows how many Food Guide Pyramid servings fit with several different calorie levels. For example, an active woman who needs about 2,200 calories a day can apply the Pyramid to choose nine servings of breads, cereals, rice, or pasta; and about six ounces of meat or alternates per day.

Figure 3.5

SAMPLE PYRAMID SERVINGS AT THREE CALORIE LEVELS

SERVINGS PER DAY	LOWER (1,600)	MODERATE (2,200)	HIGHER (2,800)
Bread Group Servings	6	9	11
Vegetable Group Servings	3	4	5
Fruit Group Servings	2	3	4
Milk Group Servings	2-3*	2-3*	2-3*
Meat Group (ounces total)	5	6	7
Total Fat (grams)	53	73	93
Total Added Sugars (teaspoons)	6	12	18

*Women who are pregnant or breastfeeding, teenagers, and young adults to age 24 need 3 servings.

What is a serving? The amount of food that counts as a serving is listed in Figure 3.6. For example, a serving of rice is ½ cup. Does this mean each of us should limit our rice intake to ½ cup per day? No. Servings are defined just to help us count the foods we eat. A **serving** is a measurement used for keeping track of amounts of food. This is different from a portion. A **portion** is the total amount of a food served or consumed at any point in time. A portion can be larger (or smaller) than a serving. To meet a total of the recommended 6-11 servings from the Bread, Cereal, Rice, & Pasta Group, you may choose to eat:

▶ 1 ounce of cereal at breakfast (1 serving),

▶ 2 slices of bread (2 servings) in a sandwich at lunch,

▶ several crackers (1 serving) for a snack, and

▶ 1½ cups of rice or pasta (3 servings) with dinner.

This would provide a total of seven servings from this group for a day.

For mixed foods, estimate food group servings of the main ingredients. For example, a generous serving of pizza would count in the bread group (crust), the milk group (cheese), and the vegetable group (tomato). A serving of beef stew would count in the meat group and the vegetable group. Both have fat—in the cheese from the pizza and in the gravy from the stew. Figure 3.7 offers more examples for counting mixed dishes, and Figure 3.8 gives Food Pyramid pointers.

Figure 3.6

SERVING SIZES FOR THE FOOD GUIDE PYRAMID

BREAD, CEREAL, RICE, AND PASTA

1 slice of bread

1 cup of ready-to-eat cereal

¹/₂ cup of cooked cereal, rice, or pasta

FRUIT

1 medium apple, banana, orange

¹/₂ cup of chopped, cooked, or canned fruit

³/₄ cup of fruit juice

MILK, YOGURT, AND CHEESE

1 cup of milk

1¹/₂ ounces of natural cheese

2 ounces of processed cheese

VEGETABLES

1 cup of raw leafy vegetables

¹/₂ cup of other vegetables, cooked or chopped raw

³/₄ cup of vegetable juice

MEAT, POULTRY, FISH, DRY BEANS, EGGS, AND NUTS

2-3 ounces of cooked lean meat, poultry, or fish

¹/₂ cup of cooked dry beans, 1 egg, ¹/₃ cup of nuts, or 2 tablespoons of peanut butter count as 1 ounce of lean meat.

COUNTING MIXED DISHES IN THE FOOD GUIDE PYRAMID

FOOD & SAMPLE PORTION	GROUP: GRAINS	VEGETABLE	FRUIT	MILK	MEAT/BEANS	FAT
Cheese pizza (2 med slices)	2½ servings	½ serving	0 servings	½ serving	0 servings	19% DV
Lasagna (1 piece 3½" x 4")	1½	½	0	½	1	23
Macaroni & cheese (1 cup, made from packaged mix)	2	0	0	½	0	30
Tuna noodle casserole (1 cup)	1½	0	0	½	2	29
Spinach quiche (1 piece)	1	½	0	½	½	40
Chicken pot pie (8 oz. pie)	2½	½	0	0	1½	43
Beef taco (2)	2½	½	0	¼	2	40
Bean & cheese burrito (1)	2½	¼	0	1	1	44
Egg roll (1)	½	¼	0	0	½	10
Chicken fried rice (1 cup)	1½	½	0	0	1	19
Rice & beans (1 cup)	1½	0	0	0	1½	17
Stuffed peppers (½ pepper)	½	1	0	0	1	19

Figure 3.7

COUNTING MIXED DISHES IN THE FOOD GUIDE PYRAMID, *CONTINUED*

FOOD & SAMPLE PORTION	GROUP: GRAINS	VEGETABLE	FRUIT	MILK	MEAT/BEANS	FAT
Beef stir-fry (1 cup)	0 servings	1½ servings	0 servings	0 servings	1½ servings	16% DV
Clam Chowder (New England) (1 cup)	½	¼	0	½	3½	8
Cream of tomato soup (2 cups)	½	1	0	½	0	7
Double cheeseburger (with mayo)	3½	½	0	½	2½	54
Italian sub (6" sub)	2	½	0	½	2½	58
Peanut butter & jelly sandwich (1)	2	0	0	0	1	22
Tuna salad sandwich (1)	2	½	0	0	2	11
Chef salad (3 cups, no dressing)	0	3	0	0	3	5
Pasta salad with vegetables (1 cup)	1½	1	0	0	0	24
Apple pie (1 slice)	2	0	½	0	0	25
Pumpkin pie (1 slice)	1½	¼	0	¼	¼	22

Note: Daily Value (DV) is a form of nutrition recommendation used in Nutrition Facts Labels. See Chapter 9 for more information.

Figure 3.8

FOOD PYRAMID POINTERS

Choose most of your foods from the grain products group (6-11 servings), the vegetable group (3-5 servings), and the fruit group (2-4 servings).

Eat moderate amounts of foods from the milk group (2-3 servings) and the meat and beans group (2-3 servings).

Choose sparingly foods that provide few nutrients and are high in fat and sugars.

BREAD, CEREAL, RICE, AND PASTA POINTERS

- To get the fiber you need, choose several servings a day of foods made from whole grains.

- Choose most often foods that are made with little fat or sugars, like bread, English muffins, rice, and pasta.

- Go easy on the fat and sugars you add as spreads, seasonings, or toppings.

- When preparing pasta, stuffing, and sauce from packaged mixes, use only half the butter or margarine suggested; if milk or cream is called for, use low fat milk.

VEGETABLE GROUP POINTERS

- Different types of vegetables provide different nutrients. Eat a variety.

- Include dark green leafy vegetables and legumes several times a week—they are especially good sources of vitamins and minerals. Legumes also provide protein and can be used in place of meat.

- Go easy on the fat you add to vegetables at the table or during cooking. Added spreads or toppings, such as butter, mayonnaise, and salad dressing, count as fat.

- Use low fat salad dressing.

FRUIT GROUP POINTERS

- Choose fresh fruits, fruit juices, and frozen, canned or dried fruit. Go easy on fruits canned or frozen in heavy syrups, and on sweetened fruit juices.

- Eat whole fruits often—they are higher in fiber than fruit juices.

- Count only 100% fruit juice as fruit. Punches, fruitades, and most fruit "drinks" contain only a little juice and lots of added sugars.

MILK, YOGURT, AND CHEESE POINTERS

- Choose skim milk and non-fat yogurt often. They are lowest in fat.

- 1½ to 2 ounces of cheese and 8 ounces of yogurt count as a serving from this group because they supply the same amount of calcium as 1 cup of milk.

- Choose part skim or low fat cheeses when available and lower fat milk desserts, like ice milk or frozen yogurt.

MEAT, POULTRY, FISH, DRY BEANS, EGGS, AND NUTS GROUP POINTERS

- Choose lean poultry without skin, fish, lean meat, and dry beans and peas often. They are the choices lowest in fat.

- Prepare meats in low fat ways by broiling, grilling, or roasting. Trim away all the fat you can see.

- Nuts and seeds are high in fat, so eat them in moderation.

Source: USDA

Figure 3.9

As explained in Chapter 1, basic food preferences and habits vary considerably among cultures. To make the Food Guide Pyramid more effective as a teaching tool, nutrition professionals have converted the Pyramid to fit other cultural and dietary habits. One example is the Mediterranean Food Pyramid. The Mediterranean Food Pyramid is based on the dietary traditions of the Mediterranean region of Europe. It has also been held up as a model for American eating practices because of its reliance on olive oil and monounsaturated fats. This pyramid also emphasizes minimal processing of foods, limiting red meats, and using plant sources for a significant portion of the diet. The Vegetarian Food Pyramid (Figure 3.9) is based on a meatless diet. Note that a person who eats a vegetarian diet will not be including meats for this group of

VEGETARIAN FOOD PYRAMID

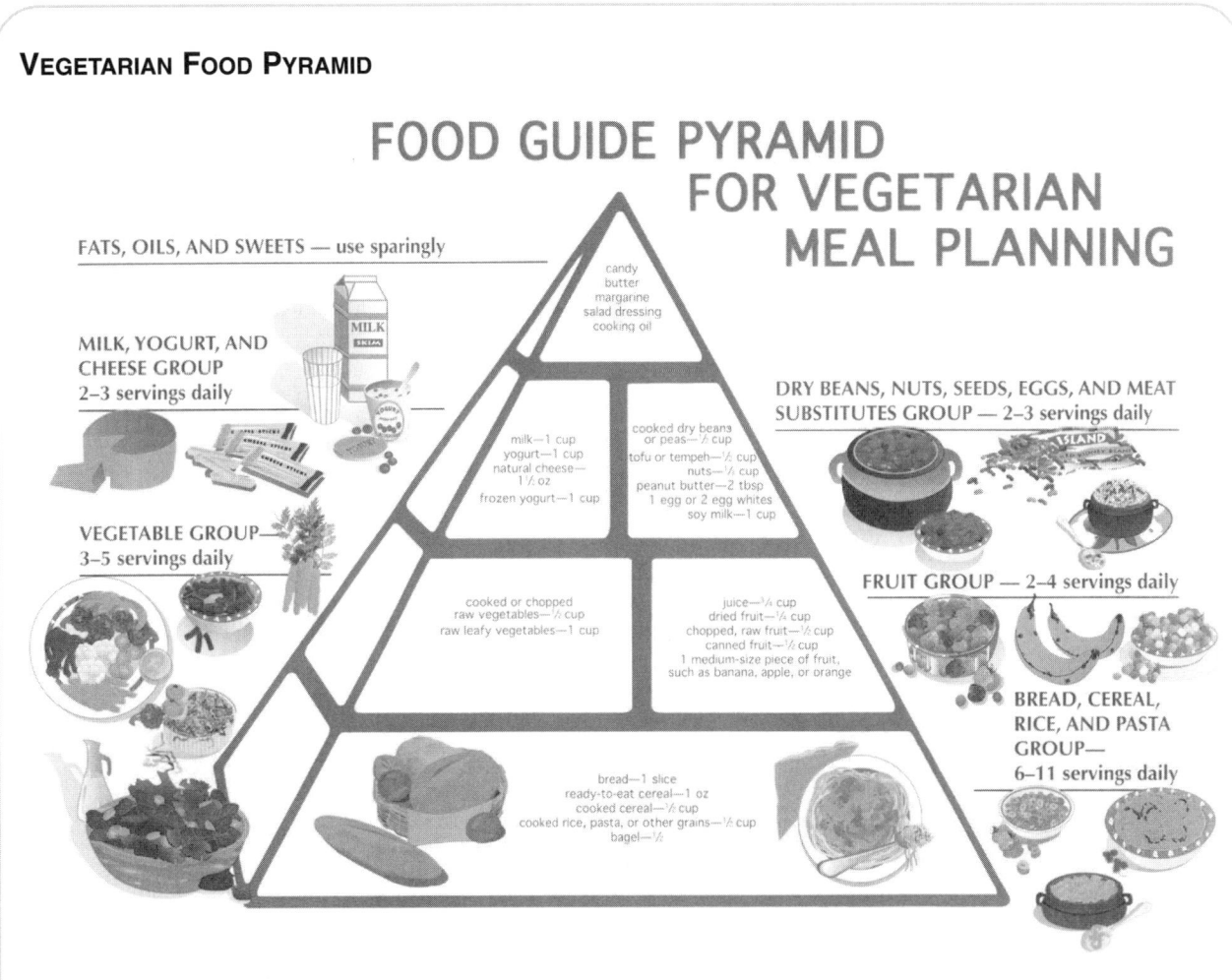

© 1997, American Dietetic Association. "Food Guide Pyramid for Vegetarian Meal Planning." Used with permission.

the Pyramid. Instead, a vegetarian diet should include meat alternatives. Meat alternatives provide significant levels of protein, as well as many of the other nutrients commonly found in meat. Examples of meat alternatives include:

- Soy milk, soy cheese, soy-based meat substitutes, or tofu
- Dried beans or peas (peas, chick peas, split peas, lentils, navy beans, red beans, lima beans, peas)
- Nuts and nut butters (peanut butter, cashews, almonds, etc.)

As mentioned in Chapter 1, some vegetarians (vegans) do not use dairy products. Thus, a vegetarian pyramid may or may not include traditional milk and cheeses in the Milk, Yogurt, & Cheese group. A vegetarian avoiding dairy products will need to obtain added protein and calcium from other sources. Often, soy milk or rice milk fortified with calcium and vitamin D, or a similar substitute becomes the staple source.

Another version of the pyramid is tailored specifically for individuals who are seeking to lose weight or maintain a healthy body weight. The Mayo Clinic Healthy Weight Pyramid (Figure 3.10) places specific limits on high-calorie foods, encourages intake of fruits and vegetables, and also includes physical activity as part of the Pyramid. The Mayo Clinic Healthy Weight Pyramid is a tool to help individuals lose weight or maintain weight. It focuses on nutritious foods that contain a small number of calories in a large amount of food—such as fruits, vegetables, legumes, poultry, fish or whole grains. Fruits and vegetables, allowed in unlimited amounts, form the foundation of the Pyramid. This pyramid also recommends healthy food choices within each food group. Candy and other processed sweets are acceptable, but in moderation—up to 75 calories daily.

There are also food pyramids designed for various cultural groups, translated into many languages, and adapted for young children. For more information, see the USDA Food & Nutrition Information Center Resource List for the Food Guide Pyramid, listed in Appendix A.

A food pyramid approach provides a simple tool that is readily understood. Most people can select their own food choices from within each food group, and make personal dietary choices that contribute to good health. The pyramid image is easy to conceptualize and makes a good educational tool as well. Note that the Food Guide Pyramid, like other food guides, is not absolute. As you will learn in later chapters, an individual's nutritional needs vary throughout the stages of life. In addition, medical conditions can affect what constitute "ideal" dietary choices for any individual. In later chapters, you will learn more about how diets may need to be modified for certain disease states.

Figure 3.10

Mayo Clinic Healthy Weight Pyramid

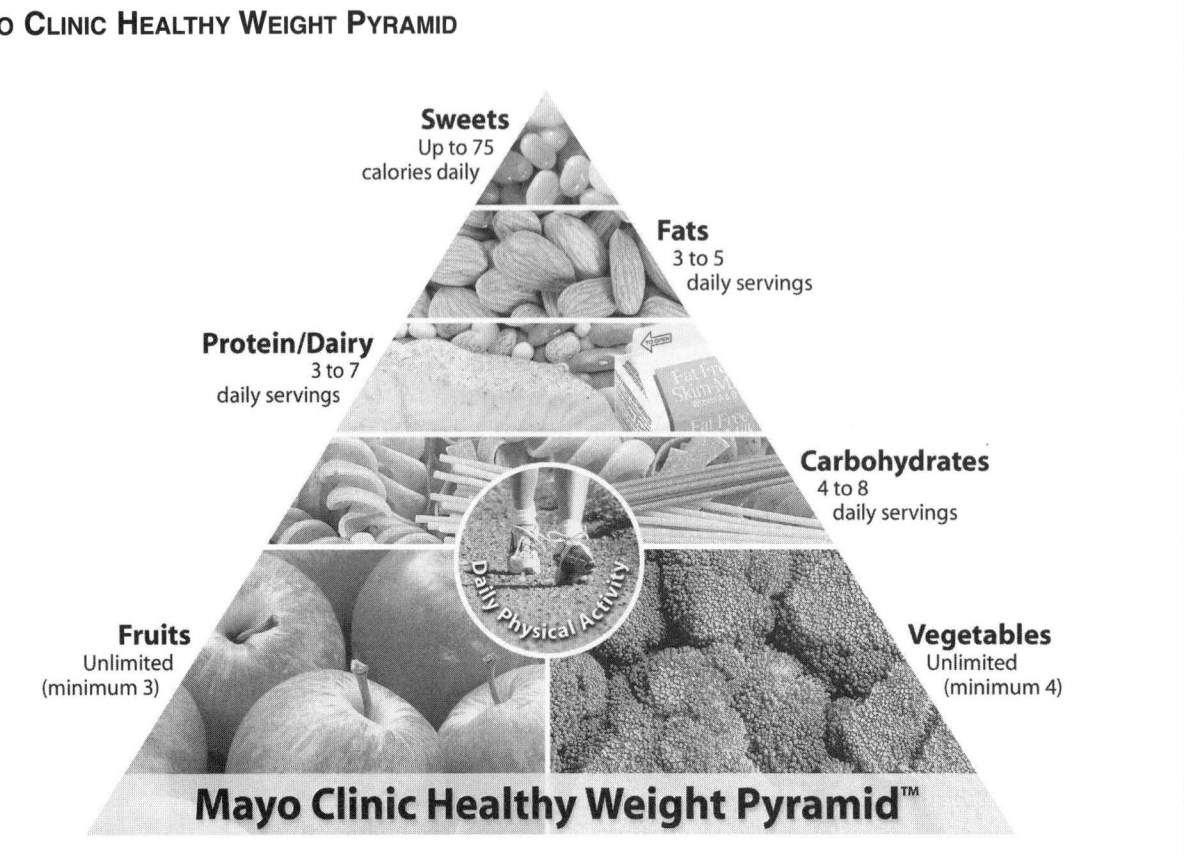

Copyright Mayo Foundation for Medical Education and Research. All rights reserved. Used with permission.

Dietary Guidelines for Americans

Dietary Guidelines for Americans (2000) represent a set of simple dietary recommendations for Americans. The first edition was released in 1980, and has now undergone several revisions by the USDA and the Department of Health and Human Services. The fifth edition was released in 2000. The next revision is already being planned by a committee of professionals, and is slated for release in 2005. The guidelines are designed to promote healthful diets. Background to the Guidelines states that: "Healthful diets contain the amounts of essential nutrients and calories needed to prevent nutritional deficiencies and excesses. Healthful diets also provide the right balance of carbohydrate, fat, and protein to reduce risks for chronic diseases, and are a part of a full and productive lifestyle. Such diets are obtained from a variety of foods that are available, affordable, and enjoyable."

Dietary Guidelines for Americans are intended for people over the age of two. The Dietary Guidelines for Americans apply to diets consumed over several days and not to single meals or foods. Background to the Guidelines further states: "Many genetic, environmental, behavioral, and cultural factors can affect health. Understanding family history of disease or risk factors—body weight and fat distribution, blood pressure, and blood cholesterol, for example—can help people make more informed decisions about actions that can improve health prospects. Food choices are among the most pleasurable and effective of these actions. Healthful diets help children grow, develop, and do well in school. They enable people of all ages to work productively and feel their best. Food choices also can help to reduce the risk for chronic diseases, such as heart disease, certain cancers, diabetes, stroke, and osteoporosis, which are leading causes of death and disability among Americans. Good diets can reduce major risk factors for chronic diseases."

Dietary Guidelines for Americans focus on an **"A-B-C" approach**: Aim for Fitness, Build a Healthy Base, and Choose Sensibly. The 10 guidelines appear in Figure 3.11. Here is more detail about the guidelines:

1. Aim for a healthy weight.
For adults and children, different methods are used to find out if weight is about right for height. For an adult, you can evaluate weight in relation to height, or Body Mass Index (BMI). The further a person's BMI is above the healthy range, the higher the weight-related risk. Someone whose BMI is above the healthy range may benefit from weight loss—especially if there are other health risk factors present, such as family history of heart disease, smoking,

Figure 3.11

DIETARY GUIDELINES FOR AMERICANS, 2000

AIM FOR FITNESS: 1. Aim for a healthy weight.

2. Be physically active each day.

BUILD A HEALTHY BASE: 3. Let the Pyramid guide your food choices.

4. Choose a variety of grains daily, especially whole grains.

5. Choose a variety of fruits and vegetables daily.

6. Keep food safe to eat.

CHOOSE SENSIBLY: 7. Choose a diet that is low in saturated fat and cholesterol and moderate in total fat.

8. Choose beverages and foods to moderate your intake of sugars.

9. Choose and prepare foods with less salt.

10. If you drink alcoholic beverages, do so in moderation.

Source: USDA and Department of Health and Human Services

sedentary lifestyle, or high blood pressure. It is possible to manage weight through balancing calories consumed with physical activity. To make it easier to manage weight, nutritionists recommend making long-term changes in eating behavior and physical activity.

2. Be physically active each day.

Physical activity involves moving the body. A moderate physical activity is an activity that requires about as much energy as walking two miles in 30 minutes. The Guidelines recommend at least 30 minutes (adults) or 60 minutes (children) of moderate physical activity most days of the week, preferably daily. They advise choosing activities that are enjoyable, and doing them regularly. Physical activity and nutrition work together for health. For example, physical activity increases the amount of calories used. For those who have intentionally lost weight, being active makes it easier to maintain the weight loss. The Guidelines suggest:

- Choose physical activities that fit in with your daily routine, or choose recreational or structured exercise programs, or both.
- Consult your healthcare provider before starting a new vigorous physical activity plan if you have a chronic health problem, or if you are over 40 (men) or 50 (women).

3. Let the Pyramid guide your food choices.

The Food Guide Pyramid described earlier in this chapter is part of the Dietary Guidelines for Americans. It provides a model for selecting foods.

4. Choose a variety of grains daily, especially whole grains.

Foods made from grains (like wheat, rice, and oats) help form the foundation of a nutritious diet. They provide vitamins, minerals, carbohydrates (starch and dietary fiber), and other substances that are important for good health. Grain products are low in fat, unless fat is added in processing, in preparation, or at the table. Whole grains differ from refined grains in the amount of fiber and nutrients they provide, and different whole grain foods differ in nutrient content, so choose a variety of whole and enriched grains. Tips:

- Combine whole grains with other tasty, nutritious foods in mixed dishes.
- Prepare or choose grain products with little added saturated fat and a moderate or low amount of added sugars. Also, check the sodium content on the Nutrition Facts Label.

5. Choose a variety of fruits and vegetables daily.

Eating plenty of fruits and vegetables of different kinds, as part of the healthful eating patterns described by these guidelines, may help protect against many chronic diseases. It also promotes healthy bowel function. Fruits and vegetables provide essential vitamins and minerals, fiber, and other substances that are important for good health. Most people, including children, eat fewer servings of fruits and vegetables than are recommended. The Guidelines suggest:

- Choose fresh, frozen, dried, or canned forms and a variety of colors and kinds.
- Choose dark-green leafy vegetables, orange fruits and vegetables, and cooked dry beans and peas often.

6. Keep food safe to eat.

Foods that are safe from harmful bacteria, viruses, parasites, and chemical contaminants are vital for healthful eating. Tips include:

- Clean. Wash hands and surfaces often.
- Separate. Separate raw, cooked, and ready-to-eat foods while shopping, preparing, or storing.
- Cook. Cook foods to a safe temperature.
- Chill. Refrigerate perishable foods promptly.
- Check and follow the label.
- Serve safely. Keep hot foods hot and cold foods cold.
- When in doubt, throw it out.

7. Choose a diet that is low in saturated fat and cholesterol and moderate in total fat.

Saturated fats increase the risk for coronary heart disease by raising the blood cholesterol. In contrast, unsaturated fats do not increase blood cholesterol. Eating too much of any type of fat can provide excess calories. Here is some advice:

- Limit use of solid fats, such as butter, hard margarines, lard, and partially hydrogenated shortenings. Use vegetable oils as a substitute.
- Choose fat free or low fat dairy products, cooked dry beans and peas, fish, lean meats and poultry.
- Focus on the lower sections of the Food Pyramid.
- Use the Nutrition Facts Label to help choose foods lower in fat, saturated fat, and cholesterol.

8. Choose beverages and foods to moderate your intake of sugars.

During digestion, all carbohydrates except fiber break down into sugars. Sugars and starches occur naturally in many foods that also supply other nutrients. Examples of these foods include milk, fruits, some vegetables, breads, cereals, and grains. Foods containing added sugars provide calories, but may have few vitamins and minerals. In the US, the number-one source of added sugars is regular soft drinks. Sweets and candies, cakes and cookies, and fruit drinks and fruitades are also major sources of added sugars. The Guidelines suggest:

- Choose sensibly to limit your intake of beverages and foods that are high in added sugars.
- Get most of your calories from grains (especially whole grains), fruits and vegetables, low fat or non-fat dairy products, and lean meats or meat substitutes.
- Take care not to let soft drinks or other sweets crowd out other foods you need to maintain health, such as low fat milk or other good sources of calcium.
- Between meals, eat few foods or beverages containing sugars or starches. If you do eat them, brush your teeth afterward to reduce the risk of tooth decay.
- Drink water often.

9. Choose and prepare foods with less salt.

Many people can reduce their chances of developing high blood pressure by consuming less salt. Only small amounts of salt occur naturally in foods. Most of the salt we eat comes from foods that have salt added during food processing or during preparation in a restaurant or at home. Here are some tips:

- Choose sensibly to moderate your salt intake.
- Choose fruits and vegetables often. They contain very little salt unless it is added in processing.
- Read the Nutrition Facts Label to compare and help identify foods lower in sodium—especially prepared foods.
- Use herbs, spices, and fruits to flavor food, and cut the amount of salty seasonings by half.
- If you eat restaurant foods or fast foods, choose those that are prepared with only moderate amounts of salt or salty flavorings.

10. If you drink alcoholic beverages, do so in moderation.

Alcoholic beverages supply calories but few nutrients. Alcoholic beverages are harmful when consumed in excess, and some people should not drink at all. Taking more than one drink per day for women or two drinks per day for men (12 ounces of regular beer, 5 ounces of wine, or 1.5 ounces of 80-proof distilled spirits) can raise the risk for motor vehicle crashes, other injuries, high blood pressure, stroke, violence, suicide, and certain types of cancer. Even one drink per day can slightly raise the risk of breast cancer. Alcohol consumption during pregnancy increases risk of birth defects. Here are the suggestions:

- If you choose to drink alcoholic beverages, do so sensibly and in moderation.

- Limit intake to one drink per day for women or two per day for men, and take with meals to slow alcohol absorption.

- Avoid drinking before or when driving, or whenever it puts you or others at risk.

The 5 A Day Concept

The **5 A Day program** is jointly sponsored as a public and private collaboration by the National Cancer Institute and the Produce for Better Health Foundation (PBH), a nonprofit consumer education foundation representing the fruit and vegetable industry. The concept originated with the Food Guide Pyramid's suggested dietary intake of at least two servings of fruit and three servings of vegetables each day. This has led to a concept originally dubbed, "5 A Day for Better Health," intended to promote consumer awareness that eating at least five servings of fruits and vegetables represents a sound dietary habit. Recently, the concept has been called 5 to 9 A Day to reflect the idea that five to nine daily servings of fruits and vegetables are advisable.

Educational materials, recipes, and tips for including fruits and vegetables in the diet are all available through several 5 A Day websites (see Appendix A). The 5 A Day Program focuses on several key areas to further the goal of increasing consumption of fruits and vegetables for all Americans. These include supporting the educational efforts of health and extension agencies throughout the US, working for change in the areas of policy, supporting nutrition education, conducting and evaluating research, promoting communications, and working with industry and other partners. Figure 3.12 offers a "report card" identifying benefits of fruits and vegetables.

Figure 3.12

BENEFITS OF EATING FRUITS AND VEGETABLES

The following is a "report card":

CONDITION	STRENGTH OF EVIDENCE	ASSESSMENT OF EVIDENCE
Cancer	Substantial for some sites	Convincing for many cancers
Cardiovascular Disease	Growing use of biomarkers	Convincing
Hypertension	Few diverse trials	Convincing as adjunct
Stroke	Growing	Promising
COPD and Lung Function	Growing	Highly suggestive
Diabetes	Limited	Potential, plausible mechanisms
Obesity	Sparse direct data	Convincing as adjunct
Longevity	Limited	Plausible
Bone Health	Few human studies	Plausible
Aging and Cognition	Few human studies	Plausible
Neurodegenerative Disease	Limited human data	Plausible
Skin Health and Wrinkling	Sparse	Watching
Diverticulosis	Strong	Convincing
Arthritis	Sparse	Watching
Birth Defects	Substantial, proven	Most convincing
Cataracts	Needs clinical trial	Suggestive

© 2003 Produce for Better Health Foundation. Reprinted with permission.

DIETARY MODIFICATIONS

Today's nutrition advice indicates a need to make some adjustments to the usual American diet. Here are more tips for making changes for each of the macronutrients.

Carbohydrate

The Dietary Guidelines for Americans recommend using sugars only in moderation. Foods containing large amounts of refined sugars should be eaten in moderation by most healthy people and sparingly by people with low calorie needs. For very active people with high calorie needs, sugars can be an additional source of calories. The following tips can help reduce sugar in the diet:

▶ Instead of regular soft drinks or powdered drink mixes, choose diet soft drinks, 100% fruit juices, bottled waters such as seltzer, or iced tea made without added sugar or with nonnutritive sweeteners.

- Instead of sweet desserts such as cake, emphasize fruits in desserts. Fresh fruit can be baked (as in baked apples), poached (as in poached pears), broiled, or made into compote. Choose canned fruits that are packed in fruit juice (not syrup).

- Make your own cakes, cookies, pies, and other baked goods and reduce the sugar by one-quarter to one-third. It usually does not affect the quality of the product. Use recipes that contain fruits to sweeten, and sweet spices such as cinnamon, nutmeg, and cloves.

- Try a cookie that uses less sugar, such as graham crackers, vanilla wafers, ginger snaps, or fig bars.

- Choose 100% pure fruit juices. They do not contain added sugars. Products labeled as fruit drinks, fruit beverages, or flavored drinks usually contain only small amounts of fruit juice and much refined sugar.

- Choose unsweetened breakfast cereals. Choose cereals with less than four grams of sugar per serving, unless the sugar comes from a dried fruit such as raisins. Top cereals with fresh fruit.

- Jams, jellies, and pancake syrup contain considerable amounts of refined sugar. For less refined sugar and calories, select jams and jellies made without (or with less) sugar, and pancake syrup labeled "reduced calorie." Other toppings for toast or pancakes are chopped fresh fruit, applesauce, part-skim ricotta cheese, and fruit.

- Instead of sweetened breakfast pastries such as Danish, try a bagel, English muffin, roll, or fruited muffin.

- Use less refined sugars in coffee, tea, cereals, etc., or use sugar substitutes.

- Try fresh or dried fruit for a sweet snack instead of candy.

Carbohydrates should provide approximately 60% of daily calories, with 50% coming from complex carbohydrates: starch and fiber. The easiest way to increase dietary starch is to follow the Food Guide Pyramid.

General recommendations for fiber intake are from 20 to 35 grams daily. The Daily Value used for Nutrition Facts Labeling is 25 grams. For children, use the "age + 5" rule, which recommends that children consume an amount of fiber equal to their age plus an additional 5 grams of fiber. Unfortunately, the average American takes in less than 20 grams of fiber a day. Figure 3.13 lists good sources of fiber. When increasing fiber intake, do so slowly to avoid problems with cramps, diarrhea, and excessive gas. Also, it's important to chew foods well and drink at least 8 to 10 glasses of water each day, because fiber takes water out of the body with it. Fiber-rich foods are not recommended for acute diseases of the gastrointestinal tract such as diverticulitis, ulcerative colitis, and inflammatory bowel disease (discussed in Chapter 6).

Figure 3.13

GOOD SOURCES OF FIBER

BREAKFAST CEREALS
Bran-type cereals

Raisin Bran-type cereals

Whole wheat breakfast cereals

Whole oat breakfast cereals

BREADS AND PASTAS
Whole wheat bread

Bran muffin

Whole wheat pasta

VEGETABLES
Broccoli

Brussels sprouts

Cabbage

Carrots

Cauliflower

Peas

Potatoes with skin

Spinach

Sweet potatoes

FRUITS
Apple

Banana

Blackberries

Blueberries

Cherries

Dates

Figs

Grapefruit

Kiwi fruit

Orange

Pear

Prunes

Raspberries

Strawberries

DRIED BEANS AND PEAS
All cooked beans and peas

Fat

The Dietary Guidelines for Americans recommend a diet moderate in total fat, and low in saturated fat and cholesterol. Guidelines generally suggest that no more than 30% of daily calories should come from fat. Figure 3.14 gives some examples of fat levels corresponding to various calorie levels. Additional recommendations include:

▶ No more than 10% of total calories should be in the form of saturated fat.

▶ Polyunsaturated fats and monounsaturated fats are normally each about 10% of total calories.

▶ Limit trans-fatty acids.

▶ Cholesterol intake should be less than 300 milligrams daily.

Figure 3.14

RECOMMENDED FAT AND SATURATED FAT INTAKE

TOTAL DAILY CALORIES	SATURATED FAT	TOTAL FAT
1,200	13 grams	40 grams
1,500	17	50
1,800	20	60
2,000	22	67
2,200	24	73
2,400	27	80
2,600	29	86
2,800	31	93
3,000	33	100

Total fat is 30% of total calories; saturated fat is 10% of total calories.

This advice does not apply to infants and toddlers below the age of two years. After that age, children should gradually adopt a diet that, by about five years of age, contains no more than 30% of calories from fat. As they begin to consume fewer calories from fat, children should replace these calories by eating more grain products, fruits, vegetables, low fat milk products or other calcium-rich foods, beans, lean meat, poultry, fish, or other protein-rich foods.

Meat, poultry, fish, and shellfish contain saturated fat and/or cholesterol. Luckily, some choices are quite low in saturated fat. In general, poultry is low in saturated fat, especially when the skin is removed. When buying fresh ground turkey or chicken, find a product that says "light meat" or "breast" on the label. Poultry products that include the skin and/or dark meat and are much higher in fat. Goose and duck are also high. Most fish is lower in saturated fat and cholesterol than meat and poultry. Fatty fish (such as salmon and tuna) are rich in omega-3 fatty acids which may protect against heart disease and certain forms of cancer. Shellfish varies in cholesterol content.

Figure 3.15 lists lean cuts of meat. High-fat processed meats, such as many luncheon meats and sausages, provide a hefty 60 to 80% of their calories from fat, much of which is saturated. Other examples of these processed meats are bacon, bologna, salami, hot dogs, and sausage. In some cases, these processed meats are made from turkey or chicken and are lower in fat. Look for low fat processed meats. Organ meats, like liver, sweetbreads, and kidneys are relatively low in fat. However, these meats are high in cholesterol.

Figure 3.15

LEAN CUTS OF MEAT

BEEF	VEAL	PORK	LAMB
Eye of the round	Shoulder	Tenderloin	Leg-shank
Top round	Ground veal	Sirloin	
	Cutlets	Top loin	
	Sirloin		

Source: National Institutes of Health

When cooking meats, poultry, and fish, use cooking methods that use little or no fat, such as roasting, broiling, grilling, boiling, stir frying or poaching. Do not fry. When making pan gravy, refrigerate the drippings first so the fat will solidify and can be removed. One may also extend meat with pasta or vegetables for hearty dishes. For less saturated fat and cholesterol and more variety, dried beans or legumes are an excellent meat alternative.

Although many people believe that meats have the highest cholesterol and saturated fat content, dairy products can also be high in saturated fat and cholesterol. As dairy products are often added to foods like casseroles, cakes, or pies, it's easy to eat a significant amount of them without knowing it. Both 1% and skim milk provide much less saturated fat and cholesterol and fewer calories than whole milk, as shown in Figure 3.16.

Often, when people cut back on meat, they replace it with cheese, thinking they are cutting back on their saturated fat and cholesterol. They couldn't be more wrong. Because most cheeses are prepared from whole milk or cream, they are also high in saturated fat and cholesterol. Cheeses are particularly high in saturated fat (Figure 3.17). Fortunately, manufacturers offer low fat versions of cheese favorites like cheddar, Swiss, and mozzarella. They use skim milk and vegetable oils to replace some of the cream and other fat. The result is reduced fat or fat free cheese. (Please see Chapter 9 for terms used on food labels and their exact definitions.)

Americans love ice cream. Ice cream is made from whole milk and cream and therefore contains a considerable amount of saturated fat and cholesterol. Some frozen desserts such as ices, popsicles, and sorbet are generally made without fat. Ice milk contains less fat and saturated fat than regular ice cream, as does frozen low fat yogurt. With the wide variety of frozen desserts, it's a good idea to read nutrition labels.

Egg yolks are high in cholesterol. The average large egg yolk contains 213 milligrams of cholesterol, about two-thirds of the suggested daily intake. For less cholesterol and fat, use egg substitutes with less than 60 calories per

Figure 3.16

Figure 3.17

COMPARISON OF MILK

	TOTAL FAT	SATURATED FAT	CHOLESTEROL	CALORIES
Skim milk	0.4 grams	0.3 grams	4 milligrams	86
1% milk	2.6	1.6	10	102
2% milk	4.7	2.9	18	121
Whole milk	8.2	5.1	33	150

Source: National Institutes of Health

POULTRY, MEAT, AND CHEESE: A COMPARISON

FOOD	SATURATED FAT	CHOLESTEROL	TOTAL FAT
Roasted chicken, no skin, light meat, 3 ounces	1 gram	64 milligrams	4 grams
Beef, top round, broiled, 3 ounces	3	73	8
Natural cheddar, 1 ounce	6	30	9

Source: National Institutes of Health

one-quarter cup serving, or egg whites, which contain no cholesterol. Two egg whites can be substituted for one egg in recipes.

Choose vegetable oils high in polyunsaturated fats, such as corn oil, safflower oil, and sunflower oil, or monounsaturated fats, such as olive oil and canola oil. Whipped margarines (and whipped butter) contain fewer calories because air is whipped into them. Products labeled as light margarine, diet margarine, and margarine spread have water added to them so they contain less fat and fewer calories. Fat free margarines are even available. Reduced fat and fat free versions of salad dressings and mayonnaise contain less fat and saturated fat. (See Chapter 9 for labeling terms.)

Most breads and bread products contain only small amounts of fat, with less than two grams per slice or serving—that is, if we don't spread margarine or mayonnaise on them. Some breads typically have significant fat added in their preparation. Examples include biscuits, croissants, cornbread, and muffins. Also note that most granolas are high in fat. Commercial cakes, pies, cookies, donuts, and pastry are often high in fat, saturated fat, and calories. In addition, some are quite high in cholesterol. Tasty alternatives include angel food cake, sponge cake, fig bars, ginger snaps, and baked goods specially made with little or no fat. Recipe substitution ideas appear in Figure 3.18. Many desserts

Figure 3.18

LOWER FAT BAKING SUBSTITUTIONS

INSTEAD OF	USE
1 cup shortening	2/3 cup vegetable oil
1 whole egg	2 egg whites
1 cup sour cream	1 cup reduced-fat sour cream
1 cup whole milk	1 cup skim milk
1 tablespoon cream cheese	1 tablespoon Baker's cheese or Neufchatel cheese
1 cup cream	1 cup low fat yogurt
1 ounce baking chocolate	3 tablespoons cocoa and 1 tablespoon vegetable oil
Some of the butter or oil in a baked product	Fruit-based butter and oil replacements

can also be made with less fat. Simply reduce the fat called for by one-fourth to one-third the original amount.

Protein

According to surveys conducted by the USDA, 14 to 18% of calories in the American diet come from protein. The recommended level is closer to 10-12% of calories. Eating too much protein has no benefits. It will not result in bigger muscles, stronger bones, or increased immunity. In fact, eating excess protein as meat may add excessive fat and calorics. It may also lead to increased calcium losses from the body and kidney disease. The best way to manage protein intake is to follow the Food Guide Pyramid. Also note that many of the recommendations for reducing dietary fat and saturated fat go hand-in-hand with achieving a moderate protein intake. The key reductions come from limiting meat intake to Pyramid Guidelines. A vegetarian eating plan, if applied well, accomplishes this too. A vegetarian, however, needs to avoid substituting high-fat dairy products for meats.

DIETARY REFERENCE INTAKES (DRIs)

Since 1941, the Food and Nutrition Board of the National Academy of Sciences has been preparing recommendations on nutrient intakes for Americans. Contemporary studies address topics ranging from the prevention of classical nutritional deficiency diseases to the reduction of risk of chronic diseases such as osteoporosis, cancer, and cardiovascular disease. In partnership with Health Canada, the Food and Nutrition Board has responded to these developments by making fundamental changes in its approach to setting nutrient reference values. This partnership issued the first of its new standards in 1997. Dietary Reference Intakes is the inclusive name being given to the new approach.

Dietary Reference Intakes (DRIs) is a generic term used to refer to four types of reference values: **Estimated Average Requirement**, **Recommended**

Dietary Allowance, **Adequate Intake**, and **Tolerable Upper Intake Level**. Reference intakes are designed for various age and gender groups, because nutrient needs vary from childhood through adulthood, and some needs vary between males and females.

Estimated Average Requirement (EAR). The EAR is the intake value that is estimated to meet the requirement defined by a specified indicator of adequacy in 50% of a specific group (age and gender group). A **requirement** is how much is needed in the diet to prevent symptoms of deficiency. A **deficiency** is the illness that occurs over time when a nutrient is not present in adequate amounts. For example, not eating enough vitamin C causes scurvy. Not having enough vitamin D causes rickets. Scurvy and rickets are examples of nutrient deficiency illnesses. At the EAR level of intake, 50% of the specified group would not have its needs met. In other words, if everyone consumed exactly the EAR levels of nutrients, some people would actually develop nutrient deficiencies. Thus, the EAR is designed only for setting a benchmark for baseline nutrient requirements. An EAR is *not* intended for use in evaluating an individual's dietary intake.

Recommended Dietary Allowance (RDA). A Recommended Dietary Allowance (RDA) is the amount of a nutrient that is adequate to meet the known nutrient needs of practically all healthy persons. Contrary to popular belief, an RDA is not a minimum daily requirement. It is a dietary recommendation. To develop RDAs, scientists first reviewed research studies that indicated what minimum levels of nutrients might be required to prevent nutrient deficiencies. Then, they padded the requirements to account for additional factors that might affect requirements. They also padded the numbers to account for the difference between the amount of a nutrient consumed and the amount the body can actually use. (As explained in Chapter 4, our bodies do not always use 100% of what we eat.) These scientists used statistics to calculate individual variations in nutrient needs, and projected figures that would address the needs of most healthy people. Thus, an RDA is truly a recommendation about how much of a nutrient to consume through food. If everyone consumed exactly the RDA levels of nutrients, very, very few people in that group would develop nutrient deficiencies. Also, RDAs are for healthy individuals. RDAs do not always apply to someone who is suffering from a chronic illness or who has special medical conditions. Unlike the EAR, an RDA is a goal for individuals.

Adequate Intake (AI). For some nutrients, we simply don't know enough to set a meaningful RDA. We lack the scientific research that backs up the calculation of requirements. When this is the case, we use an Adequate Intake value. For example, we do not have a great deal of information about the physiological requirements for choline. Instead of setting an RDA, experts have designated an AI for choline. An AI represents a scientific judgment. We cannot be certain that an AI covers the nutrient needs of groups or individuals, but the AI value seems to be a reasonable point of reference based on what we know. When the only standard we have for a nutrient is an AI, it is fine to apply the AI to both groups and individuals.

Tolerable Upper Intake Level (UL). The UL is the maximum level of daily nutrient intake that is unlikely to pose risks of adverse health effects. ULs have been developed for some nutrients as safety guidelines. For example, these points of reference are helpful in determining whether the doses of nutrients contained in nutritional supplements represent safe intakes.

As you might guess, setting dietary reference intakes is a complex task. Use of statistics is critical to the job. Scientists are working to develop figures we can refer to when assessing individuals' diets, when planning menus, and more. Due to the enormity of this undertaking, the Dietary Reference Intake project has been divided into seven nutrient groups, and one to two groups of nutrients are reported on each year. Please see Appendix D for the DRI charts.

PROTECTING NUTRIENTS IN FOODS

The best-planned diet can go a bit awry if foods lose their nutrients during storage, cooking, and service. Exchange with air and/or water often allows foods to lose nutrients. Water-soluble vitamins are particularly susceptible to escaping from foods. Minerals and fat-soluble vitamins tend to be more stable, but can also be lost. Heat can also destroy vitamins, as can a very alkaline (high) pH. What can happen? Vitamin C can gradually escape from fruit or vegetables stored too long, even in the refrigerator. Nutrients including vitamins A, C, E, K, and the B vitamins are often destroyed through exposure to air. Vitamins and minerals may also leach out into water during soaking or boiling. Figure 3.19 offers tips for protecting foods from unnecessary nutrient losses.

FOOD OR SUPPLEMENTS?

A common nutritional question concerns nutritional supplements. Should you rely on a balanced diet or pills to ensure good nutrition? In the medical setting, sometimes the question arises differently. A patient may be obtaining all or some nutrients through a liquid feeding tube into the gastrointestinal tract. Or, a patient may receive nutrition through an intravenous solution. When all nutrition is received by vein, this is called **total parenteral nutrition (TPN)**. Interestingly, maintaining patients on TPN for extended periods of time has helped us identify nutrients and better understand nutrient needs. In theory, scientists today can formulate solutions, beverages, or pills that provide needed nutrients. In practice, however, there are a few limitations worth noting. While nutrition science is quite advanced, we are only beginning to understand the many components of foods that are active in the human body. The emerging concept of functional foods makes this quite evident; see *Nutrition in the News* at the end of this chapter. Beyond vitamins, minerals, protein, lipids, and carbohydrates, foods provide other natural chemicals. Some appear to offer health benefits. Already, some functional ingredients in foods have been incorporated into nutritional supplements. But this is not a complete answer for

TIPS FOR PROTECTING NUTRIENTS

▶ Minimize storage time. Do not store foods longer than necessary.

▶ Keep foods wrapped or covered in storage.

▶ Do not soak foods in water unless absolutely necessary. If you need to soak a food, use as little water as possible. If practical, add the water to your product (e.g. a soup).

▶ Cut and cook vegetables in large pieces to minimize contact between surface area and air.

▶ To cook vegetables, steam rather than boil. This helps them retain nutrients.

▶ Cook vegetables as soon as possible after cutting.

▶ Use raw vegetables (rather than cooked) as practical.

▶ Avoid adding baking soda to vegetables during cooking. Some people use this practice to retain color. However, it destroys thiamin and vitamin C.

▶ Avoid overcooking food, as heat can destroy vitamins (especially vitamin C). Cook just until tender.

▶ Before cooking rice, do not rinse it.

▶ Do not brown uncooked rice before adding water. This destroys thiamin.

▶ After cooking rice, pasta, or other grain-based foods, do not rinse; just drain.

▶ Store food away from light or in dark containers. This is important for milk, since riboflavin, a B vitamin in milk, is destroyed by light.

▶ In foodservice operations, cook food as close to service times as possible. Cook in small batches as appropriate. For example, steamed vegetables may be prepared in small batches throughout an extended meal service time.

▶ Minimize holding time as possible. Keep foods covered during holding.

Source: USDA

sound nutrition. The bottom line is that real food is preferable to chemical formulations. In real food, provided through a balanced diet and based on established dietary guidance, we can obtain necessary nutrients, as well as compounds we may not understand very well as yet. Real food also gives people pleasure, as explained in Chapter 1. In addition, real food offers fiber (not present in all supplemental products), and water. It provides a sense of satiety or fullness when we eat it.

Nutritional supplements can be important for an individual who wishes to ensure adequate nutrition, or who needs to correct a deficiency. Iron supplements, for example, may be important to supplement dietary intake of iron. Iron-deficiency anemia is common in the US, and it is not easy for everyone to consume adequate iron through food. Calcium is another nutrient that may be worth supplementing—especially for adult women. The AI level is not easy for every woman to achieve, and calcium plays a role in preventing osteoporosis. These are just examples of situations in which supplementation may be useful.

However, it's prudent to consider supplements as what they are—*supplements*—not *replacements* for healthy eating habits. It is also important to review DRIs for nutrients, and pay particular attention to the UL levels for nutrients. Excessive supplementation of some nutrients can cause health problems.

In all, a diet is complex. So much information about nutrition bombards us that it can be challenging to make dietary choices. Reliance on the Food Pyramid and the Dietary Guidelines for Americans is an excellent way to assure a healthy diet, given all that we know today. For menu planning and in-depth assessment, the DRIs offer science-based standards of reference.

FUNCTIONAL FOODS PROVIDE BENEFITS BEYOND BASIC NUTRITION

Functional Foods are foods that may provide a health benefit beyond basic nutrition. The good news with functional foods is that what you do eat may be more important for your health than what you don't eat. Examples include everything from fruits and vegetables to fortified or enhanced foods. Biologically active components in functional foods impart health benefits or desirable physiological effects. Functional attributes of many traditional foods are being discovered, while new food products are being developed with beneficial components.

DEMAND

Consumer interest in the relationship between diet and health has increased the demand for information on functional foods. Rapid advances in science and technology, increasing healthcare costs, changes in food laws affecting label and product claims, an aging population and rising interest in attaining wellness through diet are among the factors fueling U.S. interest in functional foods. Credible scientific research indicates many potential health benefits from food components. These benefits could expand the health claims now permitted by the Food and Drug Administration (FDA).

SCIENTIFIC CRITERIA

Many academic, scientific and regulatory organizations are considering ways to establish the scientific basis to support claims for functional components or the foods containing them. The FDA regulates food products according to their intended use and the nature of claims made on the package. Two types of statements or claims are allowed on food and dietary supplement labels:

1. Structure and function claims describing effects on normal function of the body.
2. Disease risk reduction (health) claims implying a relationship between components in the diet and a disease or health condition, as approved by the FDA and supported by significant scientific agreement.

A large body of credible scientific research is needed to confirm the benefits of any particular food or component. For functional foods to deliver their potential public health benefits, consumers must have a clear understanding of and a strong confidence level in the scientific criteria that are used to document health effects and claims. The scientific community is in the early stages of understanding the potential for functional foods.

Functional foods are an important part of wellness that includes a balanced diet and physical activity. Consumers should consume a wide variety of foods, including the examples listed on the following page. These examples are not "magic bullets." The best advice is to include foods from all of the food groups, which would incorporate many potentially beneficial components.

EXAMPLES OF FUNCTIONAL COMPONENTS*

Class/Components	Source*	Potential Benefit
CAROTENOIDS		
Alpha-carotene	carrots	neutralizes free radicals which may cause damage to cells
Beta-carotene	various fruits, vegetables	neutralizes free radicals
Lutein	green vegetables	contributes to maintenance of healthy vision
Lycopene	tomatoes, tomato products (ketchup, sauces, etc)	may reduce risk of prostate cancer
Zeaxanthin	eggs, citrus, corn	contributes to maintenance of healthy vision
COLLAGEN HYDROLYSATE		
Collagen Hydrolysate	gelatine	may help improve some symptoms associated with osteoarthritis
DIETARY FIBER		
Insoluble fiber	wheat bran	may reduce risk of breast and/or colon cancer
Beta glucan**	oats	may reduce risk of cardiovascular disease (CVD)
Soluble fiber**	psyllium	may reduce risk of CVD
Whole Grains**	cereal grains	may reduce risk of CVD
FATTY ACIDS		
Omega-3 fatty acids—DHA/EPA	tuna; fish, marine oils	may reduce risk of CVD & improve mental, visual functions
Conjugated Linoleic acid (CLA)	cheese, meat products	may improve body composition, may decrease risk of certain cancers
FLAVONOIDS		
Anthocyanidins	fruits	neutralize free radicals, may reduce risk of cancer
Catechins	tea	neutralize free radicals, may reduce risk of cancer
Flavanones	citrus	neutralize free radicals, may reduce risk of cancer
Flavones	fruits/vegetables	neutralize free radicals, may reduce risk of cancer
GLUCOSINOLATES, INDOLES, ISOTHIOCYANATES		
Sulphoraphane	cruciferous vegetables (broccoli, kale), horseradish	neutralizes free radicals, may reduce risk of cancer
PHENOLS		
Caffeic acid Ferulic acid	fruits, vegetables, citrus	antioxidant-like activities, may reduce risk of degenerative diseases; heart disease, eye disease

EXAMPLES OF FUNCTIONAL COMPONENTS, *CONTINUED*

PLANT STANOLS/STEROLS

Stanol/Sterol ester**	corn, soy, wheat, wood oils	may reduce risk of coronary heart disease (CHD) by lowering blood cholesterol levels

PREBIOTIC/PROBIOTICS

Fructo-oligosaccharides (FOS)	Jerusalem artichokes, shallots, onion powder	may improve gastrointestinal health
Lactobacillus	yogurt, other dairy	may improve gastrointestinal health

SAPONINS

Saponins	soybeans, soy foods, soy protein-containing foods	may lower LDL cholesterol; contains anti-cancer enzymes

SOY PROTEIN

Soy Protein**	soybeans, soy-based foods	25 grams per day may reduce risk of heart disease

PHYTOESTROGENS

Isoflavones— Daidzein, Genistein	soybeans, soy-based foods	may reduce menopause symptoms, such as hot flashes
Lignans	flax, rye, vegetables	may protect against heart disease and some cancers; may lower LDL cholesterol, total cholesterol and triglycerides

SULFIDES/THIOLS

Diallyl sulfide	onions, garlic, olives, leeks, scallions	may lower LDL cholesterol, helps to maintain healthy immune system
Allyl methyl	cruciferous vegetables trisulfide, Dithiolthiones	may lower LDL cholesterol, helps to maintain healthy immune system

TANNINS

Proanthocyanidins	cranberries, cranberry products, cocoa, chocolate	may improve urinary tract health; may reduce risk of CVD

*Examples are not an all-inclusive list.

**FDA approved health claim established for component.

© International Food Information Council (IFIC) Foundation. Reprinted with permission.

- Nutrition scientists today devote a great deal of research to nutritional excess and imbalance.

- Sound nutrition and weight management may reduce risks for heart disease, hypertension, diabetes, cancer, joint problems, and more.

- Various food guides provide shortcuts or easy-to-use tools that consumers can use to direct their own food choices.

- The Food Guide Pyramid is a visual tool for managing intake of various food groups to meet sound nutrition principles.

- Dietary Guidelines for Americans (2000) represent a set of simple dietary recommendations for Americans, and they incorporate the Food Guide Pyramid.

- The 5 A Day program promotes intake of fruits and vegetables.

- Functional foods are foods that may impart a health benefit beyond basic nutrition.

- General recommendations for fiber intake are from 20 to 35 grams daily.

- Guidelines generally recommend that no more than 30% of daily calories should come from fat, with no more than 10% coming from saturated fat. Recommended cholesterol intake is less than 300 milligrams daily.

- Dietary Reference Intakes (DRIs) is a generic term used to describe four types of reference values: Estimated Average Requirement, Recommended Dietary Allowance, Adequate Intake, and Tolerable Upper Intake Level. Reference intakes are designed for various age and gender groups, because nutrient needs vary from childhood through adulthood, and some needs vary between males and females.

- A variety of factors allow foods to lose nutrients. Water soluble vitamins are most susceptible. Sound practices during storage and preparation can minimize nutrient losses.

Adequate Intake (AI): an estimate of reasonable intake, used when requirements are not precisely known

Deficiency: the illness that occurs over time when a nutrient is not present in adequate amounts

Dietary Guidelines for Americans: a set of simple dietary recommendations for Americans, first released in 1980 by the USDA and the Department of Health and Human Services

Dietary Reference Intakes (DRIs): a generic term used to describe four types of nutritional reference values: Estimated Average Requirement, Recommended Dietary Allowance, Adequate Intake, and Tolerable Upper Intake Level

Estimated Average Requirement (EAR): an average intake value that is estimated to meet the requirement of half the people in a group

Five a Day program: a concept developed by the National Cancer Institute and the Produce for Better Health Foundation to promote consumption of fruits and vegetables

Food Guide Pyramid: A practical guide about how to eat. It classifies foods into five groups, with each group's position on the pyramid reflecting the number of servings recommended per day by the US Department of Agriculture (USDA) and the Department of Health and Human Services.

Obese: having a BMI of 30 or greater

Overweight: having a BMI of 25-29.9

Portion: the total amount of a food served or consumed at any point in time

Recommended Dietary Allowance (RDA): the amount of a nutrient that is adequate to meet the known nutrient needs of practically all healthy people

Requirement: the amount of a nutrient needed in the diet to prevent symptoms of deficiency

Risk factor: a habit, trait, or condition of any individual that is associated with an increased chance of developing a disease

Serving: a measurement used for keeping track of amounts of food

Tolerable Upper Intake Level (UL): the maximum level of daily nutrient intake that is unlikely to pose risks of adverse health effects

Total parenteral nutrition (TPN): the provision of all nutrition by vein

1. According to a Surgeon General's Report on Nutrition and Health in 1988, a key nutritional concern in the US is:

   A. Vitamin A deficiency
   B. Potassium deficiency
   C. Nutrient excesses
   D. Reliance on too many organic foods

2. Obesity and overweight result from:

   A. Eating too much carbohydrate
   B. Following a vegetarian diet
   C. An imbalance between calorie consumption and physical activity
   D. Eating genetically engineered foods

3. An advantage of the Food Pyramid for teaching others about nutrition is that it:

   A. Is easy to understand
   B. Focuses on eating more meat
   C. Limits intake of starchy foods to ½ cup per meal
   D. Helps people add up vitamin content of foods

4. Which of the following is true about the 5 A Day Concept?
   A. It limits fruit and vegetable consumption to five servings per day
   B. It limits meat consumption to five ounces per day
   C. It limits egg consumption to five per day
   D. It encourages fruit and vegetable consumption of at least five servings per day

5. Which of the following is NOT one of the Dietary Guidelines for Americans?
   A. Aim for a healthy weight.
   B. Let the Pyramid guide your food choices.
   C. Avoid high-carbohydrate foods.
   D. Choose and prepare foods with less salt.

6. An RDA is:
   A. The minimum requirement for a nutrient
   B. The amount of a nutrient that is adequate to meet the known nutrient needs of practically all healthy persons
   C. The maximum amount of a nutrient a person can safely consume
   D. The amount of a nutrient that will cause deficiency

7. A UL is:
   A. The minimum requirement for a nutrient
   B. The amount of a nutrient that is adequate to meet the known nutrient needs of practically all healthy persons
   C. The maximum amount of a nutrient a person can safely consume
   D. The amount of a nutrient that will cause deficiency

8. An EAR may be applied to:
   A. Individuals and groups
   B. Groups only
   C. Individuals only
   D. Children only

9. Which of the following would NOT be a good way to reduce saturated fat in your diet?
   A. Substitute dried beans for meat
   B. Remove skin from chicken before cooking it
   C. Use roasting, broiling, grilling, boiling, or poaching as cooking methods for meat
   D. Eat more cheddar and Swiss cheeses

10. Recommended protein consumption for healthy adults is about:
   A. 5-7% of total calories
   B. 10-12% of total calories
   C. 20-30% of total calories
   D. 50-55% of total calories

An understanding of how digestion occurs helps a dietary manager plan and modify menus for individuals who have unique needs.

After completing this chapter, you should be able to:

- Define the term digestion and relate it to nutrition.
- Identify the organs involved in digestion.
- Distinguish between mechanical and chemical breakdown of foods.
- Describe the process of digestion for carbohydrates, and identify where it occurs.
- Describe the process of digestion for fat, and identify where it occurs.
- Describe the process of digestion for protein, and identify where it occurs.
- Explain the concepts of absorption and availability of nutrients.

SYSTEMS OF THE HUMAN BODY

Digestion occurs through the digestive system. The body is made up of systems. Each has a purpose. The word **system** describes groups of organs working together to perform functions. Systems are made up of organs. Organs are made up of body tissues. In turn, tissues are made up of cells. *Cells* are the basic unit of life, and the building blocks of the human body. Each cell has a cell membrane that surrounds and protects the cell. Most cells also have a nucleus, which directs the work going on in the cell. The body contains many types of cells, such as nerve cells, bone cells, muscle cells, and fat cells. Each type of cell has a unique structure related to what it does in the body.

Tissues are groups of similar cells that work together to perform a certain function. For example, epithelial tissue lines many body surfaces, and one of its functions is to protect the body. *Organs* are made of several kinds of tissue. Examples of body organs include the liver, stomach, intestines, gallbladder, kidney, brain, and heart. Even skin is considered an organ. Organs work together as part of body systems. Systems include:

- The digestive system, which digests food
- The circulatory system, which circulates blood and lymph (a body fluid)
- The musculoskeletal system, essential for body movement
- The nervous and endocrine (hormone) systems, which control body functions
- The respiratory system, responsible for breathing
- The immune system, which protects against illness and infection
- The reproductive system, responsible for new life
- The urinary system, which excretes waste (urine)

The Digestive System

When we eat food, it goes through three different processes: digestion, absorption, and metabolism. **Digestion** is the process through which the body converts food into nutrients and eliminates solid wastes. To understand digestion, it's helpful to review the anatomy, which is called the gastrointestinal tract. The **gastrointestinal tract (GI tract)** is like a hollow tube running down the middle of the body (Figure 4.1). It starts with the mouth, which is connected in turn to the throat or pharynx, esophagus, stomach, small intestines, large intestine, rectum, and anus, where solid wastes leave the body. Figure 4.2 lists the organs involved in digestion.

Body cells cannot use a steak, or an apple, or a slice of bread for food. Instead, they need food in its smaller chemical units, as nutrients. Thus, to convert food into nutrients, the body needs to break it down into smaller components. This

Figure 4.1

THE GASTROINTESTINAL TRACT

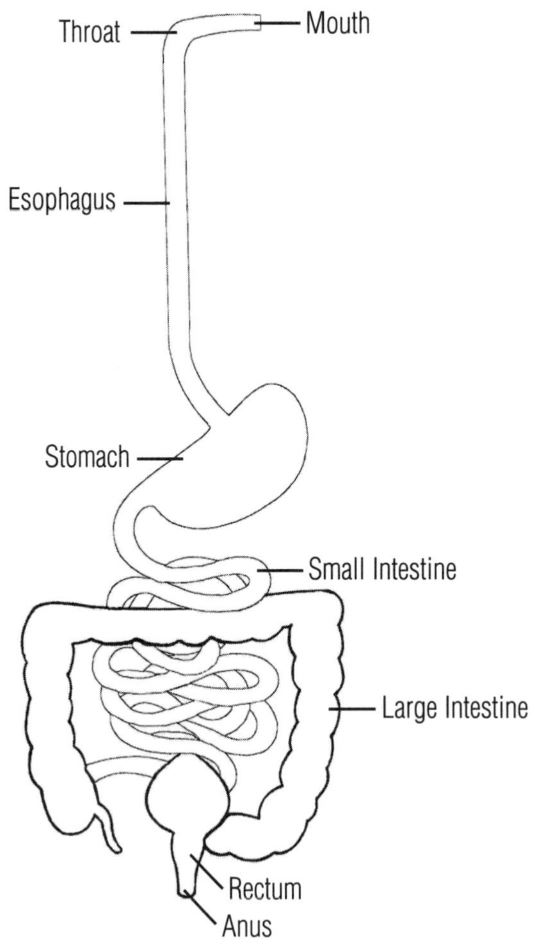

Figure 4.2

ORGANS IN THE DIGESTIVE SYSTEM

ORGAN	WHAT HAPPENS HERE
Mouth	Chewing and mixing of food with salivary fluids
Esophagus	Delivers swallowed food to the stomach
Stomach	Food is churned and mixed with hydrochloric acid and pepsin for further breakdown. The food mixture that leaves the stomach is called chyme. Alcohol and certain drugs are absorbed from the stomach.
Duodenum (first part of the small intestines)	Mixes food with secretions from the liver and pancreas to neutralize stomach acid and further digest food. Much absorption of food occurs here.
Jejunum (second part of the small intestines)	Continues chemical digestion. Much absorption of food occurs here.
Ileum (third part of the small intestines)	Re-absorbs bile salts used to digest fats earlier in the small intestines.
Colon	Absorbs water and vitamins. Collects indigestible residue (waste) to form feces.
Rectum	Controls release of waste (feces)
Liver	Produces bile, a chemical that emulsifies fat, i.e. it breaks fat down into smaller globules so that digestive enzymes can go to work.
Gallbladder	Stores bile and secretes it into the duodenum during digestion
Pancreas	Produces many digestive enzymes

is part of what digestion is about. Essentially, the body takes food apart so that it can use the pieces to re-build exactly what it needs for life.

During the process of digestion, food is broken down two ways: mechanically and chemically. **Mechanical breakdown** is the physical breaking of food into smaller pieces. In the digestive system, this is the job of the mouth, the esophagus, and the stomach. The first part is obvious. When we chew food, we break it into smaller bites. Teeth, tongue, and jaws all help with this process. The next forms of mechanical breakdown are invisible to us. As food moves through the esophagus towards the stomach, strong muscular action breaks it down a little bit more. When food is in the stomach, it is churned into even smaller pieces.

Chemical breakdown of food occurs with the help of digestive enzymes. *Enzymes* are substances that speed up chemical reactions and help in the breakdown of complex nutrients. Enzymes break complex proteins into simpler amino acids. They break starch into sugar, and reduce complicated sugars to simple sugars such as glucose. Enzymes also break large fat molecules down to fatty acids and glycerol. Figure 4.3 lists some of the digestive enzymes.

Figure 4.3

EXAMPLES OF DIGESTIVE ENZYMES

NAME OF ENZYME	WHERE IT IS	WHAT IT DOES
Salivary amylase	Mouth (made by salivary glands)	Breaks down starch and complex sugars
Pepsin	Stomach	Breaks down protein
Lipases	Secreted by the pancreas into the small intestines	Break down fat
Proteases	Secreted by the pancreas into the small intestines	Break down protein

The digestive system starts with the mouth or oral cavity. The tongue, which extends across the floor of the mouth, moves food around the mouth during chewing and rolls it into a ball to be swallowed. There are 32 permanent teeth in the mouth that grind and break down the food. Chewing is important because it breaks the food up into smaller pieces so that enzymes can get in and do their job. Saliva, a fluid secreted into the mouth from the salivary glands, not only produces amylase to begin breakdown of starches. It also lubricates the food so that it may readily pass down the throat and esophagus. The mucous-like substance in saliva coats food and helps to form a mass of chewed food called a **bolus**. Food in the form of a bolus can safely be swallowed.

How does swallowing work? There are two steps. In the first step, the tongue pushes the bolus back towards the pharynx, or the back of the oral cavity (see Figure 4.4). Then, an involuntary muscular contraction pushes the bolus into the esophagus. *Involuntary* means that this occurs automatically, as a reflex. We do not consciously control this step. During this second step, the body automatically closes the respiratory passages, so that we will not breathe in food. Anatomically speaking, a muscular flap called the *epiglottis* covers the trachea, the passageway to the lungs. From time to time, this process doesn't work. You can probably think of times when a little bit of food or drink has accidentally entered your respiratory system. This is called aspiration. In a healthy person, the result is coughing to clear it out.

Food enters the esophagus, a muscular tube about 10 inches long that connects the throat to the stomach. Food is propelled down the esophagus by rhythmic contractions of circular muscles in the wall of the esophagus. These contractions are called *peristalsis*. Peristalsis also helps break up food into smaller and smaller particles. You might want to think of it as squeezing a marble (the bolus) through a rubber tube. Food passes down the esophagus through the *lower esophageal sphincter (LES)*, a muscle that relaxes and contracts to move food from the esophagus into the stomach. The LES works like a gatekeeper into the stomach. Normally, it allows only a one-way movement. When a person experiences heartburn, the LES has mistakenly allowed acid stomach contents to shoot back up into the esophagus. This backflow of stomach

Figure 4.4

ANATOMY INVOLVED IN SWALLOWING

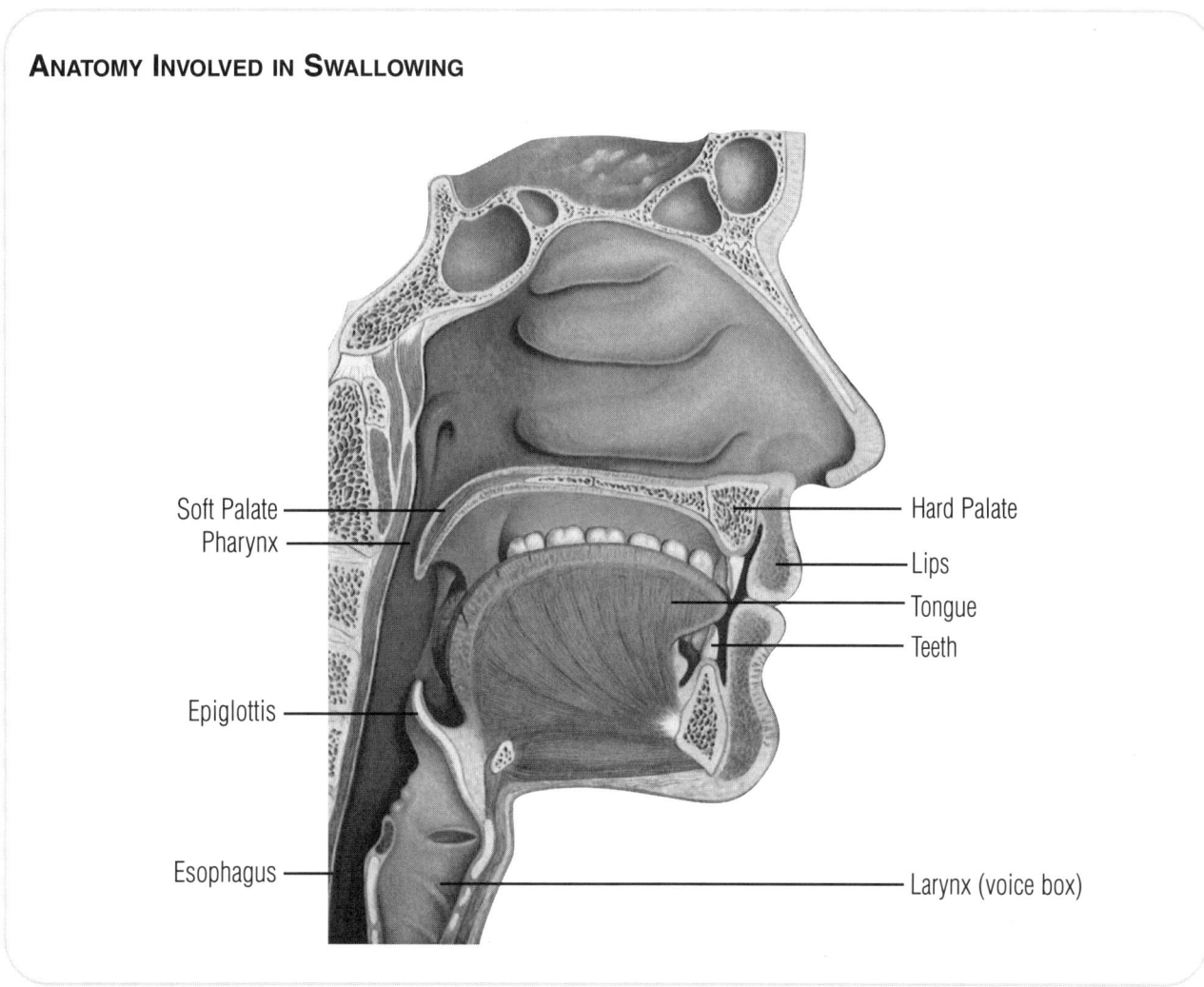

Soft Palate
Pharynx
Epiglottis
Esophagus

Hard Palate
Lips
Tongue
Teeth
Larynx (voice box)

contents is also called *reflux*. (Note that heartburn actually has nothing to do with the heart. It acquires its name because the discomfort sufferers feel is close to the position of the heart.)

The stomach is a muscular sac that holds about one liter of food. It is lined with a mucous membrane. Within the folds of the mucous membranes are digestive glands that make the enzyme pepsin, as well as hydrochloric acid. Hydrochloric acid makes stomach contents very acid (pH about 2.0, more acid than vinegar), which activates the pepsin for protein digestion. Hydrochloric acid also destroys harmful bacteria, and increases the ability of calcium and iron to be absorbed. People sometimes wonder why the stomach does not digest itself. The stomach has several forms of protection from these strong chemicals. First, it has a mucous lining that can neutralize hydrochloric acid. Second, it keeps the enzyme pepsin ready in a safer state called pepsinogen. Only after food arrives does it release acid and make pepsin active.

The stomach churns food so that it can be passed into the first part of the small intestines in small amounts because the small intestines can't process too much food at one time. When the food is ready, it reaches a liquid consistency known as *chyme*. The stomach functions like a holding tank and takes approximately two to six hours to empty. A high amount of fat in a meal slows stomach emptying. Little absorption of nutrients takes place here. However, this is the site where alcohol and aspirin are absorbed.

Another specialized muscle called the *pyloric sphincter* allows chyme to travel from the stomach into the small intestines. The small intestines are about 20 feet long and have three parts: the *duodenum*, the *jejunum*, and the *ileum*. They are called the small intestines because their diameter is smaller than that of the large intestine. Like the mouth and the stomach, the small intestines add digestive juices to food. These juices include enzymes and other chemicals produced by the pancreas. One of the chemicals is sodium bicarbonate, which simply neutralizes the acid chyme arriving from the stomach. Next is an array of digestive enzymes that convert protein to amino acids and small groups of amino acids. The duodenum, about one foot long, receives the digested food from the stomach. A small organ above the intestines, the pancreas, releases enzymes into the duodenum to help digest carbohydrate, protein, and fat.

Before enzymes can work on fat, however, the fat must be broken down into smaller parts. This is the job of *bile*, a compound produced by the liver and stored in the *gallbladder*. The gallbladder releases bile into the small intestines. Bile works like detergent, to emulsify fat. What does this mean? Imagine that your hands are greasy from rubbing oil on a turkey, or changing oil in your car. You cannot rinse the fat off your hands with water. You use soap or detergent to split fat globules into smaller parts so you can wash them away. Bile works quite similarly. Its action produces smaller pieces of fat, so that enzymes can get at them and digest the fat.

In the wall of the duodenum—and throughout the entire small intestines—are tiny, fingerlike projections called *villi*. The muscular walls mix the chyme with the digestive juices and bring the nutrients into contact with the villi for absorption. Most nutrients pass through the villi of the duodenum and jejunum into either the blood or lymph vessels, where they are transported to the liver and to the cells of the body. The duodenum connects with the second section, the jejunum, which connects to the ileum.

The large intestine or *colon*, which is four to five feet long, extends from the end of the ileum to the rectum. Water and some minerals are absorbed here. In addition, healthful bacteria in the colon actually manufacture vitamin K, as well as some biotin and folic acid. The body absorbs and uses these nutrients. One of the functions of the large intestine is to receive and store the waste products of digestion; in other words, it handles the material that has not entered the blood or lymph vessels. The waste accumulated here includes indigestible fiber from foods. Bacteria that are naturally present in the colon ferment some of the fiber, producing gases. Indigestible fiber also attracts and holds water. This makes stools softer and helps prevent constipation. The large intestine stores waste material until it is released as solid feces, through the anus, the lower opening of the gastrointestinal tract.

Before the body can use any of the nutrients present in food, the nutrients must pass through the walls of the gastrointestinal tract through a process called **absorption**. Nutrients pass through the cells of the intestinal tract into the circulatory system. Two parts of the circulatory system are involved: blood and lymph. The blood and lymph are two body fluids that circulate throughout the body, delivering needed products to the cells for use. Sugars and amino acids travel into the blood, while fatty acids enter the body through the lymphatic system. Remember that fat and water do not mix. The blood is largely water-based. This is why fat cannot enter the bloodstream. Lymphatic fluid, on the other hand, can hold and carry fat. If nutrients are not absorbed into the blood or lymph at some point along the gastrointestinal tract, they are excreted in the feces.

As the blood and lymph circulate nutrients through the body, cells begin to use the nutrients in a process called metabolism. **Metabolism** refers to all the chemical processes in a cell by which nutrients are used to support life. Metabolism involves building substances (called *anabolism*) or breaking down substances (called *catabolism*). Nutrients such as glucose are split into smaller units in a catabolic reaction that releases energy to maintain body temperature or to perform work within the cell. Anabolism is the opposite of catabolism. It is the process of building substances, such as proteins, from their components.

AVAILABILITY OF NUTRIENTS

An important aspect of nutrition is the *bioavailability* of nutrients. The term bioavailability describes how well a nutrient is absorbed and used by the body. When the process of digestion and absorption is complete, the amount of a nutrient a body *actually has* may differ from the amount *consumed*. For example, the body typically absorbs only about 10% of dietary iron. If the iron is from a meat source (a form called *heme iron*), absorption may rise to about 25%. Interestingly, studies demonstrate that individuals who have iron deficiency absorb iron more efficiently.

In addition, presence of other nutrients in the intestinal tract can have positive or negative effects on absorption. Vitamin C, for instance, seems to promote iron absorption. A person taking an iron supplement along with a glass of orange juice may enjoy better absorption and a higher bioavailability of the nutrient. Conversely, high amounts of magnesium in the gastrointestinal tract may interfere with absorption of iron and calcium. A natural compound in dark leafy green vegetables called *oxalate* can also slow down iron absorption. To absorb fat-soluble vitamins, the body generally needs some fat in the intestinal tract, too. In a food-based diet, this is easy to accomplish, because fat-soluble vitamins appear in conjunction with dietary fat.

Even after absorption, various factors affect how well the body can use nutrients. For example, alcohol counteracts the effects of vitamin B6 in metabolism. Many drugs, too, can affect the metabolism of nutrients. Some increase bioavailability; some decrease it.

Gastrointestinal illness can affect bioavailability of nutrients, as well. If the intestines are inflamed and intestinal villi are damaged, as in Crohn's disease, adequate nutrient absorption may not take place. In another example, a poorly functioning pancreas may fail to make enough of the critical enzymes needed for digestion of protein and fat, leading to poor bioavailability of protein and fat in the body. In cases of illness, an average diet that is adequate in protein, fat, carbohydrate, vitamins, and minerals may nevertheless not be adequate to maintain good nutritional status. This is due to reduced absorption and reduced bioavailability of nutrients. For healthy people, the RDA levels of nutrients address ordinary factors that influence nutrient bioavailability. It's important for a dietary manager to know, however, that established nutrient standards may not always fit the bill under various medical conditions. Thus, individual screening and assessment (described in Chapter 8) are important to help a dietary manager address the unique needs of each client. Likewise, communication with medical staff and a dietitian can help assure that meals leaving the kitchen are nutritionally adequate for the population being served.

Key Points

▶ To use the nutrients in food, the body must first break food down into its components through the process of digestion.

▶ Digestion occurs throughout the gastrointestinal tract, which spans from the mouth to the anus.

▶ Mechanical breakdown of food occurs through chewing, through peristalsis in the esophagus, and through churning in the stomach.

▶ Chemical breakdown of food occurs in part through the work of enzymes.

▶ Chemical breakdown of starch begins in the mouth with salivary amylase, and continues in the small intestines with the help of pancreatic enzymes.

▶ Chemical breakdown of protein begins in the stomach, with the work of pepsin, and continues in the small intestines, with the help of pancreatic enzymes.

▶ Chemical breakdown of fat begins in the small intestines, with the help of pancreatic enzymes.

- Bile, produced by the liver and stored in the gallbladder, helps break fat into smaller globules so that enzymes can digest the fat.

- Carbohydrate, in the form of sugars, is absorbed from the small intestines into the bloodstream.

- Protein, mostly in the form of amino acids, is absorbed from the small intestines into the bloodstream.

- Fat is absorbed into the lymphatic system.

- In the body, nutrients are used in many body processes which together constitute metabolism.

- How well the body can use nutrients from the diet is called bioavailability.

Key Terms

Absorption: the process by which nutrients pass through the cells of the intestinal tract into the circulatory system

Bolus: a mass of chewed food formed in the mouth

Chemical breakdown: the use of digestive enzymes to break down complex nutrients

Digestion: the process through which the body converts food into nutrients and eliminates solid wastes

Gastrointestinal tract (GI tract): a hollow tube running down the middle of the body from the mouth to the anus

Mechanical breakdown: the physical breaking of food into smaller pieces

Metabolism: the chemical processes in a cell by which nutrients are used to support life

System: group of organs working together to perform functions

Review Questions

1. A group of organs working together to perform a function is called a(n):
   A. Cell
   B. Tissue
   C. Enzyme
   D. System

2. Which of the following is NOT an example of an organ?
   A. Pancreas
   B. Skin
   C. Chyme
   D. Stomach

3. The purpose of salivary amylase is to:
   A. Begin digestion of starch into sugars
   B. Begin digestion of protein into amino acids
   C. Prevent absorption of bacteria into the circulatory system
   D. Neutralize stomach acid

4. Alcohol is absorbed from the:
   A. Stomach
   B. Esophagus
   C. Duodenum
   D. Colon

5. The purpose of bile is to:
   A. Break starch into smaller units
   B. Break fat into smaller units
   C. Break protein into smaller units
   D. Break minerals into smaller units

6. Breakdown of starch begins in the:
   A. Mouth
   B. Pharynx
   C. Stomach
   D. Small intestines

7. Breakdown of protein begins in the:
   A. Mouth
   B. Pharynx
   C. Stomach
   D. Small intestines

8. An organ that produces enzymes to break down proteins and fats is the:
   A. Pharynx
   B. Small intestines
   C. Pancreas
   D. Colon

9. A term that describes nutrients passing through the walls of the intestines into the circulatory system is:
   A. Digestion
   B. Absorption
   C. Metabolism
   D. Anabolism

10. Typically, a person absorbs about:
    A. 10-25% of dietary iron
    B. 30-40% of dietary iron
    C. 50-75% of dietary iron
    D. 95-100% of dietary iron

Nutrition needs vary throughout the life cycle. It is up to a dietary manager to acknowledge and address the specialized nutrition needs of each client group.

After completing this chapter, you should be able to:

- Define the term *life cycle*, and explain why nutrition needs can change during the life cycle.
- Explain how the nutrition needs of infants and children are unique.
- Explain how the nutrition needs of adolescents are unique.
- Explain how the nutrition needs of pregnant and lactating women are unique.
- Explain how the nutrition needs of the elderly are unique.
- Recommend general menu modifications to address nutrition needs in various stages of the life cycle.
- Identify key elements of school meal regulations.
- Define nutritionally *at risk* populations.

LIFE CYCLE AND NUTRITION

As you've learned in earlier chapters, nutrition provides the fuel for body processes. Besides imparting forms of energy to sustain life, nutrients in food contribute to a stunning array of metabolic processes. Without adequate nutrition, some of these processes may not occur, or may not work well. Chapter 4 describes the basic concepts of anabolism and catabolism. Nutrients provide many of the building blocks for body tissue. In addition, some nutrients serve as co-enzymes or "stimulators" in metabolic processes. Protein and minerals often provide the building blocks for body tissues. Breaking down unneeded byproducts of metabolism and being able to work them out of the system also require nutrients.

As you might guess, metabolism changes throughout a person's life. Biological priorities shift throughout the life cycle. The term **life cycle** describes the series of stages in any individual's life—from early infancy through late maturity. While the basic nutrients and their functions remain constant through a lifetime, their amounts may change. In addition, other developmental factors affect how a person actually eats. In this chapter, we'll examine how stages of the life cycle interplay with nutrition.

NUTRITION DURING PREGNANCY

Pregnancy is not really the time to "eat for two." As a matter of fact, a mother who eats for just one and one-half will gain too much weight! The current recommendation is for women of normal weight to gain between 25 and 35 pounds during pregnancy. Underweight women should gain 28 to 40 pounds, and overweight women should gain 15 to 25 pounds. These weights are the most appropriate to produce a baby of optimal size: between six and one-half to nine pounds. In addition, optimal weight gain supports a healthy outcome. Inadequate weight gain during pregnancy is associated with premature birth. Overweight women run a higher risk for pregnancy-related complications, such as hypertension, gestational diabetes (a blood sugar disorder that occurs during pregnancy), and stillbirths.

Most women gain approximately three pounds during the first three months (also called the first trimester) and one pound a week thereafter. A woman's weight gain is distributed as follows for a total weight gain of 22 to 28 pounds:

Fetus . . . . 6½ to 9 pounds

Placenta . . . . 1½ pounds

Amniotic fluid . . . . 2 pounds

Increase in size of uterus, breast, & blood volume . . . . . 9 pounds

Fat. . . . . 2-8 pounds

The developing infant is called a *fetus*. The *placenta* is a new organ that develops in the first month of pregnancy and provides an exchange of nutrients and wastes between the fetus and the mother. The *amniotic fluid* is the fluid surrounding the fetus. This stage of development does require increased amounts of some nutrients:

Energy. During the second trimester, women should eat an additional 340 calories per day. During the third trimester, women should eat approximately 425 more calories per day.

Protein. The RDA for protein during pregnancy is 25 grams higher than usual. Many American adults already exceed the RDA for protein, so this may not require special attention. However, a woman who follows a vegetarian diet or eats very little meat and dairy products may need to increase sources of protein in the diet.

Essential Fatty Acids. Research suggests that essential fatty acids may be particularly important for healthy growth in the fetus. The omega-3 and omega-6 fatty acids available in vegetable oils, nuts, seeds, and fish may help promote development.

Iron. The RDA for iron in pregnancy takes a big jump, from 18 mg (non-pregnant female) to 27 mg per day. All this iron is essential for producing the extra blood volume required to nourish a developing fetus. Note that blood volume increases 50% during pregnancy. In addition, the fetus actually stores up iron during development, so that after birth, an infant has adequate iron stores to last about four to six months. This places hefty demands on a woman's body.

SOURCES OF IRON

Shellfish like shrimp, clams, mussels, and oysters

Lean meats (especially beef), liver* and other organ meats*

Ready-to-eat cereals with added iron

Turkey dark meat (remove skin to reduce fat)

Sardines**

Spinach

Cooked dry beans (such as kidney beans and pinto beans), peas (such as black-eyed peas), and lentils

Enriched and whole grain breads.

*Very high in cholesterol

**High in sodium

Read food labels for brand-specific information.

Thus, an iron supplement is recommended during pregnancy. Usually iron is prescribed for two reasons: it's almost impossible to meet the increased need for iron through diet alone, and many women enter pregnancy with borderline stores and may even be anemic. Sources of iron appear in Figure 5.1.

Folate. The need for folate increases 50% during pregnancy. It is needed to sustain the growth of new cells and the increase in blood volume during pregnancy. Folate is critical in the first four to six weeks of pregnancy (when most women don't even know they are pregnant) because the neural tube, the tissue in the embryo that develops into the brain and spinal cord, forms at this time. Without enough folate, birth defects of the brain and spinal cord, such as spina bifida, can occur. In spina bifida, parts of the spinal cord are not fused together properly, so gaps are present. Because of the importance of folate during pregnancy and the difficulty most women encounter trying to get adequate folate through diet, the Food and Drug Administration has required manufacturers of certain foods to fortify them with folate. Women eating folate-fortified foods should not assume that these foods will meet all their folate needs. They should still seek out folate-rich foods, such as leafy green vegetables (spinach, cabbage, romaine), oranges and orange juice, dry beans, peas, and lentils.

Calcium. Inadequate calcium intake by pregnant women can result in fetal bone development at the expense of the mother's bone health. A pregnant woman with inadequate calcium intake may actually lose calcium from her own bones to build the baby's bones. While the RDA for calcium does not change for pregnancy, maintaining adequate intake becomes particularly critical. Along with calcium, a pregnant woman needs adequate intakes of other nutrients that

Figure 5.2

DAILY FOOD GUIDE FOR PREGNANCY AND LACTATION

FOOD GROUP	SERVINGS	SERVING SIZE
Meat/meat alternate	6 during pregnancy to include	1 oz cooked lean meat, poultry, or fish
	1 serving legumes	1 egg
	6 during lactation	1 oz cheese
		1/4 cup cottage cheese
		1/2 cup dried beans or peas
		2 T peanut butter
Milk	3 during pregnancy	1 cup milk, yogurt, pudding, or custard
	4 during lactation	1-1 1/2 oz cheese
		1-1 1/2 cups cottage cheese
Vegetables	3+ during pregnancy and lactation	1/2 cup cooked or juice
		1 cup raw
Fruits	2+	Portion commonly served, such as a medium apple or banana
Grain	6+ during pregnancy and lactation	1 slice whole grain or enriched bread
		1 cup ready-to-eat cereal
		1/2 cup cooked cereal or pasta
		1/2 bagel or hamburger roll
		6 crackers
		1 small roll
		1/2 cup rice or grits
Fats and sweets*		Includes butter, margarine, salad dressings, mayonnaise, oils, candy, sugar, jams, jellies, syrups, soft drinks, and any other fats, or sweets

* In general, the amount of these foods to use depends on the number of calories you require. Get essential nutrients in the other food groups first before choosing foods from this group.

help build bones and teeth: vitamin D, phosphorous, and magnesium. Most women rely on milk and other dairy products to maintain calcium intake. A woman whose diet does not include these may be a candidate for calcium supplementation. Sources of calcium appear in Chapter 2.

Figure 5.2 provides a Daily Food Guide for pregnant and lactating women. The increased demand for some nutrients can be met through a balanced diet of fruits, vegetables, whole grains, lean meats, and low fat dairy products. A simple approach is to add one extra serving from each food group to account for added nutrient needs. The following tips can help in planning menus for pregnant women:

- Offer a varied and balanced selection of nutrient-dense foods. When there is such an increased need for so many nutrients, empty calories are rarely an acceptable choice.
- In addition to traditional meat entrees, provide some entrees based on legumes and/or grains and dairy products.
- Avoid frying foods and using rich sauces.
- Use low fat milk and milk products.
- Use assorted fruits and vegetables in all areas of the menu, including appetizers, salads, entrees, and desserts.
- Use iodized salt to provide adequate iodine.
- Offer some iron-rich foods such as meats, egg yolk, seafood, green leafy vegetables, legumes, dried fruits, and whole grain and enriched breads and cereals.
- Offer foods rich with fiber such as legumes, whole grains, fruits, and vegetables.
- Use folate-fortified breads and cereals.

Various medical experts, including the Surgeon General of the US, advise pregnant women to avoid alcohol during pregnancy. Alcohol can cause fetal alcohol syndrome, which exhibits itself as facial malformations and impaired development in children. Alcoholic beverages contain the following warning label:

> *Government Warning: According to the Surgeon General, women should not drink alcoholic beverages during pregnancy because of the risk of birth defects.*

Dieting, particularly low-carbohydrate dieting, is not appropriate during pregnancy and may result in deformities. It has not been shown that caffeine and sugar substitutes adversely affect the fetus, but it is recommended to use these substances in moderation. Furthermore, use of herbal supplements can be especially hazardous during this critical time, as some may interfere with hormonal balance or affect the developing fetus. A pregnant woman considering use of herbal supplements should first seek advice from a qualified health professional.

During pregnancy, several diet-related changes and complaints are common, as outlined below.

Nausea and vomiting. This condition, commonly referred to as "morning sickness" (it really occurs at any time of day), may be due to hormonal changes during pregnancy. It is generally mild and limited to the first 17 weeks of pregnancy. Dietary advice in the past has concentrated on frequent, small, carbohydrate-rich meals. For many women, this dietary advice doesn't work. Recent advice allows women to eat whatever food they think will stay down.

Taste changes and cravings. Pregnant women commonly report changes in taste and smell, which probably result from hormonal changes. Some women develop an enhanced taste for salty foods, or crave sweets and dairy products. Conversely, some pregnant women develop aversions (intense dislikes) to foods such as alcoholic beverages, caffeinated drinks, or meats. Cravings and aversions do not necessarily reflect actual physiological needs. Most likely, they simply reflect changes in sensitivity of taste and smell.

Constipation. Constipation is not uncommon, due in part to the gastrointestinal tract slowing down and relaxing. This can be counteracted with increased fiber (20-35 gm/day), adequate fluid, and regular exercise.

Heartburn. Heartburn is a common complaint because of the growing fetus crowding the stomach. Also, the muscle that controls the passage of food from the esophagus into the stomach relaxes, causing the acidic stomach contents to be regurgitated back into the esophagus. This is called heartburn, even though it has nothing to do with the heart. Possible solutions include eating small and frequent meals, eating slowly and in a relaxed atmosphere, avoiding caffeine, and not lying down after eating. Also, it might help pregnant women with heartburn to sleep with their heads elevated.

Lactation

Lactation, also called breastfeeding, provides a way for the mother's body to continue nourishing an infant after birth. Along with nutrients in optimal forms for use by the infant's body, human milk provides immune factors that help protect a baby from illness early in life. Breastfeeding supports healthy emotional and psychological development for an infant, too. For mothers who have just given birth, there are nutrition advantages to breastfeeding. First, making milk, a type of anabolism, requires extra energy. Along with sound dietary choices and exercise habits, this can help a mother gradually lose any excess weight. Second, shaping up is enhanced by the hormonal action of breastfeeding. As an infant feeds during early weeks after birth, the mother's body produces hormones that contract the uterus. Finally, breastfeeding delays the return of menstruation. In turn, this helps a mother recover her iron stores (ordinarily depleted through monthly blood loss).

Lactation substantially increases the mother's needs for many nutrients, such as protein, calcium, phosphorus, and magnesium, as these nutrients are secreted into the milk. Because a mother typically produces less milk during the second six months of an infant's life (about 20 ounces per day versus 25 ounces per day in earlier months), nutrition needs for that period may be somewhat lower. During lactation, mothers need 500 extra calories a day, and plenty of fluids. If the mother is not eating well, the quantity of milk may be adversely affected. Small amounts of caffeine are acceptable. Very little or no alcohol is advised.

NUTRITION AND FEEDING INFANTS

The nutrient needs of a newborn are very high due to a rate of growth that will never again be duplicated. Babies actually triple their weight by the end of the first year; weight doubles in just the first four months. For the first four to six months, the only food necessary is mother's milk or infant formula. Figure 5.3 provides feeding guidelines for this period. Breast milk is the food of choice for infants. Besides the benefits listed above, breast milk provides some protection from later development of food allergies, asthma, and possibly even cardiovascular disease. As compared with bottle-feeding, breastfeeding promotes better tooth and jaw alignment, too.

Infant formula is made to resemble breast milk (except formula has added vitamin D, and breast milk doesn't), and all formulas must meet nutrient standards set by the American Academy of Pediatrics. Formulas come in three different forms: ready-to-feed, liquid concentrate, and powdered. Infant feedings must be handled in a sanitary manner to prevent contamination and foodborne illness. If a baby is allergic to the protein in milk-based commercial formulas, there are other special formulas, such as soy-based formulas, that can be used. Supplemental fluoride drops are recommended for infants receiving breast milk or formulas prepared with non-fluoridated water. Fluoride is important to form healthy, strong teeth that are resistant to decay. Breast-fed babies also may need vitamin D supplementation, as breast milk is a poor source.

A baby is ready to eat semisolid foods such as hot cereal when he can sit up and open his mouth for them. This usually occurs between four and six months of age. Some other signs that the baby is ready to begin spoon-feeding are when the baby:

- has doubled his/her birth weight, or
- drinks more than a quart of formula per day, or
- often seems hungry.

Figure 5.3

FOOD GUIDE FOR INFANTS

AGE	FOOD	AMOUNT
0-4 months	Breast milk or formula*	21-29 oz formula, 5-8 feedings daily or 6-8 nursings
4-6 months	Breast milk or formula	27-39 oz formula, 4-6 feedings daily or 4-5 nursings
	Iron-fortified infant cereal (usually starts at 5 months)	Give 1 T with mother's milk/formula to start. Start with rice cereal. Give once to twice daily. Can work up to 1½ T twice daily.
	Strained vegetables and fruits (usually starts at 6 months; do vegetables first)	Give 1-2 tsp once to twice daily. First fruits can be be applesauce, pears, peaches, and bananas. First vegetables can be carrots, squash, and sweet potatoes. Slowly increase to 2 T twice daily.
	Fruit juice (vitamin C fortified, non-acid) (usually starts at 5 months)	Start with 2 oz watered-down juice, usually apple juice. Limit fruit juice to ½ cup daily.
6-9 months	Breast milk or formula	30-32 oz formula, 3-5 feedings daily or 3-5 nursings
	Iron-fortified infant cereal	3 T plus mother's milk/formula twice daily
	Strained fruits & vegetables	3 T twice daily
	Strained plain meats	1 to 2 T twice daily
	Crackers, plain toast	When baby has teeth, offer these foods or teething biscuit after other foods are eaten.
9-12 months	Breast milk or formula	24-32 oz formula, 3-4 times daily or 3-4 nursings
	Fruit juice (vitamin C fortified)	½ cup daily
	Iron-fortified infant cereal	3-4 T plus mother's milk/formula twice daily
	Vegetables, cut up	3-4 T twice daily
	Fruits, cut up	3-4 T twice daily
	Meats, cut up	2-3 T twice daily
	Egg yolk (usually at 10 months)	Mix with a little milk or add to cereal
	Egg white (usually at 12 months)	1 egg=1 serving of meat
	Bread and bread products	½ slice four times daily

*Physician may request iron-fortified formula by third or fourth month.

Avoid the following foods in the first year because of possible allergic reactions: chocolate, nuts, berries, tomatoes, shellfish.

Although some parents think feeding the baby solids will help the baby to sleep through the night, feeding a baby solid foods before she is ready can create problems, because the baby's digestive system is not ready for food. Feeding solids early also increases the risk of allergies and may encourage overfeeding. Although eating solid food is certainly simple for an adult, it involves a number of difficult steps for the baby. First the infant must have enough muscular control to close the mouth over a spoon, scrape the food from the spoon with the lips, and then move the food from the front to the back of the tongue. A child will gag when he can't swallow well enough to get the food from the back of the tongue into the pharynx. The food guide for infants in Figure 5.3 shows the order in which foods should be introduced. The first solid food is iron-fortified baby cereal mixed with breast milk or formula. Usually rice cereal is offered first because it is the grain least likely to cause an allergic reaction. Cereals should not be put in the infant's bottle. Once the baby is accustomed to various cereals, strained vegetables and fruits may be introduced. New foods should be added to the infant's diet one at a time (and in small quantities) so that if there is an allergic reaction, we will know which food caused it. Babies adjust differently to new tastes and new textures. If the baby does not like a certain food, offer it a week or two later. Always try new foods when the baby is hungry, such as at the beginning of the meal. While solid foods should not be introduced too early, it is important to introduce them when an infant is ready. A child who is not weaned appropriately may miss iron-rich foods in the diet and later develop iron-deficiency anemia.

Fruit juice that is fortified with vitamin C can be started about the fifth month. Although some babies get two or more bottles a day of apple juice (or other type of juice), it is a good idea to limit juice to one-half cup or four fluid ounces daily. Sometimes a baby who drinks too much juice starts drinking less mother's milk or formula. Another problem can occur when a baby goes to sleep with a bottle in her mouth. The natural sugars in the juice can cause devastating tooth decay, which is called *nursing bottle syndrome*. This can also result from sleeping with a bottle of formula in the mouth, as formula also contains carbohydrate, which favors tooth decay. By 10 months of age, an infant may be ready to begin drinking juice from a cup. Fruit-flavored beverages and soft drinks should not be given because the baby needs the vitamin C found in most juices. If during an illness such as vomiting and diarrhea, a physician recommends feeding the baby an electrolyte replacement beverage, the beverage is appropriate only during the illness. Once the illness is resolved, the extra nutrients in these products may make the baby sick.

Before a baby can move on to finger foods, he has to be able to eat lumpy foods, control the location of the food in his mouth, move his jaw up and down to mash it, and control swallowing. At seven to 10 months, a baby learns to grasp objects and can try picking up pieces of finger foods to transfer to the mouth. About this time infants can also start eating protein foods. Poultry and fish must be very tender, and meat will have to be chopped or cut very fine. Between 10 and 12 months of age, many infants are eating table foods with the family. At this time it is also appropriate to let a child start learning to drink from a cup. It takes time, but sooner or later the child will get the idea.

Several foods should be avoided during the first year. Honey may be contaminated with harmful bacteria, and may cause foodborne illness. Infants represent one of the groups that is most highly susceptible to foodborne illness, so this is not an advisable risk. Certain foods cause choking because they are just the right size to lodge in the throat and cause choking. Examples include nuts, raisins, hot dogs, popcorn, grapes, and chunks of apple. The American Academy of Pediatrics recommends no hot dogs, peanuts, or hard candy until age three. If hot dogs are offered later, they should be sliced like coins. Certain foods are apt to cause allergies: milk, eggs, wheat, nuts, chocolate, and shellfish. Whole milk may be offered after 12 months of age, but not earlier, according to the American Academy of Pediatrics.

NUTRITION FOR CHILDREN

Around the age of one year, the growth rate decreases significantly, and corresponding to this change, a child's appetite normally diminishes. At the beginning of childhood, the one-year-old learns to walk, jump, and run. Baby fat starts to disappear and muscles and bones undergo significant development. Until adolescence, growth will now come in spurts during which the child will grow and eat more. You can count on a yearly weight gain of four to six pounds and an increase in height of about three inches per year until age seven, and then just two inches until the adolescent growth spurt. Figures 5.4 and 5.5 show growth grids for boys and girls that compare the child's height and weight to national percentiles. These are commonly used by physicians as an indicator of the child's overall nutritional health, but are only reference points.

Between the ages of one and three, a child needs approximately 1,300 calories a day. Between ages four and six, needs jump to 1,800 calories and then to 2,000 calories for children between the ages of seven and 10. Growth, of course, increases the demand for all nutrients. Protein, calcium, phosphorus, magnesium, and zinc are of particular importance. Some of the nutrients taken in during childhood will actually be stored and used for the upcoming growth spurt. Foods containing few nutrients, such as cookies, should not be encouraged during childhood; they contribute to poor nutrition and possible obesity. Even though the first cow's milk for an infant (12+ mos.) should be whole milk, the USDA recommends gradually changing from whole milk to lower fat dairy products such as 2%, 1%, or fat free milk by age five.

After the first birthday, as a child's physical capabilities and desire for independence increase, he or she will become more capable of feeding himself. By 18 months, many children can successfully use a spoon without too much

Figure 5.4

GROWTH GRID FOR GIRLS

2 to 20 years: Girls
Stature-for-age and Weight-for-age percentiles

NAME _____

RECORD # _____

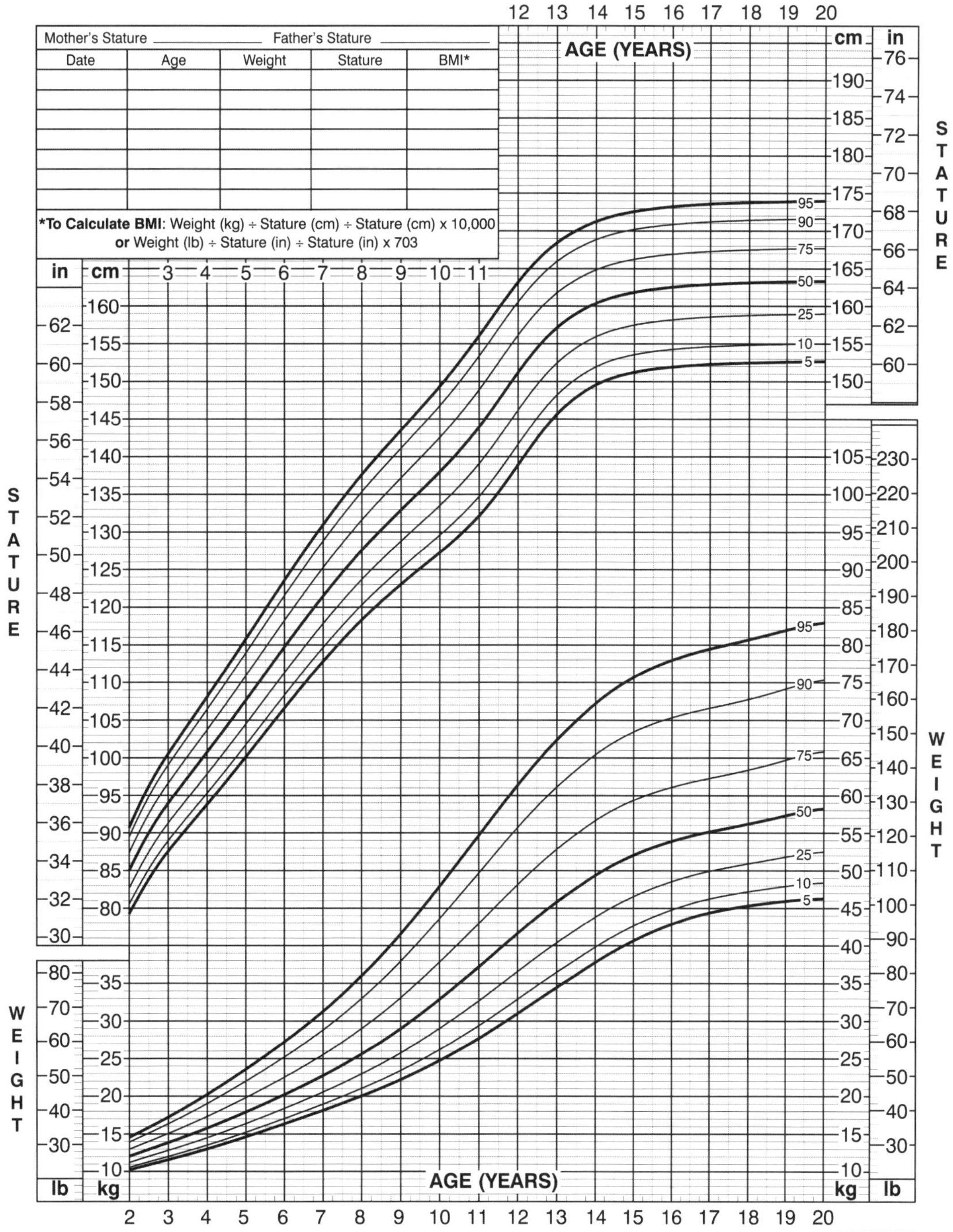

Mother's Stature _____ Father's Stature _____				
Date	Age	Weight	Stature	BMI*

***To Calculate BMI:** Weight (kg) ÷ Stature (cm) ÷ Stature (cm) x 10,000
or Weight (lb) ÷ Stature (in) ÷ Stature (in) x 703

AGE (YEARS)

12 13 14 15 16 17 18 19 20

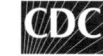

Published May 30, 2000 (modified 11/21/00).
SOURCE: Developed by the National Center for Health Statistics in collaboration with
the National Center for Chronic Disease Prevention and Health Promotion (2000).
http://www.cdc.gov/growthcharts

CDC
SAFER·HEALTHIER·PEOPLE™

Figure 5.5

GROWTH GRID FOR BOYS

2 to 20 years: Boys
Stature-for-age and Weight-for-age percentiles

NAME _____

RECORD # _____

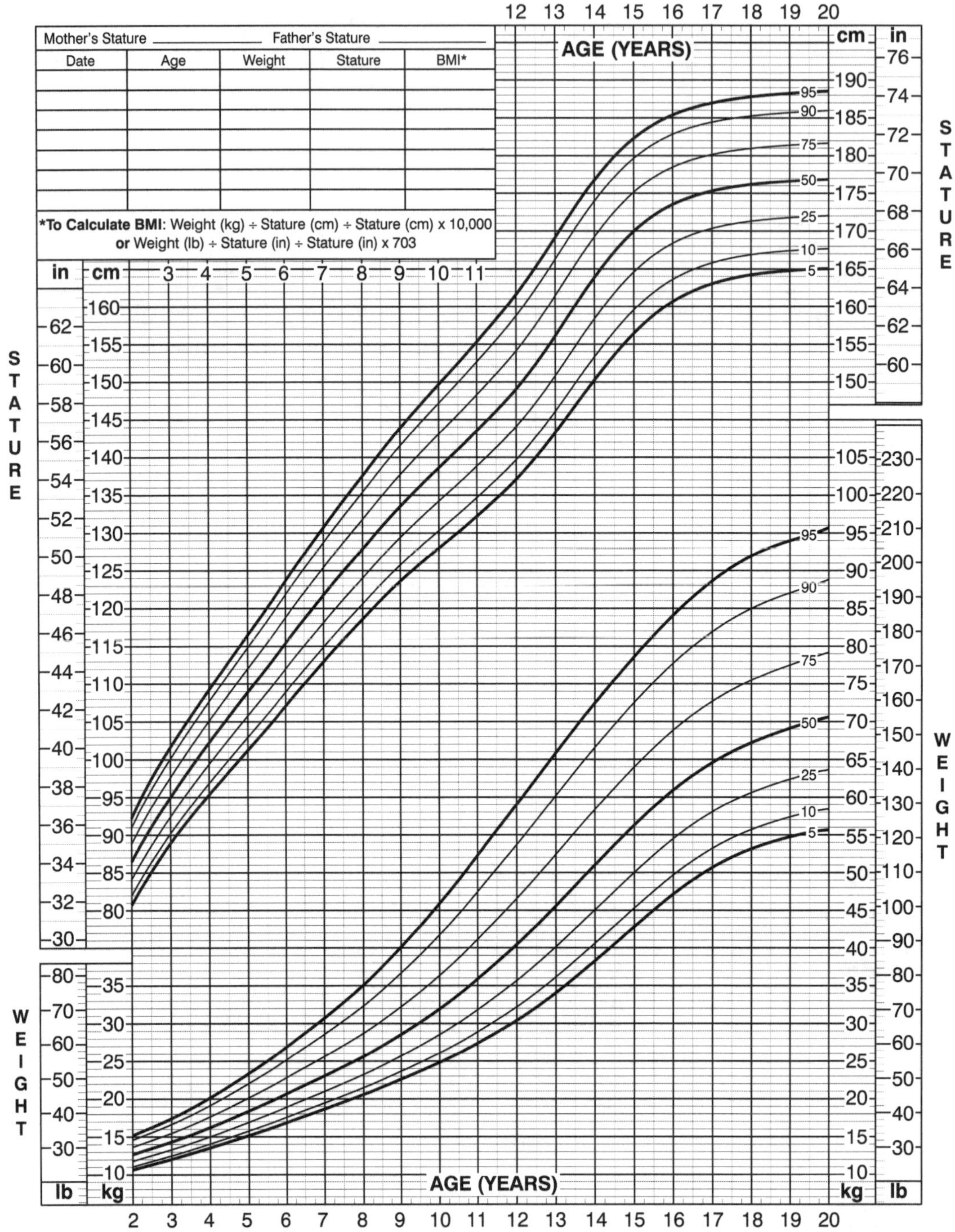

*To Calculate BMI: Weight (kg) ÷ Stature (cm) ÷ Stature (cm) x 10,000
or Weight (lb) ÷ Stature (in) ÷ Stature (in) x 703

Published May 30, 2000 (modified 11/21/00).
SOURCE: Developed by the National Center for Health Statistics in collaboration with
the National Center for Chronic Disease Prevention and Health Promotion (2000).
http://www.cdc.gov/growthcharts

CDC
SAFER · HEALTHIER · PEOPLE™

spilling. However, exploring food with fingers is an important part of a child's development, so plenty of finger food that a child can handle without utensils is appropriate. By 24 months, most of the child's teeth are in and most children can drink well from a cup.

Preschoolers exhibit some food-related behaviors that may alarm parents. For example, many toddlers go through food jags, when they want to eat just one food continually. Preschoolers also often pick at foods or refuse to eat vegetables or drink milk. Lack of variety and erratic appetites are typical of this age group. There are several things parents can do to deal with their preschoolers' food habits:

- Make mealtime relaxing. Don't nag, bribe, force, or cajole a child to eat.
- Offer food in child-friendly portions. For a preschooler, the USDA suggests a typical portion size is about ⅔ of the usual adult portion. An even smaller portion may encourage a child to try a new food.
- Let the child participate in food selection and preparation. Figure 5.6 lists ideas for involving children in meal preparation.
- Make sure the child has appropriately sized utensils and can reach the table comfortably.

A young child may not be ready to sit through an entire meal. Also, most children will eat when they're hungry and stop eating when they're full. Both preschoolers and school-age children learn about eating by watching others: their parents, their friends, and their teachers. During childhood, television viewing habits may be quite relevant to nutrition. Research demonstrates that children who watch a lot of television are more apt to be overweight. Research also confirms that many school-age children are significantly overweight and not physically fit. What can parents do to start their children on a nutritious eating path? Here is some advice for parents:

- Be a good role model by eating a well-balanced and varied diet.
- Have nutritious food choices readily available at home.
- Serve a regular, nutritious breakfast. Children need breakfast to be able to concentrate and perform well at school.
- As much as possible, maintain regular family meals. Family meals are an appropriate time to model healthy eating habits and try out new foods.
- Try to get children involved in planning meals, buying the food, and preparing food. This is a great way to teach them food and nutrition basics.
- Limit television watching and encourage physical activity instead.

Figure 5.6

IDEAS FOR INVOLVING CHILDREN IN MEAL PREPARATION

Children have to be shown and taught how to do these activities. Each child has his or her own pace for learning, so give it time and the skills will come.

2-year-olds:

- Wipe table tops
- Snap green beans
- Scrub vegetables
- Wash salad greens
- Tear lettuce or greens
- Play with utensils
- Break cauliflower
- Bring ingredients from one place to another

3-year-olds: Can do what 2-year-olds do, plus...

- Wrap potatoes in foil for baking
- Shake liquids in covered container
- Knead and shape yeast dough
- Spread soft spreads
- Pour liquids
- Place things in trash
- Mix ingredients

4-year-olds: Can do all that 2- and 3-year-olds do, plus...

- Peel oranges or hard cooked eggs
- Mash bananas using fork
- Move hands to form round shape
- Set table
- Cut parsley or green onions with dull scissors

5- to 6-year-olds: Can do all that 2-, 3-, and 4-year-olds do, plus...

- Measure ingredients
- Use an egg beater
- Cut with blunt knife

Source: USDA Tips for Using the Food Guide Pyramid for Young Children

Menu Planning for Preschoolers

There are several factors that make planning a menu for preschoolers challenging. A child's mouth is more sensitive to hot and cold than an adult's, so serve foods warm, not hot. Avoid strong-flavored and highly salted foods because children have more taste buds than adults, so these foods may taste too strong to them. Smooth textured foods such as pea soup or mashed potatoes should not have any lumps, because children often find this disturbing. Offer simply prepared foods and avoid mixed dishes if the child prefers separate foods on the plate. Additionally, try to make sure each meal includes:

- at least one soft or moist food that is easy to chew,
- at least one crisp or chewy food (important for developing chewing skills), and
- at least one colorful food, such as carrot sticks.

Vegetables are more likely to be accepted if served raw and cut up as a finger food. If serving celery, however, be sure to take off the strings. When serving cooked vegetables, it is better to serve them undercooked. For children who won't eat vegetables, you can also hide vegetables in tomato sauce on spaghetti, on pizza, and in chili. Soups and casseroles are great places to add vegetables.

Most preschoolers love carbohydrate-rich foods, including cereals, breads, and crackers, as they are easy to hold and chew. Use them often as snack foods. Cut fruit and vegetables also make good snacks. Also let the preschooler spread peanut butter on crackers or use a spoon to eat yogurt. Snacks are important to preschoolers because they need to eat more often than adults to get the nutrients they need.

Before the age of four, at which time the skills to cut up food start to develop, serve foods in bite-size pieces that are either eaten as finger foods or with a spoon or fork. For example, cut meat into strips or use ground meat, cut fruit into wedges or slices, cut sandwiches into quarters, and serve pieces of raw vegetables instead of a mixed salad. Other good finger foods include cheese cut into sticks, wedges of hard-boiled eggs, dry ready-to-eat cereal, fish sticks, arrowroot biscuits, and graham crackers.

Menu Planning for School-Age Children

Among elementary school-age children, a few more nutritional considerations apply. Energy needs vary, depending on a child's age, size, activity, and pattern of growth. In general, though, it's important to understand that the entire growth process involves building new tissue at a rapid rate. This places many key nutrients in high demand, including protein, calcium, and iron. As a child grows, total protein requirements grow, too. The need for calcium remains stable at 800 mg per day from one year of age until 11 years of age, when it increases again. Consuming an adequate amount of calcium is very important at this time (and beyond), as it is essential for healthy bone growth. Adequate calcium in early years may also prevent osteoporosis in later years. Milk and milk products are an important source of calcium. Iron needs range from roughly 8 to 10 mg per day. According to current research, iron may be critical for brain development and functioning, as well as for red blood cell formation. Slight iron deficiency, before it reaches a stage that would be diagnosed as iron-deficiency anemia, may reduce attention span and intellectual performance. It may even have long-term effects on intellectual development.

Many school-age children eat most of their food from home, so if a wide variety of well-liked nutritious foods is available, it is more likely that the child will have a balanced and adequate diet. Good snack choices are important for school-age children, as they do not always have the desire or the time to sit down and eat. Snacks can include fresh fruits and vegetables, juices, breads, unsweetened cereals, popcorn, tortillas, muffins, milk, yogurt, cheese, pudding, custard, sliced meats and poultry, eggs, or peanut butter.

Another concern in childhood years is the prevalent concern of hyperactivity, or attention deficit disorder (ADD). This is characterized by difficulty in paying attention and a certain amount of impulsive behavior. The condition is poorly understood, and both parents and educators find cause for concern when a child is diagnosed with ADD. While pharmaceutical treatments are common, so is the belief that ADD is a nutritional disorder—and that the "right" diet can cure it. Dietary approaches include avoiding sugar and avoiding food colorings. Unfortunately, there is no dietary quick-fix for ADD, and research has not confirmed the value of any dietary treatments for this condition.

NUTRITION FOR ADOLESCENTS

The beginning of adolescence is marked by a growth spurt that results in physically mature adults. Most girls are in this rapid growth spurt by age 11. For boys, this spurt starts later, usually between 12 and 13 years of age. The growth spurt ends at about age 15 for girls and age 19 for boys. Both boys and girls get taller and heavier. Boys put on twice as much muscle as girls, while girls deposit more fat. During the adolescent growth spurt, approximately 20% of adult height and 50% of ideal body weight are gained.

Whereas parents are the main providers of food for young children, adolescents make many of their own food decisions. Of course, it helps to have healthy foods available to them to eat at home. Eating patterns of adolescents are influenced by peers, lifestyles, body image, popular media, and food preferences. Meal skipping (usually breakfast and/or lunch) and snacking are common. Although snack foods can be nutritious and make a contribution to the overall diet, popular teen snack foods may gravitate towards the top of the Food Pyramid, including choices such as chips, cookies, candies, soft drinks, and ice cream. Eating disorders often start during adolescence. *Anorexia nervosa*, self-induced starvation and highly distorted body image, is particularly common among adolescent girls. Another disorder called *bulimia* involves binge eating and forced vomiting. Both are unhealthy approaches to controlling weight and require intensive, long-term treatment.

During the adolescent growth spurt, the nutrient requirements of a young person are higher than before. The need for calcium and iron increases at age 11. More calcium is needed for growing bones and more iron is needed for the increased blood volume and muscle in both sexes. Once menstruation begins, girls also experience a higher need for iron to replace lost blood.

Adolescents need four glasses of milk (or equivalent) daily and lots of high-iron foods such as meats, egg yolk, seafood, green leafy vegetables, legumes, dried fruits, whole grain and enriched breads and cereals. Teenagers often drink empty-calorie beverages, such as soft drinks, instead of more nutritious choices such as milk or juice. Nutrients that may be lacking in an adolescent's diet include calcium, iron, vitamin A, vitamin C, and sometimes even calories and protein. Adolescent girls are at higher risk for nutritional deficiencies than boys because girls must get in more nutrients in fewer calories than boys.

In planning menus for adolescents, it's a good idea to include nutritious snack choices that are portable and can be eaten on-the-run, such as fresh fruit, individually packaged cereals, muffins, bagels, yogurt, popcorn, juices, fig bars, or oatmeal raisin cookies. Emphasize quick and nutritious breakfasts such as whole grain pancakes or waffles with fruit, juices, whole grain toast or muffins with low fat cheese, cereal topped with fresh fruits, or bagels with peanut butter. To provide protein and iron, offer lean beef, poultry, and fish. For calcium and more protein, offer low fat milk and milk products. For teenagers who are watching their weight, appropriate low-calorie options may include sugar-free beverages, diet dressings, and baked or grilled foods (rather than fried). Fresh fruits are an excellent alternative to fatty desserts. It's also a good idea to emphasize complex carbohydrates, such as assorted breads, rolls, cereals, potatoes, vegetables, pasta, rice, and legumes. Use whole grain breads and bread products as much as possible for added vitamins, minerals, and fiber. Offer good sources of vitamin A and vitamin C, such as yellow vegetables, citrus fruits, tomatoes, and leafy greens. Besides being important nutrients, these vitamins are classified as *leader nutrients*. This means where they appear, most likely other essential nutrients appear as well.

NATIONAL SCHOOL LUNCH PROGRAM

Legislation that established the National School Lunch Program was signed by President Harry Truman in 1946. Through its **National School Lunch Program**, the USDA supports nutritious, low-cost or free breakfasts and lunches to more than 25 million children each school day. School districts and independent schools that choose to take part in the lunch program receive cash subsidies and donated commodities from the USDA for each meal they serve. In return, they must serve lunches that meet Federal requirements, and they must offer free or reduced price lunches to eligible children. School food authorities can also be reimbursed for snacks served to children through age 18 in afterschool educational or enrichment programs.

School lunches must meet the applicable recommendations of the Dietary Guidelines for Americans, with no more than 30% of calories from fat, and less than 10% from saturated fat. Regulations also establish a standard for school lunches to provide one-third of the RDAs for protein, Vitamin A, Vitamin C, iron, calcium, and calories. School lunches must meet federal nutrition requirements, but decisions about what specific foods to serve and how they are prepared are up to school foodservice administrators.

The requirements originally set for school lunches stipulated that lunches must provide two ounces of meat or alternate, two or more servings of fruit and/or vegetables, one serving of bread or alternate, and eight ounces of milk. Newer requirements allow schools to move away from this food-based system to a nutrient-analysis system. Nutrient Standard Menu Planning (NSMP), or NuMenus, is one of the options available to schools to meet the Dietary Guidelines. According to the USDA, "NSMP/NuMenus requires that school meals meet a specific nutrient standard, one-third of the RDA for lunch and

Figure 5.7

WHY CHILDREN ARE "FLUNKING" HEALTHY EATING

▶ Only 2% meet all the recommendations of the Food Guide Pyramid; 16% do not meet any

▶ Less than 15% of school children eat the recommended servings of fruit

▶ Less than 20% eat the recommended servings of vegetables

▶ About 25% eat the recommended servings of grains

▶ Only 30% consume the recommended milk group servings

▶ Only 19% of girls ages 9 to 19 meet the recommended intakes for calcium

▶ Only 16% of school children meet the guidelines for saturated fat

Source: USDA. Helping Students Learn to Eat Healthy

Figure 5.8

SUPPORTING SOUND NUTRITION IN SCHOOLS

The USDA suggests that support for sound nutrition through school programs must occur at all levels—federal, state, and local. On a local level, the USDA suggests the following:

▶ Involve students and parents in developing food and nutrition policy

▶ Teach healthy eating skills in the classroom and dining areas

▶ Serve meals that meet USDA nutrition standards in the school dining areas

▶ If a la carte foods are offered, be sure they contribute to healthy eating patterns

▶ If vending machines, snack bars, and school stores are available, be sure they contain healthy snacks

▶ Schedule meals when children are hungry — not at 10 a.m. or 2 p.m.

▶ Allow adequate time for children to enjoy their meals with friends

▶ Provide sufficient serving areas to reduce the time students must wait to receive a meal

▶ Provide adequate dining space and pleasant ambiance

▶ Teach by example — adults and peers are role models

▶ Eliminate use of food as a reward

▶ Ensure financial decisions do not undermine nutrition goals

Source: USDA. Helping Students Learn to Eat Healthy

one-fourth of the RDA for breakfast, and comply with the Dietary Guidelines recommendations for levels of fat and saturated fats in meals. Under NSMP/NuMenus, the menu is evaluated through the nutrient analysis of all foods offered over a school week to ensure that meals meet specific standards for key nutrients and recommended levels of fat and saturated fat." The USDA encourages use of software for compliance with the NuMenu system, and maintains a list of software packages that support this menu planning standard. An up-to-date list is available on the USDA Healthy School Meals Resource System website, listed in Appendix A.

In 1966 the USDA established the School Breakfast Program. About 60% of schools that offer the school lunch program also offer the school breakfast program. School breakfasts must provide one-fourth of the RDAs for the same nutrients examined for lunch. Figure 5.7 lists concerns about nutrition for children and adolescents, and Figure 5.8 lists ideas for supporting sound nutrition through school decision-making.

NUTRITION FOR THE ELDERLY

Among the US population, numbers of older Americans are growing most quickly. The older population will burgeon between the years 2010 and 2030, when the baby boom generation reaches age 65. With advances in medicine, average lifespans are increasing. Population information suggests that within the next few decades, the proportion of our population over 85 will quadruple. By 2030, there will be about 70 million older persons, more than twice their number in 1998. What does all this mean for a dietary manager? Among other things, it means that a typical foodservice operation is likely to be serving more and more clients of advancing age. Numbers of elderly individuals in nursing homes are expected to triple within the next few decades. Correspondingly, the eldercare foodservice industry, which provides nutrition to older Americans through a variety of models (not just nursing homes), is growing quickly. To serve this client group well, it's essential to understand a number of changes that occur during the aging process—and the impact they have on nutrition.

Elderly is a loose term, and there is no defined age at which the body undergoes dramatic aging-related changes. What happens when we age? Metabolism changes, and body systems and organs lose their peak efficiency. The rate of decline is typically very gradual, and shows great individual variation. Both genetic and environmental factors (such as nutrition) affect the rate of aging. Conversely, changes brought about by the aging process affect nutrition status. Of particular importance are those changes that affect digestion, absorption, and metabolism of nutrients.

The basal metabolic rate (baseline energy requirement) declines between eight and 12% from age 30 to 70 and is accompanied by a 25 to 30% loss in muscle mass. Combined with a general decrease in activity level, these factors clearly indicate a need for decreased calorie intake, which generally does take place during aging. But the elderly don't have to lose all that muscle mass. Studies have shown that when the elderly do regular weight training exercises, they increase their muscular strength and basal metabolism, and improve appetite and blood flow to the brain. For more information about these benefits, see *Nutrition in the News* (A Fountain of Youth) at the end of this chapter. Overall, the functioning of the cardiovascular system declines with age. The workload of the heart increases due to atherosclerotic deposits and less elasticity in the arteries. The heart does not pump as hard as before, and cardiac output is reduced in elderly people who do not remain physically active. Blood pressure increases normally with age. Lung capacity decreases by about 40% throughout life. This decrease does not restrict the normal activity of healthy, older persons but may limit vigorous exercise. Kidney function deteriorates over time, and the aging kidney is less able to excrete waste. Adequate fluid intake is very important, as is avoiding megadoses of water-soluble vitamins because they put a strain on the kidneys to excrete them. Lastly, loss of bone occurs normally during aging, and osteoporosis is common.

Factors Affecting Nutrition Status

The nutrition status of an elderly person is greatly influenced by many variables, such as physiological factors, psychosocial factors, and socioeconomic factors, as outlined below.

Physiological Factors:

Disease. The presence of diseases, both acute and chronic, and use of modified diets can affect nutrition status. The most prevalent nutrition-related problems of the elderly are chronic conditions that require therapeutic diets. Certain chronic diseases are associated with **anorexia** or loss of appetite. Examples include gastrointestinal disease, congestive heart failure, renal disease, and cancer. Other diseases, such as stroke, are not associated with anorexia but can affect ability to eat.

Caloric intake. An individual who adjusts caloric intake downwards to accompany decline in basal energy expenditure and muscle mass faces a new challenge: that of nutrient density. With even fewer calories, nutrient-dense food choices become increasingly crucial.

Dentition. Approximately 50% of Americans have lost their teeth by age 65. Despite widespread use of dentures, chewing still presents problems for many elderly people.

Functional disabilities. Functional disabilities interfere with the ability of the elderly to perform daily tasks, such as the purchasing and preparation of food, and eating. These disabilities may be due to arthritis/rheumatism, stroke, visual impairment, heart trouble, or dementia (deterioration in mental functioning such as thinking and memory). One study reports that 39% of the elderly subjects need help food shopping and 26% need help making meals.

Taste and smell. Around age 60, there is a decline in the ability to taste and smell. The tongue's taste buds are less sensitive, and the nerves in the nose that detect aromas need extra stimulation to detect smells. That's why seniors may find ordinarily seasoned foods too bland.

Changes in the gastrointestinal tract. The movement of food through the gastrointestinal tract slows down over the years, causing problems such as constipation, a frequent complaint of older people. Constipation may also be related to low fiber and fluid intake, medications, or lack of exercise. Other frequent complaints include nausea, indigestion, and heartburn. Intestinal changes typical of aging also reduce absorption of the vitamin B12 produced in the body.

Medications. More than half of seniors take at least one medication daily and many take six or more a day. Medications often alter appetite or the digestion, absorption, or metabolism of nutrients. More information about the effects of medications appears in Chapter 8.

Thirst. Many elderly people have a diminished perception of thirst that can cause problems, especially when they are not feeling well. Because the aging kidney is less able to concentrate the urine, more fluid is lost, setting the stage for dehydration.

Psychosocial Factors:
Ability to think. Poor thinking may affect nutrition—or perhaps poor nutritional status is contributing to poor thinking. If an elderly person is confused part of the time, this can affect meal patterns.

Social support. An individual's nutritional health results in part from a series of social acts. The purchasing, preparation, and eating of foods are social events for most people. For example, elderly people may rely upon each other for a ride to the supermarket, cooking, or sharing meals. The benefits of social networks or support are largely due to the companionship and emotional support they provide. This support can have a positive effect on appetite and dietary intake.

Socioeconomic Factors:
Education. Higher levels of education are positively associated with increased nutrient intakes.

Income. Money spent on food is a significant predictor of dietary quality.

Living arrangements. The elderly, particularly women, are more likely to be widowed. The trend has been for widows and widowers in the US to live alone after the spouse dies. Research indicates that living alone is a risk factor for dietary inadequacy for older men, especially those over 75 years of age, and for women only in the youngest age group (55 to 64 years old).

Availability of federally funded meals. The availability of nutritious meals through federal programs such as Meals-on-Wheels, in which meals are delivered to the home, is crucial to the nutritional health of many elderly people. Many communities also have Senior Centers that provide meals, and educational and social programs.

NUTRITION FOR THE LATER YEARS

A survey completed for the new Nutrition Screening Initiative—targeted at improving the nutritional health status of the aging—shows that while 85% of seniors believe nutrition is important for their health and well-being, few act on their beliefs. Further, 30% admit they skip at least one meal a day. These numbers may well soar as America continues to age at an increasing rate. Studies of the elderly have shown that maintaining adequate calorie intake is vital to good nutrition. An elderly person must fit more nutrients into fewer calories. Tufts University offers a modified Food Pyramid for Older Adults, shown in Figure 5.9. The base of the pyramid suggests drinking eight 8-oz cups of water or other liquid each day to avoid dehydration. It also emphasizes consuming foods high in antioxidant vitamins to prevent free radical damage that can advance the aging process. It emphasizes vitamin D and calcium to keep bones strong, and folic acid to maintain optimal brain functioning. Also, high-fiber foods receive special attention because they can help regulate bowel functioning.

At a time when good nutrition is so important to good health, there are many obstacles to eating well, including a basic lack of nutrition knowledge. Good nutritional status helps prevent many illnesses and improve outcomes for individuals who become ill or undergo surgery. But in addition, good nutritional status can optimize body functioning and enhance quality of life. RDAs now include a category for older adults, and this has become a point of ongoing nutrition research and guidance. So far, RDAs for most nutrients are set the same as for younger adults. However, the RDA for vitamin D has been raised in an effort to prevent bone disease. What can older Americans do to eat nutritiously? Here are some ideas:

- Try to eat with other people. This usually makes mealtime more enjoyable and stimulates appetite.
- Prepare larger amounts of food and freeze some for a later time.
- If big meals are too much, eat small amounts more frequently during the day.
- If getting to the supermarket is a bother, go at a time when it is not busy or check on a delivery service.
- Use the "unit price" (price per ounce, pound, or pint) to compare the cost of different brands and package sizes. Many stores show the unit price on the shelf. Buy items on sale to cut back on cost.
- Take advantage of community meal programs for the elderly such as Meals-on-Wheels and Senior Centers.

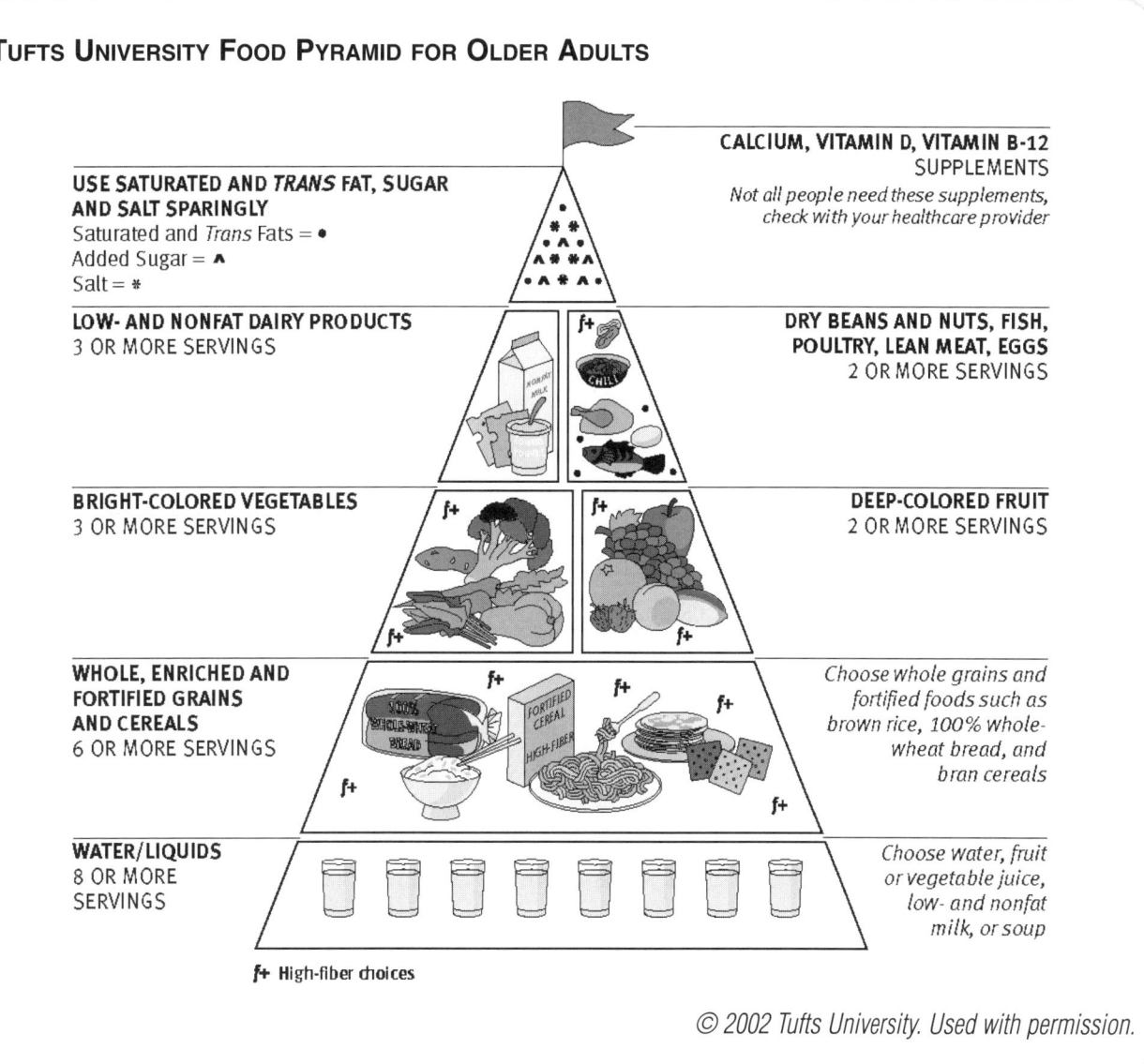

TUFTS UNIVERSITY FOOD PYRAMID FOR OLDER ADULTS

CALCIUM, VITAMIN D, VITAMIN B-12
SUPPLEMENTS
*Not all people need these supplements,
check with your healthcare provider*

USE SATURATED AND *TRANS* FAT, SUGAR
AND SALT SPARINGLY
Saturated and *Trans* Fats = •
Added Sugar = ▲
Salt = ✳

LOW- AND NONFAT DAIRY PRODUCTS
3 OR MORE SERVINGS

DRY BEANS AND NUTS, FISH,
POULTRY, LEAN MEAT, EGGS
2 OR MORE SERVINGS

BRIGHT-COLORED VEGETABLES
3 OR MORE SERVINGS

DEEP-COLORED FRUIT
2 OR MORE SERVINGS

WHOLE, ENRICHED AND
FORTIFIED GRAINS
AND CEREALS
6 OR MORE SERVINGS

*Choose whole grains and
fortified foods such as
brown rice, 100% whole-
wheat bread, and
bran cereals*

WATER/LIQUIDS
8 OR MORE
SERVINGS

*Choose water, fruit
or vegetable juice,
low- and nonfat
milk, or soup*

f+ High-fiber choices

© 2002 Tufts University. Used with permission.

MENU PLANNING FOR THE ELDERLY

Basic guidelines for menu planning for older adults need to address a range of factors, as outlined above. They need to stimulate eating through aroma, taste, and visual appeal. They need to provide nutrient-dense choices, and adapt comfortably to any physical limitations. If chewing is a problem, menus must offer softer foods. Chapter 6 presents guidelines for offering a mechanical soft diet, which may be helpful. Following are some other useful techniques and ideas for meal planning:

Meals need to be moderate in size. Older adults frequently complain when given too much food because they hate to see waste, so offering moderate portions is desirable.

Emphasize complex carbohydrate and high-fiber foods. Fruits, vegetables, whole grains, and beans are good choices. Older people requiring softer diets may have problems chewing some high-fiber foods. High-fiber foods that are soft in texture include cooked beans and peas, bran cereals soaked in milk, oatmeal, canned fruit, and cooked vegetables.

Moderate the use of fat. Use lean meats, poultry, or fish and sauces prepared with vegetable or fruit purees. Have low fat dairy products available, such as skim milk.

Offer adequate protein. Use a variety of both animal and vegetable sources. Providing protein on a budget need not be a problem. Lower-cost protein sources include dried beans and peas, cottage cheese, macaroni and cheese, eggs, liver, yogurt, nonfat dry milk, chicken, and ground beef.

Use herbs and spices to make foods flavorful. Seniors are looking for tasty foods just like anyone else, and they may need them more than ever. For more information, see *Nutrition in the News* (The Graying of the American Taste Bud) at the end of this chapter.

Variety. Offer a variety of foods, including traditional menu items, as well as ethnic and regional cuisine.

Encourage fluid intake. Fluid intake is critical, so offer a variety of beverages. Provide user-friendly service ware and personal assistance to those who need it. Beverages such as water, milk, juice, coffee, or tea, and foods such as soup, ices, and gelatin desserts contribute to fluid intake.

Vitamins and minerals. Intake of vitamin D, calcium, and zinc may be inadequate in older adults should be considered in menu planning. Meat, dairy products, and fortified cereals can provide these nutrients.

AT RISK POPULATIONS

Throughout the life cycle, you can see that people experience fluctuations in nutritional needs and priorities. Sometimes, health experts describe a group as being **at risk** for certain nutritional problems. For example, females from adolescence until menopause are at risk for iron-deficiency anemia. Body needs are high, and meeting iron needs requires careful attention to food choices. After menopause, women are particularly vulnerable to osteoporosis, as are elderly people in general. *Osteoporosis* describes a gradual loss of minerals from bones, which causes loss of height and frequent fractures. For more information about bone loss, see *Nutrition in the News* (A Fountain of Youth) at the end of this chapter. Additionally, elderly individuals are at risk for dehydration due to an imperfect thirst mechanism and the reduced efficiency of body systems.

Individuals in various states of illness are also at risk for developing nutritional problems. For example, a patient who has cancer may suffer loss of appetite, along with high nutrient needs due to the demands of a growing tumor. With various treatments, eating adequately may be difficult. Thus, a cancer patient may be at risk for developing protein calorie malnutrition. A resident of a nursing home who is unable to move about may be at risk for developing pressure ulcers (discussed in Chapter 6). Sound nutrition is crucial for protecting against this common problem. An individual who has difficulty swallowing, or one who is afflicted by Alzheimer's disease, may not be able to consume adequate amounts of food. These are two more populations at risk for developing malnutrition. When working with any population group, a dietary manager needs to consider nutritional needs and risks, and plan meals accordingly.

Interestingly, two extremes in age also present another type of food-related risk—that of foodborne illness. As you may already have learned in a food safety and sanitation course, the FDA identifies certain populations as being more susceptible to contracting foodborne illness. These include very young children and older adults. Within these groups, immune response may not be as strong as it is during other phases of the life cycle. Not only may an individual in these groups be more likely to become ill when exposed to foodborne pathogens; the individual may suffer more serious consequences as well. Pregnant women also represent a high-risk group because of the susceptibility of the fetus to insult and injury. For example, Listeria-related foodborne illness causes stillbirth. For these reasons, sound food sanitation becomes even more crucial in serving these populations.

A FOUNTAIN OF YOUTH ● FOOD INSIGHT, JANUARY/FEBRUARY 1998

It was not as simple as taking a sip from the proverbial fountain of youth, but the results were as dramatic and satisfying. And they were real.

At Tufts University, 40 women participated in research looking at the effects of strength conditioning on bone density. The results literally "turned back the clock" with regard to their bone health. And, that was not the only benefit—the women also reported increased energy, confidence and improved body composition.

Many people have a fear of growing old, and we are reminded of that fear when we look at older relatives who struggle to lift themselves out of a chair or have difficulties with stairs. No one wants to lose the physical capacity to do everyday activities with the same ease and frequency as were once enjoyed.

As recently as the early 1980s, it was a commonly held belief in the scientific community that as a person aged, the loss of muscle, bone and strength was inevitable and irreversible. This aging myth began to dispel in 1990 when research was published in The Journal of the American Medical Association (JAMA) detailing the results of high-intensity strength workouts for older individuals. The eight men and women in the study were between the ages of 86-96, and all had at least two chronic diseases. The program was based on rehabilitation medicine—"start at a safe level and gradually progress as strength increases." After eight weeks of three sessions per week, these frail nursing home residents increased their strength by an average of 175 percent and increased their walking speed and balance.

These compelling results, along with other studies that suggested strength training may increase bone density, encouraged Miriam Nelson, Ph.D., Associate Chief of the Human Physiology Laboratory at the Jean Mayer USDA Human Nutrition Research center on Aging at Tufts University, to do her own study. Her research investigated the effects of weight training on bone mass in women. Forty healthy, but sedentary, post-menopausal women (who were not taking hormones) were recruited to participate. Those in the control group were instructed to continue with their usual lifestyle, while the others traveled to Tufts for twice a week 40-minute weight lifting sessions. The results, published in JAMA in 1994, were remarkable. "After one year, the women's bodies were 15 to 20 years more youthful. They actually gained bone at an age when women typically lose bone," remarked Dr. Nelson.

Around age 40, most women start to lose approximately one-half pound of muscle a year and replace it with fat. Similar to what happened when the first astronauts floated weightlessly in space, when muscles are not used, they lose significant strength. This is called sarcopenia—from the Greek "sarco" for muscle and "penia" for loss. Sarcopenia does not kill like heart disease, nor does it come about quickly, but it can affect quality of life. However, it can be prevented through healthful eating and physical activity that includes strength conditioning. Robert Butler, M.D., director, International Longevity Center, Mount Sinai Medical Center, remarked, "Finally, a science-based program to help women of all ages live strong and vital lives."

BETTER EATING FOR BETTER AGING ● November 1999

Good nutritional habits never get old. It is important to continue eating a variety of foods to get necessary nutrients throughout the golden years. Eating well helps keep you strong and enables your body to fight diseases better.

Persons aged 65 or older are the fastest growing segment of the U.S. population. By the year 2030, the 65 and older set will number one in five. With the increasing median age of the population, a heightened awareness of the needs of this group is important.

Unfortunately, some older Americans are not getting enough nutrients to stay healthy, and may suffer from malnutrition. Malnutrition in older people is a complex condition caused by a combination of factors in their lives. This is a serious health problem for the nation's older adults. Nutrition screening programs in a wide variety of institutional and community settings have reported elder malnutrition risk rates ranging from 25% to 85%.

WHAT CAUSES POOR NUTRITION IN OLDER AMERICANS?

Older Americans may not get proper nutrients because of a variety of conditions. This can happen for many reasons.

Many older people live alone and are unable to get around as easily as they used to. One in five elders have trouble walking, grocery shopping, and preparing food as they age. This can restrict access to adequate amounts and variety of food.

Also, depression sometimes affects older adults and can impact nutritional status by contributing to a lack of desire to eat or prepare food. Declining oral health, lack of teeth or poor-fitting dentures can also affect food intake. A healthy mouth, teeth

and gums are needed to eat and poor- fitting denture s can interfere with eating. In addition, some medications and medical procedures and treatments may cause loss of appetite.

Another reason many older Americans may not get proper nutrition is because of a loss or decline in the senses of taste and smell. A large proportion of the population older than 65 years has age-related sensory losses that impair overall health, self-sufficiency, and quality of life.

All of these factors-physical, mental, economic and social factors-can interfere with eating, causing weight loss, poor nutritional status and decreased immunity to fight diseases. Understanding and addressing these problems can help improve overall health and quality of life. Given the importance of taste to health, improving the flavors of foods can lead to better nutritional status.

HOW DO WE TASTE?

The sense of taste has many components. We taste food when chemicals in foods and beverages come in contact with taste buds. Taste buds are scattered on the surface of the tongue, cheek, soft palate, the first part of the esophagus and other parts of the mouth and throat. The components in food stimulate taste buds during chewing and swallowing, and tongue movements enhance flavor sensations. Complex interactions take place within and among the taste buds-which are filled with nerves-to evaluate the major flavors, or tastes.

There are four most common tastes that we usually think of-sweet, sour, salty and bitter. But, studies show that there is much more to taste than these four components. Other taste qualities may include metallic (from iron components in

BETTER EATING FOR BETTER AGING, *CONTINUED*

medicines) and chalky (from calcium salts). There is also a taste called umami or savory that is used to describe the taste and mouth-feel of glutamate, an amino acid found in protein foods and the flavor enhancer, MSG. In addition to adding flavor to foods, we also get taste sensations, such as richness and mouth-feel, from fat.

Another player in the sense of taste is the trigeminal system, or 'free nerve endings' in the mouth and nose that connect with the brain. These nerves detect irritants such as hot chilies and black pepper; cool sensations such as mint; and carbonation.

HOW DO WE SMELL?

Smell occurs when nerve receptors in your nose send messages to your brain. The sense of smell plays an important role in perception of foods. The interaction of the oral and nasal senses blend together to give us the impression of a certain food, or increase the sensory perceptions we receive. Smells can also create emotional responses to food. This is because emotions and smell sensations overlap in your brain. Smells can create both positive and negative emotional responses to food. A positive response can improve the desire to eat, while a negative response may decrease the desire to eat.

WHAT CAUSES CHANGES IN TASTE AND SMELL?

Declining taste and smell is a normal part of the aging process for many people. Age-related impairment of the senses can be caused by many factors including environmental pollutants. As a result, taste buds and smell receptors do not function as well as in earlier years, causing a decline in the senses of taste and smell. These changes can decrease the desire for food.

In addition to normal aging processes, chronic diseases and conditions can affect the senses of taste and smell, including Parkinson's disease, diabetes mellitis, Alzheimers disease and others. Some of the medications people take can also interfere with these senses and decrease appetite as well.

CAN ANYTHING HELP TO IMPROVE THE EATING HABITS FOR OLDER AMERICANS WITH IMPAIRED TASTE AND SMELL?

Yes. Enhancing the flavors of foods can help improve eating and, subsequently, health for older Americans. Adding table salt or flavor enhancers such as monosodium glutamate (MSG); spices and herbs; or other concentrated essences and extracts to food can improve the taste and aroma of foods. These enhancements can improve food enjoyment and increase food intake, which is important for maintaining a healthy weight, a strong immune system and overall health.

It is important to remember other dietary concerns, such as hypertension (high blood pressure) when enhancing food flavors. Adding table salt may not be the best choice to enhance flavors if a low-salt (or low-sodium) diet is recommended because of high blood prressure. MSG may be a better option because it contains only one third the sodium of table salt. When small quantities of MSG are used in combination with a reduced amount of table salt during food preparation, the flavor enhancing properties of MSG allow for far less salt to be used during and after cooking. MSG brings out the best natural flavors in food and can reduce total sodium by 30-40 percent without reducing palatability.

When considering flavor enhancement for older adults, keep individual food preferences, allergies or sensitivities in mind. With an abundance of alternative combinations of spices, herbs and food ingredients, it is possible to enhance flavor while addressing individual choices and preferences.

The senses of taste and smell play an important role in eating habits. Loss of these senses can impact your health by reducing the desire to eat.

Tastes and smells are important because they bring pleasure and enjoyment to eating, which can improve the desire to eat. This, in turn, can help maintain a healthy weight and immune system, which will improve overall health.

Without the simple pleasures of taste and smell, the overall quality of life is greatly reduced.

WAYS TO ENHANCE THE FLAVORS OF YOUR FOOD

Flavor Enhancers & Concentrated Flavors

You can add flavor enhancers or concentrated flavors to food to amplify taste and smell. They are concentrated mixtures of flavor and odorous molecules that are taken from natural products or are made by a chemical process. You can buy both concentrated flavors (e.g., jellies or sauces) or flavor enhancers in the form of bouillon cubes (e.g., chicken or beef bouillon) in the supermarket. Adding flavor to food amplifies taste and aroma of food. This can help make food more palatable for someone with impaired taste and smell.

Monosodium Glutamate

When you buy MSG in the supermarket, you will find suggested uses on the container label. MSG is generally added to foods before or during cooking, much like table salt. As a general guideline, about half a teaspoon of MSG per pound of meat or four to six servings of vegetables should be sufficient. Once the proper amount is used, adding more contributes little to food flavors. A little enhancement goes a long way.

▶ Nutritional needs vary throughout the life cycle.

▶ Within each age group, a variety of factors may further influence dietary choices and habits.

▶ Pregnant women have increased needs for calories, protein, essential fatty acids, iron, folate, calcium, and other nutrients.

▶ Sound nutrition during pregnancy can have a positive effect on the growth and development of the fetus.

▶ Pregnant women should not drink alcohol, due to the risk of fetal alcohol syndrome.

▶ Lactating women and their infants enjoy nutritional advantages as well as psychological benefits.

▶ Infants should consume breast milk or an infant formula until 12 months of age. At 12 months, whole milk (cow's milk) may be introduced.

▶ Semi-solid foods may be introduced at about 4-6 months of age.

▶ Preschoolers may have erratic eating habits.

▶ Nutritious finger foods and involvement in meal preparation are appropriate for preschoolers.

▶ School-age children have high needs for protein, calcium, and iron to support growth.

▶ Eating habits of adolescents may be influenced by social factors and lifestyles, and often pose the problem of empty calories.

▶ The USDA warns that the eating habits of many children and adolescents do not match recommendations of the Food Guide Pyramid.

▶ The USDA supports nutritious, low-cost or free breakfasts and lunches through the National School Lunch Program, and nutritional guidelines apply to school menus.

▶ Aging can be associated with shifts in muscle and bone mass and other changes in metabolism.

▶ Changes in taste and smell, along with many physiological, psychosocial, and socioeconomic factors, can influence dietary intake and nutritional status among older Americans.

▶ Nutrients of particular concern for the elderly are water, vitamin D, calcium, folic acid, and fiber.

Anorexia: loss of appetite

At risk: belonging to a group or having a dietary lifestyle which tends toward nutritional problems or disease

Life cycle: the series of stages in any individual's life from early infancy through late maturity

Lactation: the production of milk in the mammary glands; also called breastfeeding

National School Lunch Program: the USDA's program supporting the provision of nutritious, low-cost or free breakfasts and lunches to more than 25 million children each school day

1. The series of stages throughout a person's life are called:

   A. Life cycle
   B. Anabolism
   C. Catabolism
   D. Enzymes

2. Recommended weight gain during pregnancy, for a woman of normal weight, is:

   A. 5-10 pounds
   B. 10-20 pounds
   C. 25-35 pounds
   D. 45-55 pounds

3. Which of the following nutrients is particularly critical during the early weeks of pregnancy to prevent brain defects and spina bifida?

   A. Simple sugar
   B. Vitamin A
   C. Magnesium
   D. Folate

4. During lactation, a mother needs approximately how many extra calories each day?

   A. 100
   B. 500
   C. 1000
   D. 1500

5. Whole milk is appropriate in an infant's diet starting at what age?

   A. 3 months
   B. 6 months
   C. 12 months
   D. 18 months

6. Which of the following is good advice about offering snacks to preschoolers?

A. Offer them frequently, as preschoolers need to eat often.
B. Avoid snacks, as they form poor eating habits.
C. Use only cooked vegetables and fruits—not raw.
D. Avoid finger foods.

7. Which of the following would be an appropriate high-iron food choice for adolescents?

A. Apple juice
B. French fries
C. Pizza
D. Hamburger on enriched bun

8. School lunches should provide how much fat?

A. 20% of calories
B. 30% of calories
C. 40% of calories
D. 50% of calories

9. The Tufts University Food Pyramid for Older Adults places what at the base?

A. Fluids
B. Whole grains
C. High-fiber fruits
D. Red meat and poultry

10. Which of the following is a good approach for menu planning for the elderly?

A. Include whole milk and fried foods to ensure adequate fat intake.
B. Limit protein intake.
C. Ensure adequate intake of vitamin D, calcium, and zinc.
D. Do not provide too much fluid, which can stress older kidneys.

Chapter 6 An Introduction to Medical Nutrition Therapy

Medical nutrition therapy is important for the prevention and/or treatment of many diseases. A dietary manager is often responsible for implementing therapeutic diets. Therefore, an understanding of health conditions and related diet planning is a cornerstone of the profession.

After completing this chapter, you should be able to:

- ▶ Outline the concepts of nutrient deficiency and nutrient excess.
- ▶ Explain the concept of therapeutic diets, and describe how these relate to body systems.
- ▶ List diseases and conditions that may require medical nutrition therapy.
- ▶ Describe common therapeutic diets, and give examples of meal plans for each.
- ▶ Define *diet manual* and explain how nutrition caregivers use it.
- ▶ Explain the policy of liberalizing modified diets in the longterm care setting.

DEFICIENCY AND EXCESS

As explained in Chapter 3, a deficiency is the illness that occurs over time when a nutrient is not present in adequate amounts. Nutrition-related problems sometimes involve inadequate amounts of nutrients, resulting in deficiency. Conversely, nutritional problems can involve too much of nutrients—particularly macronutrients. These are classified as problems of nutrient excess. Too much fat, for example, contributes to obesity and heart disease, while also increasing the risk of developing cancer. Dietary planning takes into account the actual needs of an individual or group, adjusting nutrient levels and finetuning the balance of nutrients to promote wellness. What exactly needs to be done can vary based on an individual's medical condition, and how body systems are functioning. At times, a diet helps to compensate for unhealthy shifts in the body's metabolism and functioning. We will explore these ideas in much more detail throughout this chapter.

THERAPEUTIC DIETS

As explained in Chapter 1, sometimes dietary changes are dictated by health conditions. As a group, these changes are called therapeutic or modified diets. Medical nutrition therapy is a broader term. **Medical nutrition therapy** is the nutritional assessment and treatment of a condition, illness, or injury that places an individual at risk. It involves two components: assessment of the client's nutritional status (described in Chapter 8), and treatment or intervention. Medical nutrition therapy generally focuses on individuals at risk for nutritional problems. Part of the healthcare process is to identify individuals at risk. This process, nutrition screening, is described in Chapter 8.

Treatment may include therapeutic diets, counseling, and/or the use of nutrition support. This dietary treatment goes hand-in-hand with other therapies, such as medication, surgery, physical therapy, radiation, and many others. Thus, dietary professionals work with others on the healthcare team to address the medical therapeutic needs of patients.

A therapeutic diet is a regular diet that has been adjusted to meet a client's special nutrient needs. Diets may be adjusted to control specific nutrients. Examples include calorie-controlled diets for weight loss, fat and cholesterol-controlled diets for treatment of cardiovascular disease, and sodium-controlled diets used in hypertension or renal (kidney) disease. Even water or fluid may need to be limited—or increased—based on medical conditions. Protein needs to be limited during renal failure. Furthermore, some therapeutic diets accommodate difficulties in chewing or swallowing—such as pureed diets or dysphagia diets. Others are used in treatment of problems in the digestive system. These include clear liquid diets, very low fat diets, and gluten-free diets. As you can already see, medical nutrition therapy is critical in the treatment of many diseases.

How is medical nutrition therapy effective? As an example, consider that more than one-third of the nation's healthcare costs are incurred by an elderly population. Meanwhile, it is estimated that up to approximately two-thirds of individuals admitted to nursing homes already have some form of malnutrition. Among hospital patients, this figure may be approximately one-third. Often, this malnutrition includes protein calorie malnutrition, which means that many body systems are compromised. Healthcare research proves that in a hospital, for example, appropriate nutritional intervention can reduce complications from surgery and other conditions. It can reduce length of stay, so that a patient is well and released more quickly. It can actually reduce the rate of death following illness and/or medical interventions. In a longterm care setting, nutritional care can improve health and ability to fight illness. In addition, it can improve overall quality of life. Proper nutrition can also prevent pressure sores—or speed healing of sores. Pressure sores, also known as pressure ulcers, are a major problem among nursing home residents, and are discussed later in this chapter. Research further demonstrates that medical nutrition therapy can improve outcomes and reduce healthcare costs associated with diabetes, cardiovascular disease, hypertension, renal (kidney) disease, cancer, low birth weight, and many other medical conditions. A study by Ross Laboratories determined that in hospitals, effective medical nutrition therapy can save $11,000 - $16,000 per patient, per hospital stay. From other research, the American Dietetic Association demonstrated that for every dollar spent on nutrition screening and intervention, at least $3.25 is saved.

Overall, the value of nutritional intervention is quite impressive. In a report about nutrition, the Senate Committee on Education and Labor stated that 85%

of the older population has one or more chronic conditions that have been documented to benefit from nutrition interventions. In this chapter, we will address many of the conditions in which nutrition plays a crucial role.

MEDICAL NUTRITION THERAPY OF CARDIOVASCULAR DISEASE

Cardiovascular disease is a general term that refers to diseases of the heart and blood vessels. It is the number-one cause of death in the United States. About one in four Americans has one or more of these forms of cardiovascular disease:

- Coronary artery disease
- Stroke
- High blood pressure
- Rheumatic heart disease

Coronary Artery Disease (CAD)

Most heart disease is the result of **atherosclerosis**, a process in which deposits of cholesterol and other substances accumulate on the inside of arteries. Atherosclerosis is also called hardening of the arteries. This process gradually reduces the amount of blood that can flow through an artery and also makes the artery less elastic and stretchy. Sometimes the buildup, also called *plaque*, can even close off an artery and stop blood flow completely.

Coronary artery disease (CAD) occurs when the coronary arteries, which supply blood to the heart, are clogged with atherosclerotic deposits. A heart attack occurs when the arteries that feed the heart muscle are blocked. In medical language, a heart attack is called a myocardial infarction (MI). If part of the heart muscle is denied oxygen, it dies. A piece of the heart is damaged and no longer contracts, so the heart works less efficiently. A heart attack may develop slowly or suddenly. Major symptoms and warning signs are:

- Chest discomfort that lasts several minutes or longer. This may feel like pressure, squeezing, fullness or pain.
- Discomfort in other areas of the upper body, such as one or both arms, the back, neck, jaw or stomach.
- Shortness of breath
- Breaking out in a cold sweat
- Nausea or lightheadedness

As described in Chapter 3, many of the risk factors for coronary heart disease have nutrition connections. Let's look more closely at one of these factors, high blood cholesterol, or *hyperlipidemia*. Cholesterol travels through the bloodstream in little clusters of proteins and lipids called lipoproteins. Usually, we distinguish blood cholesterol measurements into two types: LDL and HDL.

Figure 6.1

GUIDELINES FOR CHOLESTEROL LEVELS

Everyone age 20 and older should have cholesterol measured at least once every five years. It is best to have a blood test called a *lipoprotein profile*. This blood test is done after a 9- to 12-hour fast and gives information about total cholesterol, LDL (bad) cholesterol, HDL (good) cholesterol, and triglycerides—another form of fat in blood. The tables below provide guidelines for interpreting the numbers.

TOTAL CHOLESTEROL LEVEL	CATEGORY
Less than 200 mg/dl	Desirable
200-239 mg/dl	Borderline high
240 mg/dl and above	High

LDL CHOLESTEROL LEVEL	LDL CHOLESTEROL CATEGORY
Less than 100 mg/dl	Optimal
100-129 mg/dl	Near optimal/above optimal
130-159 mg/dl	Borderline high
160-189 mg/dl	High
190 mg/dl and above	Very high

For HDL, higher numbers are better. A level less than 40 mg/dl is low and is considered a major risk factor because it increases the risk of developing heart disease. HDL levels of 60 mg/dl or more help to lower the risk. Triglycerides can also raise heart disease risk. Levels that are borderline high (150-199 mg/dl) or high (200 mg/dl or more) may need treatment in some people.

Source: National Cholesterol Education Program, 2003

Low-Density Lipoproteins (LDL) or "bad cholesterol" carries most of the cholesterol in the blood. Cholesterol and fat from LDLs are the main source of dangerous buildup and blockage in the arteries. Thus, the higher the LDL cholesterol level, the greater the risk of heart disease. As a memory aid, you can also think of LDL as "L= lousy" cholesterol.

High-Density Lipoproteins (HDL) or "good cholesterol" carries cholesterol away from body organs and takes it to the liver for destruction. Think of HDL as cholesterol that is on its way out of the body. A high level of HDL is a favorable health indicator. As a memory aid, you can think of HDL as "H=healthy" cholesterol.

More than 90 million Americans have blood cholesterol levels that present risks for heart disease. Reaching and/or maintaining a normal weight, exercising, and limiting fat and cholesterol in the diet can all help adjust LDL and HDL levels to a healthier profile. Drugs are also used for this purpose. Keep in mind that the preventive goal is to reduce LDL and raise HDL. The National

Cholesterol Education Program provides guidelines for cholesterol levels, shown in Figure 6.1.

To control risk factors for heart disease, the American Heart Association recommends using the Food Guide Pyramid, described in Chapter 3. More specific nutrition advice appears in Figure 6.2.

To lower blood cholesterol (LDL) through diet, it is important to choose foods low in saturated fat. While about 30% of total calories should come from fat, only 7-10% should be in the form of saturated fat. Saturated fat is found in greatest amounts in foods from animals, such as fatty cuts of meat, poultry with the skin, whole milk dairy products, lard, and three vegetable oils (coconut, palm, and palm kernel oils). Foods low in saturated fat include dried beans, fruits, vegetables, and whole grain foods. They are also high in starch and fiber. Figure 6.3 compares saturated fat in some common food choices, and Figure 6.4 offers suggestions for choosing foods low in saturated fat and cholesterol.

AMERICAN HEART ASSOCIATION EATING PLAN

▶ Eat a variety of fruits and vegetables. Choose 5 or more servings per day.

▶ Eat a variety of grain products, including whole grains. Choose 6 or more servings per day.

▶ Include fat free and low fat milk products, fish, legumes (beans), skinless poultry and lean meats.

▶ Choose fats and oils with 2 grams or less saturated fat per tablespoon, such as liquid and tub margarines, canola oil and olive oil.

▶ Balance the number of calories you eat with the number you use each day. (To find that number, multiply the number of pounds you weigh now by 15 calories. This represents the average number of calories used in one day if you're moderately active. If you get very little exercise, multiply your weight by 13 instead of 15. Less active people burn fewer calories.)

▶ Maintain a level of physical activity that keeps you fit and matches the number of calories you eat. Walk or do other activities for at least 30 minutes on most days. To lose weight, do enough activity to use up more calories than you eat every day.

▶ Limit your intake of foods high in calories or low in nutrition, including foods like soft drinks and candy that have a lot of sugars.

▶ Limit foods high in saturated fat, trans fat and/or cholesterol, such as full-fat milk products, fatty meats, tropical oils, partially hydrogenated vegetable oils and egg yolks. Instead choose foods low in saturated fat, trans fat and cholesterol from the first four points above.

▶ Eat less than 6 grams of salt (sodium chloride) per day (2,400 milligrams of sodium).

▶ Have no more than one alcoholic drink per day if you're a woman and no more than two if you're a man. "One drink" means it has no more than 1/2 ounce of pure alcohol. Examples of one drink are 12 oz. of beer, 4 oz. of wine, 1-1/2 oz. of 80-proof spirits or 1 oz. of 100-proof spirits.

Figure 6.2

Figure 6.3

SATURATED FAT IN FOODS

Food Category	Portion	Saturated Fat
CHEESE		
Regular Cheddar cheese	1 oz	6.0 grams
Low fat Cheddar cheese	1 oz	1.2
GROUND BEEF		
Regular ground beef	3 oz cooked	7.2
Extra lean ground beef	3 oz cooked	5.3
MILK		
Whole milk	1 cup	5.1
Low fat (1%) milk	1 cup	1.6
BREADS		
Croissant	1 medium	6.6
Bagel	1 medium	0.1
FROZEN DESSERTS		
Regular ice cream	½ cup	4.5
Frozen yogurt	½ cup	2.5
TABLE SPREADS		
Butter	1 tsp	2.4
Soft margarine	1 tsp	0.7

NOTE: The food categories listed are among the major food sources of saturated for US adults and children.

Whenever possible, it is best to substitute unsaturated fat for saturated fat. Unsaturated fat is usually liquid at room temperature and can be either monounsaturated or polyunsaturated. Examples of foods high in monounsaturated fat are olive and canola oils. Those high in polyunsaturated fat include safflower, sunflower, corn, and soybean oils. Experts also advise limiting trans-fatty acids in the diet. These fats raise total cholesterol and LDL cholesterol. Trans-fatty acids are produced as oils are partially hydrogenated (partially solidified) to make margarine. They appear in many types of stick margarines, and are also ingredients in some commercial baked goods. New FDA labeling regulations require manufacturers to show trans-fatty acid content on Nutrition Facts Labels, beginning in 2006.

Figure 6.4

CHOOSING FOODS LOW IN SATURATED FAT AND CHOLESTEROL

Meat, Poultry, Fish, and Shellfish

BUYING TIPS:

- Choose lean cuts of meat. Look for meats labeled "lean" or "extra lean". Eat moderate portions—no more than about 6 ounces a day. (A 3 ounce portion is about the size of a deck of cards).

- Limit organ meats like liver, sweetbreads, and kidneys. Organ meats are high in cholesterol, even though they are fairly low in fat.

- Limit high fat processed meats like bacon, bologna, salami, hot dogs, and sausage. Some chicken and turkey hot dogs are lower in saturated fat and total fat than pork and beef hot dogs. There are also "lean" beef hot dogs that are low in fat and saturated fat. Usually, processed poultry products have more fat and cholesterol than fresh poultry. To be sure, check the nutrition label on deli products to find those that are lowest in fat and saturated fat.

- Try fresh ground turkey or chicken made from white meat, like the breast.

- Limit use of goose and duck. They are higher in saturated fat, even with the skin removed.

- Choose shellfish only occasionally. Squid, shrimp, and oysters are fairly high in cholesterol; scallops, mussels, and clams are low.

- Buy canned fish packed in water, not oil.

PREPARATION TIPS:

- Trim fat from meat and remove skin from poultry before eating.

- Bake, broil, microwave, poach, or roast instead of frying. If frying, use a nonstick pan and nonstick cooking spray or a small amount of vegetable oil to reduce the fat.

- When roasting meat, place the meat on a rack so the fat can drip away.

- Brown ground meat and drain well before adding other ingredients.

- Use fat free ingredients like fruit juice, wine, or defatted broth to baste meats and poultry.

Dairy Foods

BUYING TIPS:

- Choose skim or 1% milk, rather than 2% or whole milk.

- When looking for hard cheese, select versions that are labeled fat free, reduced fat, low fat, light, or part skim.

- When shopping for soft cheeses, choose low fat (1%) or nonfat cottage cheese, farmer cheese, pot cheese, or part skim or light ricotta.

- Use low fat or nonfat yogurt; try it in recipes or as a topping.

- Try low fat or fat free sour cream or cream cheese blends for spreads, toppings, or in recipes.

PREPARATION TIPS:

- Try low fat cheese in casseroles, or try a sharp flavored regular cheese and use less than the recipe calls for. Save most of the cheese for the top.

- Use skim, 1%, or evaporated skim milk for cream soups or white sauces.

CHOOSING FOODS LOW IN SATURATED FAT AND CHOLESTEROL, *CONTINUED*

Eggs

BUYING TIPS:
- Eggs are included in many processed foods and baked goods. Look at the nutrition label to check the cholesterol content.

- Try egg substitutes.

PREPARATION TIPS:
- Substitute two egg whites for one whole egg in recipes. (Egg whites are cholesterol-free.) Or, use egg substitutes.

Fruits and Vegetables

BUYING TIPS:
- Buy fruits and vegetables often—fresh, frozen, or canned. They have no cholesterol and most are low in saturated fat. Also, most fruits and vegetables, except avocados, coconut, and olives, are low in total fat.

PREPARATION TIPS:
- Use fruits as a snack or dessert.

- Prepare vegetables as snacks, side dishes, and salads. Season with herbs, spices, lemon juice, or fat free or low fat mayonnaise. Limit use of regular mayonnaise, salad dressings, and cream, cheese, or other fatty sauces.

Breads, Cereals, Pasta, Rice, and Dry Peas and Beans

BUYING TIPS:
- Use whole grain breads, rolls, and cereals often.

- Limit baked goods made with large amounts of fat, especially saturated fat, such as: croissants, biscuits, doughnuts, butter rolls, muffins, coffee cake, Danish pastry. Avoid baked goods listing palm, palm kernel, and coconut oils as ingredients. These oils are high in saturated fats, even though they are vegetable oils.

- Choose ready-to-eat cereals often. Most are low in saturated fat, except for granola, muesli, or oat bran types made with coconut or coconut oil.

- Buy dry peas and beans often.

PREPARATION TIPS:
- Try pasta or rice in soups, or with low fat sauces as main dishes or casseroles.

- Stretch meat dishes with pasta or vegetables for hearty meals.

- Bake homemade muffins and quick breads using unsaturated vegetable oils; substitute two egg whites for each egg yolk, or use egg substitutes. Experiment with substituting applesauce for oil or cut back the amount of oil in the recipe. For each two cups of flour, only ¼ cup of vegetable oil is necessary.

- Use dry peas and beans as the main ingredient in casseroles, soups, or other one-dish meals.

Foods high in starch and fiber are excellent substitutes for foods high in saturated fat. These foods—breads, cereals, pasta, grain, fruits, and vegetables—are low in saturated fat and cholesterol. They are also usually lower in calories. In addition, research indicates that some forms of fiber may help reduce blood cholesterol (LDL) levels. Specifically using plant-based sources for much of the dietary protein is beneficial in reducing (LDL) cholesterol. In addition, some research indicates that meat-based protein, even aside from its fat content, may stimulate (LDL) cholesterol levels. So, reducing meat-based protein is a good idea. Other nutritional factors that can favorably influence blood cholesterol include omega-3 fatty acids, found primarily in fish, garlic, and green tea.

Dietary cholesterol also can raise blood cholesterol levels, although usually not as much as saturated fat. High cholesterol foods include egg yolks, liver, the fat in meats and poultry, shellfish, and dairy fat (cream, whole milk, regular cheeses, etc.). Cholesterol is found only in foods of animal origin. Cholesterol intake of less than 300 mg per day is recommended.

Experts also advise maintaining a healthy weight. People who are overweight tend to have higher blood cholesterol levels than people of a healthy weight. Overweight adults with an "apple" shape—bigger (pot) belly—tend to have a higher risk for heart disease than those with a "pear" shape—bigger hips and thighs. For anyone who is overweight, losing even a little weight can help to lower LDL and raise HDL. Being physically active also helps with weight management, while lowering LDL.

When treatment of blood cholesterol becomes challenging, some practitioners use a Step II diet approach. A Step I diet incorporates the dietary advice described above. A more aggressive Step II diet limits saturated fat to less than 7% of total calories, and dietary cholesterol to less than 200 mg per day.

Drug Treatment

Drug treatment is considered appropriate for adults who have a high LDL level, especially if they also have other CAD risk factors. Drugs referred to as bile acid *sequestrants*, such as cholestyramine, are approved for use in clients with high LDL levels who don't respond to dietary changes alone. Constipation is the most common side effect. Niacin-containing drugs such as Niacor and Nicolar are also used to bring down cholesterol levels. Side effects, which may include flushing, itching, and upset stomach, limit its use for some people. Statins, such as Mavacor (lovastatin), are used in addition to medical nutrition therapy to reduce elevated total and LDL cholesterol. Side effects are generally minimal, but may include constipation, abdominal pain, nausea, and bloating. Other drugs are available. A doctor's decision about which drug to prescribe will be based primarily on an assessment of a client's risk factors, and the potential side effects of the drugs. Physicians measure client's LDL levels four to six weeks after starting drug therapy and again at three months to see whether the therapy is effective.

Stroke

Stroke is the third leading cause of death in the US, after heart disease and cancer. About 500,000 Americans have a stroke each year. Of these, 150,000 people die while another 200,000 are left with some disability. A **stroke** occurs when blood vessels bringing oxygen to the brain burst or become clogged. The interruption of blood flow to the brain stops body functions and damages nerve cells. The brain must have a continuous supply of blood rich in oxygen and nutrients for energy. If deprived of blood flow for more than a few minutes, brains cells die. The functions these cells control—such as speech, muscle movement, or comprehension—die with them.

The majority of strokes are caused by blockages in the arteries that supply blood to the brain. The blockages may be caused by a clot, also called *thrombus*, that forms on the inner lining of a brain or neck artery already partly clogged by atherosclerotic plaque. A blood clot formed in another part of the body may also cause a stroke. Usually a wandering clot like this—called an *embolus*—breaks off from plaque in an artery wall, or originates in the heart. The most serious kinds of stroke occur not from blockage, but from hemorrhage. A *hemorrhage* occurs when a spot in a brain artery weakened by disease—usually high blood pressure or atherosclerosis—ruptures and leaks blood. If an artery inside the brain ruptures, it is called a *cerebral hemorrhage*. Sometimes, hemorrhage may be caused by an *aneurysm*, a section of the artery wall so thin that it may balloon out and burst, especially when high blood pressure is present.

Warning signs and symptoms of stroke include:

- Sudden numbness or weakness of the face, arm or leg, especially on one side of the body
- Sudden confusion, trouble speaking or understanding
- Sudden trouble seeing in one or both eyes
- Sudden trouble walking, dizziness, loss of balance or coordination
- Sudden, severe headache with no known cause

Effects of a stroke can range in severity from a slight one-sided facial sagging that disappears within two weeks, to inability to walk, inability to talk, or loss of control of bodily functions. Some stroke victims have trouble chewing and/or swallowing foods. In addition, some experience poor orientation, e.g. inability to find food on the plate. Both factors can place individuals at risk for malnutrtion. The kind of disability a stroke victim is left with depends on the location and extent of brain damage. The brain is resourceful. After brain swelling goes down following a stroke, small blood vessels around the blocked area enlarge to allow more blood flow to the damaged section. Some incapacitated cells may recover partially or completely. In many cases, other brain cells can assume the functions of the damaged ones.

An incident involving physical symptoms that lasts less than 24 hours and leaves no permanent disability is called a *transient ischemic attack (TIA)* or "mini-stroke". Some individuals have repeated attacks of TIAs without any serious consequences, but these symptoms should not be ignored and need immediate medical attention.

Hypertension

Hypertension is a medical condition involving chronic high blood pressure. High blood pressure means that the heart has to pump harder than it should to get blood to all the parts of the body. Because high blood pressure usually doesn't give early warning signs, it is known as the "silent killer." Hypertension raises chances of experiencing a stroke, a heart attack, and kidney problems. The higher the blood pressure, the greater the risk. An estimated 60 million people, more than a third of the adult population, have hypertension. Each year half a million strokes and over a million heart attacks result from hypertension.

Blood pressure is expressed as a fraction, such as 120/80 millimeters of mercury (abbreviated as "mmHg"). The numerator (120) is called the *systolic pressure*—the pressure of blood within arteries when the heart is pumping. The denominator (80) is called the *diastolic pressure*—the pressure in the arteries when the heart is resting between beats. A typical blood pressure for a young adult might be 120/80 mmHg. Hypertension Stage 1 (see Figure 6.5) is the most common form of high blood pressure. To be diagnosed as hypertensive, a person has had at least two to three readings performed on each of three separate visits.

Figure 6.5

BLOOD PRESSURE LEVELS FOR ADULTS

CATEGORY	SYSTOLIC (in mmHg)		DIASTOLIC (in mmHg)	RESULT
Optimal	less than 120	*and*	less than 80	Good for you!
Normal	less than 130	*and*	less than 85	Keep an eye on it.
High-Normal	130-139	*or*	85-89	Your blood pressure could be a problem. Make needed changes in what you eat and drink, get physical activity, and lose extra weight. If you also have diabetes, see the doctor.
Hypertension Stage 1	140-159	*or*	90-99	
Hypertension Stage 2	160-179	*or*	100-109	
Hypertension Stage 3	180 or higher	*or*	110 or higher	

If systolic and diastolic pressures fall into different categories, overall status is the higher category.

Source: National Heart, Lung, and Blood Institute, 2003

When persistently elevated blood pressure is due to a medical problem, such as hormonal abnormality or an inherited narrowing of the aorta (the largest artery leading from the heart), it's called *secondary hypertension*. This means the high blood pressure is secondary to another condition. The causes of most cases of hypertension are unknown, however. These cases are known as *essential hypertension*. Because the cause remains a mystery, essential hypertension cannot be cured. But it can be controlled. Treatment of clients with hypertension is long-term and includes lifestyle modifications and possibly medications. Lifestyle modifications include weight reduction, increased physical activity, medical nutrition therapy, moderation of alcohol intake, and tobacco avoidance.

When lifestyle modifications do not succeed in lowering blood pressure enough, drugs are the next step. Reducing blood pressure with drugs clearly decreases the incidence of cardiovascular death and disease. Two classes of antihypertensive drugs—diuretics and beta blockers—are common for initial drug therapy. *Diuretics* are a class of blood pressure medications that cause increased urine output. Some cause an increased excretion of potassium in the urine, and a client may need to eat high potassium foods. Beta blockers reduce the heart rate, so that the heart puts out less blood.

Medical Nutrition Therapy

Often, nutritional advice for hypertension includes suggestions about sodium intake. Sodium is the main mineral in salt. The current recommendation is to reduce sodium intake to less than 2,400 mg of sodium daily. Interestingly, reducing dietary sodium is not effective for everyone who has hypertension. Scientists estimate that about half of people with hypertension are sensitive to sodium. For them, reducing dietary sodium may be very effective.

One level teaspoon of salt provides about 2,300 milligrams of sodium. However, most people do not obtain the majority of their sodium by adding salt to foods. In fact, about 75% of our dietary sodium is added to food during processing and manufacturing. Figure 6.6 lists sodium content of many foods. Besides salt, common sources of sodium in the diet are:

- Processed foods with salt or other sodium-containing compounds added.
- Other sodium-containing compounds, such as baking soda, baking powder, monosodium glutamate (MSG), and soy sauce.
- Foods in which sodium is naturally present. Milk and milk products are somewhat high in sodium.
- In some areas, the water supply supplies 10% of an individual's daily sodium consumption. Sodium is often present in water that has gone through a water softening device.
- Some medications, such as some antacids

Figure 6.6

Sodium Content of Foods

Food Group	Sodium (mg)
GRAINS AND GRAIN PRODUCTS	
Cooked cereal, rice, pasta, unsalted, ½ cup	0–5
Ready-to-eat cereal, 1 cup	100–360
Bread, 1 slice	110–175
VEGETABLES	
Fresh or frozen, cooked without salt, ½ cup	1–70
Canned or frozen with sauce, ½ cup	140–460
Tomato juice, canned ¾ cup	820
FRUIT	
Fresh, frozen, canned, ½ cup	0–5
LOW FAT OR FAT FREE DAIRY FOODS	
Milk, 1 cup	20
Yogurt, 8 oz	160
Natural cheeses, 1½ oz	110–450
Processed cheeses, 1½ oz	600

Food Group	Sodium (mg)
NUTS, SEEDS, AND DRY BEANS	
Peanuts, salted, ⅓ cup	120
Peanuts, unsalted, ⅓ cup	0–5
Beans, cooked from dried, or frozen, without salt, ½ cup	0–5
Beans, canned, ½ cup	400
MEATS, FISH, AND POULTRY	
Fresh meat, fish, poultry, 3 oz	30–90
Tuna canned, water pack, no salt added, 3 oz	35–45
Tuna canned, water pack, 3 oz	250–350
Ham, lean, roasted, 3 oz	1,020
SOUPS	
Canned chicken rice soup, 1 cup	814
Canned chicken noodle, "healthy", 1 cup	460

Source: National Heart, Lung, and Blood Institute

A typical sodium restricted diet is described as a No Added Salt diet or a 4 Gram Sodium diet, which typically eliminates table salt and very high sodium foods, such as processed meats, regular canned soups, and other high sodium processed foods. Another more restricted approach is a 2 Gram Sodium diet, which includes the previous limitations while also limiting milk to 2 cups per day, and limiting regular breads and starchy foods. Low sodium breads, cereals, and other grain products may become part of this diet. Figure 6.7 shows how to convert between milligrams and grams, and Figure 6.8 lists tips for reducing sodium in the diet. Figure 6.9 lists nutrient labeling guidelines for sodium.

Figure 6.7

Do the Math: Grams or Milligrams

To convert grams of sodium to milligrams or milligrams of sodium to grams, use the following examples.

1 gram sodium = 1,000 milligrams sodium

2 grams sodium = _____ milligrams sodium
2 grams x 1,000 = 2,000 milligrams sodium

2.3 grams sodium = _____ milligrams sodium
2.3 grams x 1,000 = 2,300 milligrams sodium

3,500 milligrams sodium = ____ grams sodium
3,500 milligrams ÷ 1,000 = 3.5 grams sodium

Figure 6.8

Tips for Reducing Sodium Intake

- Choose low or reduced sodium, or no-salt-added versions of foods and condiments when available.
- Buy vegetables fresh, plain frozen, or canned with no salt added.
- Use fresh poultry, fish, and lean meat, rather than canned, smoked, or processed types.
- Choose ready-to-eat breakfast cereals that are lower in sodium.
- Limit cured foods (such as bacon and ham), foods packed in brine (such as pickles, pickled vegetables, olives, and sauerkraut), and condiments (such as MSG, mustard, horseradish, catsup, and barbecue sauce). Limit even lower sodium versions of soy sauce and teriyaki sauce. Treat these condiments like table salt. Replace pickles and olives with fresh lettuce, greens, or tomatoes.
- Replace high sodium cheeses and peanut butter with low sodium varieties.
- Use spices instead of salt. In cooking and at the table, flavor foods with herbs, spices, lemon, lime, vinegar, or salt free seasoning blends. Start by cutting salt in half.
- Cook rice, pasta, and hot cereals without salt. Cut back on instant or flavored rice, pasta, and cereal mixes, which usually have added salt.
- Choose convenience foods that are lower in sodium. Cut back on frozen dinners, mixed dishes such as pizza, packaged mixes, canned soups or broths, and salad dressings, as these often have a lot of sodium.
- Rinse canned foods, such as tuna, to remove some sodium.
- Use unsalted pretzels or crackers, or fresh fruits and vegetables to replace salty snack foods.
- Use fresh or frozen vegetables instead of canned, or choose low sodium canned foods.

Compiled from National Heart, Lung, and Blood Institute and other sources

Figure 6.9

NUTRIENT LABEL CLAIMS FOR SODIUM

Sodium free	Less than 5 mg of sodium
Very low sodium	35 mg or less of sodium
Low sodium	140 mg or less of sodium
Reduced or less sodium	At least 25% less sodium than the usual food product
Light in sodium	At least 50% less sodium than the usual food product

DASH Diet

To treat hypertension, the National High Blood Pressure Education Program, stemming from the National Institutes of Health, suggests an approach called the **DASH Diet**. DASH stands for: Dietary Approaches to Stop Hypertension.

A DASH diet limits sodium to 2,400 mg per day (or 1,500 in a more aggressive version). It boosts potassium to at least 3,500 mg per day. This is because the balance between potassium and sodium can make a difference in blood pressure. Research suggests that boosting potassium while reducing sodium—to create a high ratio of potassium to sodium—has a beneficial effect on blood pressure. In general, many fruits and vegetables are good sources of potassium. Milk and meats also provide significant amounts of potassium. The National Institutes of Health also suggests limiting alcohol consumption to no more than 1 ounce of ethanol (e.g., 24 oz beer, 10 oz wine, or 2 oz 100-proof whiskey) per day in most men and to no more than 0.5 ounce per day in women. Very much in accordance with other dietary guidance for health, a DASH diet includes plenty of fresh fruits and vegetables, as well as low fat or fat free dairy products. Note that dairy products are rich sources of calcium. Calcium appears to have a protective role in managing hypertension, so maintaining adequate calcium intake is important. Guidelines for following a DASH Diet appear in Figure 6.10.

Note that limiting sodium does not mean sacrificing flavor. Often, reducing sodium intake requires some adjustment and adaptation. People who have become accustomed to reduced sodium intake may find that they begin to enjoy other flavors in foods more. Figure 6.11 lists some ideas for creating herb blends useful as replacements for salt. In addition, many excellent cookbooks provide advice for seasoning foods with herbs and spices.

Figure 6.10

GUIDELINES FOR FOLLOWING A DASH DIET

The DASH eating plan shown below is based on 2,000 calories a day. The number of daily servings in a food group may vary from those listed, depending on your caloric needs. Use this chart to help you plan your menus or take it with you when you go to the store.

Food Group	Daily Servings*	Serving Sizes	Examples & Notes	Significance of Each Food Group to the DASH Eating Plan
Grains & grain products	7–8	1 slice bread 1 oz dry cereal** ½ cup cooked rice, pasta, or cereal	Whole wheat bread, English muffin, pita bread, bagel, cereals, grits, oatmeal, crackers, unsalted pretzels and popcorn	Major sources of energy & fiber
Vegetables	4–5	1 cup raw leafy vegetable ½ cup cooked vegetable 6 oz vegetable juice	Tomatoes, potatoes, carrots, green peas, squash, broccoli, turnip greens, collards, kale, spinach, artichokes, green beans, lima beans, sweet potatoes	Rich sources of potassium, magnesium, & fiber
Fruits	4–5	6 oz fruit juice 1 medium fruit ¼ cup dried fruit ½ cup fresh, frozen, or canned fruit	Apricots, bananas, dates, grapes, oranges, orange juice, grapefruit, grapefruit juice, mangoes, melons, peaches, pineapples, prunes raisins, strawberries, tangerines	Important sources of potassium, magnesium, & fiber
Low fat or fat free dairy foods	2–3	8 oz milk 1 cup yogurt 1½ oz cheese	Fat free (skim) or low fat (1%) milk, fat free or low fat buttermilk, fat free or low fat regular or frozen yogurt, low fat and fat free cheese	Major sources of calcium & protein
Meats, poultry, & fish	2 or less	3 oz cooked meats, poultry, or fish	Select only lean; trim away visible fats; broil, roast, or boil instead of frying; remove skin from poultry	Rich sources of protein & magnesium
Nuts, seeds, & dry beans	4–5 per week	⅓ cup or 1½ oz nuts 2 Tbsp or ½ oz seeds ½ cup cooked dry beans	Almonds, filberts, mixed nuts, peanuts, walnuts, sunflower seeds, kidney beans, lentils, peas	Rich sources of energy, magnesium, potassium, protein, & fiber
Fats & oils†	2–3	1 tsp soft margarine 1 Tbsp low fat mayonnaise, 2 Tbsp light salad dressing 1 tsp vegetable oil	Soft margarine, low fat mayonnaise, light salad dressing, vegetable oil (such as olive, corn, canola, or safflower)	DASH has 27% of calories as fat, including fat in or added to foods

GUIDELINES FOR FOLLOWING A DASH DIET, *CONTINUED*

Food Group	Daily Servings*	Serving Sizes	Examples & Notes	Significance of Each Food Group to the DASH Eating Plan
Sweets	5 per week	1 Tbsp sugar 1 Tbsp jelly or jam, ½ oz jelly beans, 8 oz lemonade	Maple syrup, sugar, jelly, jam fruit-flavored gelatin, jelly beans, hard candy, fruit punch, sorbet, ices	Sweets should be low in fat

*Servings are weekly where noted

**Equals ½ – 1¼ cups, depending on cereal type. Check the product's Nutrition Facts Label.

†Fat content changes serving counts for fats and oils: For example, 1 Tbsp of regular salad dressing equals 1 serving; 1 Tbsp of a low fat dressing equals ½ serving; 1 Tbsp of a fat free dressing equals 0 servings.

Source: National Heart, Lung, and Blood Institute

HERB BLENDS TO REPLACE SALT

These can be placed in shakers and used instead of salt:

Saltless surprise: 2 tsp garlic powder and 1 tsp each of basil, oregano, and powdered lemon rind (or dehydrated lemon juice). Put ingredients into a blender and mix well. Store in glass container, label well, and add rice to prevent caking.

Pungent salt substitute: 3 tsp basil, 2 tsp each of savory (summer savory is best), celery seed, ground cumin seed, sage, and marjoram, and 1 tsp lemon thyme. Mix well, then powder with a mortar and pestle.

Spicy saltless seasoning: 1 tsp each of cloves, pepper, and coriander seed (crushed), 2 teaspoons paprika, and 1 T rosemary. Mix ingredients in a blender. Store in airtight container.

Source: FDA

Figure 6.11

Congestive Heart Failure

Another common disease of the circulatory system is called **congestive heart failure (CHF)**. Atherosclerosis and hypertension can both lead to this condition, in which the heart itself weakens. In an effort to provide adequate circulation throughout the body, the heart works harder and harder, but is not highly effective. The heart beats faster and becomes enlarged. This can lead to fluid retention in the body, as well as a certain degree of malnutrition. Malnutrition occurs as the blood fails to deliver adequate oxygen and nutrients to body tissues. Due to excess fluid, however, an individual with CHF may not look malnourished. Experts estimate that at least 5 million Americans have CHF, and the National Institutes of Health project that this condition may become a new epidemic. Dietary treatment typically includes a sodium restricted diet, e.g. 2 Gram Sodium diet. This is because the body may not be able to rid itself of extra sodium, and sodium can contribute to fluid retention. A fluid restriction may also be necessary. Dietary treatments for underlying conditions, such as atherosclerosis and hypertension, are also recommended. If a client is over-weight, effective weight management may also reduce the burden on the heart.

Chronic Obstructive Pulmonary Disease (COPD)

Chronic obstructive pulmonary disease (COPD) is group of diseases that includes chronic bronchitis, emphysema and asthmatic bronchitis. These afflictions reduce the airflow out of the lungs. The most common symptom is shortness of breath. COPD is a leading cause of disability and death in the US, and 90% of cases result from smoking. COPD can cause malnutrition, due to loss of appetite, changes in taste, or gastrointestinal distress. In addition, COPD can make the body work harder to breathe. This increases energy (calorie) needs from day to day. In some cases, protein calorie malnutrition occurs as the body breaks down muscle to provide energy. Body wasting and decreased resistance to infection can result.

Nutritional care for a client with COPD targets maintaining adequate nutritional status without overfeeding. Too much food makes the body produce excess carbon dioxide, which can be difficult for lungs to exhale. In acute breathing problems, or when a client is on a ventilator (breathing machine), nutritionists sometimes increase the percentage of calories from fat. When the body uses fat, it needs less oxygen and produces less carbon dioxide, as compared with a high carbohydrate diet. Thus, a high fat diet (e.g. 50% of calories from fat) reduces the load on the lungs. For a client with COPD, it is also important to maintain adequate intake of nutrients such as vitamins A and C to help guard against infection. Fluid retention around the lungs may be a problem. If so, dietary fluid restriction may be needed. Clients who experience difficulties in eating com-fortably require common-sense support, which may include small, frequent meals and a diet planned around foods the client enjoys and tolerates well.

Diabetes Mellitus

Diabetes mellitus is a metabolic disorder in which the body cannot use glu-cose properly. Either there is an insufficient level of insulin, or the insulin is ineffective. *Insulin* is a hormone (a chemical messenger) made by the pancreas, an organ located near the liver. Insulin enables glucose in the blood to enter the body's cells, where it is burned for energy. Without glucose, the cells are deprived of energy. In diabetes, too much glucose accumulates in the blood. This condition is called **hyperglycemia**, which means high blood sugar. Ironically, with all this excess "food" in the bloodstream, body cells are starved for energy. The kidneys remove the extra glucose by dumping it into the urine, a condition called **glycosuria**. When not treated, diabetes can result in weight loss, insatiable hunger (called *polyphagia*), unquenchable thirst (called *polydip-sia*), frequent urination (called *polyuria*), dehydration, weakness, and fatigue. Although diabetes is popularly called "sugar diabetes," it is not caused by sugar. High sugar levels in the blood and urine are a result, not a cause, of diabetes.

Diabetes is a serious disease. It is the seventh leading cause of death in the US, and prevalence is on the rise. More than 6% of the US population has diabetes. That's about 17 million people. The American Diabetes Association estimates that about one-third of people with diabetes have not had the condition diagnosed. The life expectancy for people with diabetes is only two-thirds that of the general population. Poorly controlled diabetes can, over time, result in extensive damage throughout the body, affecting kidneys, heart, blood vessels, nerves, and vision. Diabetes is the nation's leading cause of kidney failure and adult blindness. And, because of its damaging effect on blood vessels and nerves of the lower limbs, it can require amputations of toes, feet, or legs. Having diabetes increases the risk of having a stroke or heart disease by two to four times. It is hardly surprising that this is a very expensive disease that costs the nation over $39.8 billion each year in healthcare costs, time lost from work, and Social Security disability payments (2003 estimates).

Diagnosis and Classification of Diabetes

Diagnosis of diabetes is generally dependent upon a laboratory test called a *fasting blood glucose (FBS)*. In this test, the glucose concentration in the blood is measured after an eight to 12-hour overnight fast. A normal fasting blood glucose is less than 120 mg/dl (milligrams per deciliter). A diagnosis of diabetes is generally made after testing on two occasions has revealed concentrations over 126 mg/dl. Physicians may also perform an *oral glucose tolerance test (GTT)* to better understand how the body handles glucose. This begins with a fasting blood glucose measurement. Next, a patient receives a concentrated glucose drink. At intervals afterwards, a technician keeps re-testing blood glucose. This provides a pattern of glucose levels that demonstrates the body's response.

There are three categories of diabetes: Type 1, Type 2, and gestational diabetes. Each one will be discussed in this section.

Type 1 diabetes occurs when a group of cells in the pancreas, called the beta cells, is unable to make insulin. Clients with Type 1 diabetes must depend on insulin injections to control their disease. Researchers say that Type 1 is actually an auto-immune illness. This means that special cells in the body whose job is to fight disease go awry. They destroy cells in the pancreas that make insulin. This is determined by genetics. Type 1 diabetes and other auto-immune illnesses tend to run in families. The National Institutes of Health is already testing a vaccine that may prevent this disorder. Only 5-10% of Americans with diabetes have Type 1. Type 1 usually begins in childhood. Classic symptoms of Type 1 diabetes appear abruptly and include excessive thirst, urination, hunger, and weight loss.

The most immediately life-threatening aspect of Type 1 diabetes is called *ketosis*, or the presence of dangerous chemicals called *ketones* in the blood. Because the cells don't have enough glucose to burn for energy, they start burning fat. In the process of burning fat for energy, they produce ketones.

Presence of ketones in the blood is unnatural, and begins to disturb the delicate chemical balance of the bloodstream. If not managed, this condition can lead to coma or even death.

Most cases of diabetes, from 90 to 95%, are classified as **Type 2 diabetes**. Some clients with Type 2 require insulin, but most do not. In this form of the disease, an individual's pancreas does make insulin but the cells are not as sensitive to it; the body cells don't use the insulin. Type 2 tends to strike adults over 30. As the population gets older, the percentage of people with diabetes increases. At least 80% of those with Type 2 diabetes are obese. Obesity is a risk factor for Type 2 diabetes, as is advanced age and family history. Symptoms of Type 2 match the symptoms for Type 1, but they are often overlooked because they tend to come on gradually and are less pronounced. Other symptoms that may signal the presence of Type 2 diabetes are tingling or numbness in the lower legs, feet or hands; skin or genital itching; and gum, skin, or bladder infections that recur and are slow to clear up.

Gestational diabetes is a condition characterized by abnormal glucose tolerance during pregnancy. It begins during the second half of pregnancy and ends after delivery. Most women are tested between the 24th and 28th week of gestation for diabetes. Some individuals with gestational diabetes require insulin, but most can use diet alone as a control.

Some practitioners also classify a condition called *pre-diabetes*, or impaired glucose tolerance. In this condition, blood glucose levels are higher than normal but not high enough for a diagnosis of diabetes. Some individuals with this condition may eventually develop Type 2 diabetes. This may apply to nearly 16% of adults aged 40 to 74.

Diabetes Management

Diabetes is not curable; it has to be managed. Treatment is designed to maintain as near-normal blood glucose levels as possible (referred to as *glycemic control*). Studies show that control of the blood sugar levels slows the progression of the complications of diabetes. People with diabetes juggle three factors to maintain near-normal blood glucose levels:

- Insulin or oral glucose-lowering medications
- Food
- Exercise

The guiding principle is that food (especially carbohydrate) increases blood glucose levels, while insulin and exercise lower them. When these three factors are not balanced properly, hyperglycemia can result, with uncomfortable symptoms and the ongoing risk of complications. Occasionally, these three factors become unbalanced in the other direction, causing low blood sugar, or **hypoglycemia**. Characterized by dizziness and weakness, hypoglycemia may occur when medications or exercise are in excess and/or there is not enough food consumed. In other words, factors at play are reducing blood sugar levels too well. Treatment for hypoglycemia is quick administration of foods containing glucose that is absorbed quickly, such as orange juice or corn syrup.

In some healthcare facilities, a diabetes management team may provide care for clients. This team usually includes a registered dietitian, a registered nurse, a physician, and other healthcare professionals, along with the client. Together, team members perform an assessment, set goals, implement a nutrition intervention, and evaluate and monitor results. Client education for individuals with diabetes is termed *diabetes self-management education (DSME)*. Many clients are taught conventional or intensive management, including the proper use of insulin or hypoglycemic agents, diet, exercise, and other aspects of self-care.

Insulin and Oral Hypoglycemic Agents

When the body is not producing enough insulin, a physician may prescribe insulin. Insulin, a protein, is normally injected several times each day. It can't be taken by mouth because the digestive enzymes will digest it. People with diabetes normally give themselves insulin by subcutaneous injection (below the skin) at different sites. Insulin may also be administered through an insulin pump, which delivers small doses to the body on a continual basis. The pump is surgically inserted through the abdomen. Sometimes, insulin preparations are combined in a drug regimen. Preparations of insulin vary by how quickly they act and for how long. Types of insulin include:

> **Rapid-acting insulin:** starts working in 5-20 minutes and finishes working in 3-5 hours. Examples include Humalog and Novolog.

> **Short-acting insulin:** starts working in 30 minutes and finishes working in 5-8 hours. Examples include Regular (R) insulin.

> **Intermediate-acting insulin:** starts working in 1-3 hours and finishes working in 16-24 hours. Examples include NPH (N) and Lente (L) insulin.

> **Long-acting insulin:** starts working in 4-6 hours and finishes working in 24-28 hours. Examples include Ultralente (U) insulin.

> **Very long-acting insulin:** starts working in 1 hour and finishes working in 24 hours. This type provides even control of blood glucose for 24 hours at a time. Examples include Lantus.

Oral hypoglycemic agents are drugs taken by mouth to lower blood glucose levels in individuals with Type 2 diabetes. Some also stimulate the body to produce more of its own insulin. Oral hypoglycemic agents are used only for Type 2 diabetes. Examples include: Glucophage, Metformin, Glyset, Precose, Prandin, Starlix, and Glucovance. How these medicines work varies; each is a little bit different. Some need to be taken with meals, while others do not. With some, it is important to avoid alcohol, which may cause stomach upset. Some varieties of oral hypoglycemic medicines come in an extended release form, which provides fairly even control of blood sugar over a long period of time. Typically, these are taken once per day. Other medicines may be prescribed for two or three doses per day, taken at specific times. With insulin as well as with oral medicines, meals must be planned in conjunction with a medication schedule to optimize control and prevent hypoglycemia. For example, a dose of medicine that has fairly rapid action on blood glucose could lead to hypoglycemia for a client who does not eat a meal shortly afterwards.

Medical Nutrition Therapy

The goals of medical nutrition therapy are as follows:

- Maintain as near-normal blood glucose levels as possible.
- Achieve optimal blood lipid levels.
- Provide enough calories to maintain or attain reasonable weight.
- Prevent and treat short-term and long-term complications of diabetes.
- Improve overall health through proper nutrition.

A diabetic diet needs to be custom-tailored to the individual based on type of diabetes, medication(s), nutritional status and needs, weight management objectives, medical treatment goals, food preferences, culture, age, ability to understand the diet, and lifestyle. Meal planning approaches include the Food Guide Pyramid, Exchange Lists, and Carbohydrate Counting. In any plan, recommendations are to provide a caloric breakdown as follows:

- 50-60% of total calories from carbohydrate, with up to 10% of total calories being from sugar (The remainder should come from high starch foods, which are more nutrient-dense.)
- 30% of total calories from fat, with no more than 10% of total calories from saturated fat
- 15-20% of total calories from protein

Food Guide Pyramid

The Food Guide Pyramid can provide an excellent resource for meal planning. In addition to following Pyramid guidelines, individuals with diabetes should:

- Eat meals and snacks at regular times every day.
- Eat about the same amount of food each day.
- Try not to skip meals or snacks.
- Check blood sugar about 1.5-2 hours after eating to be sure they are not overdoing carbohydrates. The American Diabetes Association suggests 180 mg/dl as a good upper limit for this.

The American Diabetes Association also offers a list of tips and suggestions for managing diabetes using the Food Guide Pyramid. For more information, visit their website, listed in Appendix A.

Exchange System

The exchange system classifies foods into groups according to how much protein, fat, and carbohydrate they contain. Serving sizes are specified, too. These groups are called **exchange lists**. This creates a system in which foods within any given group can be swapped or *exchanged* for others in the same group. Any of these trades provides about the same amount of protein, fat, and carbohydrate. Of course, with these three macronutrients being equal, calories are about equal, too. The exchange system is a tool for managing a diet that has a controlled amount of each macronutrient, in controlled proportions, such as 15% protein, 30% fat, and 55% carbohydrate. Detailed Exchange Lists for Meal Planning appear in Appendix B. There are seven exchange lists: starch, fruit, milk, other carbohydrates, vegetables, meat and meat substitutes, and fat. A nutrition caregiver sets up an appropriate meal plan in consultation with the client. A typical plan lists how many exchanges of each food group may be eaten at each meal and snack. An exchange plan requires education for the client and others involved in meals. It requires a client to keep careful track of food at every sitting, and to measure food—at least until serving sizes become familiar. As with the Food Guide Pyramid, this system does not require one exchange or serving per meal. For example, an individualized exchange diet may call for two servings from the starch group, one serving from the fruit group, and one-half serving from the milk group at breakfast. Translated into food, this might be:

- 1 whole English muffin (2 exchanges)
- ½ cup of orange juice (1 exchange)
- ½ cup of skim milk (½ exchange)

One challenge of using the exchange system is that many people do not eat single foods. Instead, they mix and combine foods into stews, casseroles, fajitas, pizza, and much more. Learning to count combination dishes requires education and sometimes nutritional analysis. The American Diabetes Association provides references for counting combination foods in an exchange system. In an exchange system, some basic advice still holds true: It's important to choose a variety of foods to provide needed nutrients.

Carbohydrate Counting

For clients who want more freedom and more flexibility than the exchange system, carbohydrate counting may work well. This approach was one of the meal planning methods used in the Diabetic Control and Complications Trial (DCCT) conducted by The National Institutes of Health from 1983-93. The total amount of carbohydrate is more important than where it comes from. The key is keeping the total carbohydrate content of the meal the same. Foods high in carbohydrate include:

rice	fruit juice	cake
pasta	starchy vegetables	pie
breads	milk	chocolate
cereals	milk products	table sugar
crackers	candy	honey
fruit	cookies	syrup

Carbohydrate grams can be counted by reading nutrition labels, using tables of nutrient content of foods, or using the exchange lists. In the exchange lists, one exchange of starch, fruit, or milk each has about 15 grams of carbohydrate. One exchange of each of these foods is called one carbohydrate choice. A meal plan can then be worked out that sets a specific number of carbohydrate choices at each meal or snack for the day.

For an individual who needs 1,800 calories, 225-270 grams of carbohydrate would be needed to meet the 50-60% of daily caloric intake from carbohydrate. This would mean 15-18 carbohydrate choices per day would be divided for the meals and snacks needed. The total number of meals and snacks, as well as the timing, is based on the individual's nutritional needs, lifestyle, and type of medication. Anyone following a carbohydrate counting plan needs to recognize that this is only a part of a healthful eating scheme. By focusing on carbohydrate alone, some clients may forget about limiting fat, or consuming adequate vitamins, minerals, and fiber. The Food Guide Pyramid, Dietary Guidelines for Americans, or similar guidance helps address overall wisdom in developing a healthy diet.

Exercise

A physician needs to approve an exercise program before a person with diabetes starts the program. This is because when an individual with uncontrolled diabetes (indicated by blood glucose levels of 240 to 300 mg/dl) exercises, the liver releases additional glucose and the hyperglycemia worsens. On the other hand, individuals with good blood glucose control (under 150 to 180 mg/dl) can benefit in many ways from exercising. Exercise lowers blood glucose levels because muscle cells use more glucose. Regular exercise results in greater sensitivity of the body to insulin and increases glucose tolerance. Exercise is especially helpful in decreasing cardiovascular risk factors and promoting weight loss. Some individuals with Type 2 diabetes gradually achieve better blood glucose control through weight loss. Individuals using conventional management are usually advised to eat a snack with 10-15 grams of carbohydrate before moderate exercise of an hour or less.

Monitoring

In order to keep an eye on how well the client is maintaining glycemic control, caregivers monitor the following variables:

- Blood sugar levels: People with diabetes routinely do self-monitoring of blood glucose (SMBG) by pricking the skin and then applying a drop of blood to a reagent strip. A glucose meter will read the sugar in the blood and display the blood glucose level. How often a person with diabetes does SMBG depends on the type of diabetes, the degree of glycemic control, and the treatment regimen (medication, diet, exercise).
- Blood lipid levels to include total cholesterol, LDL, HDL, and triglycerides.
- Glycosylated hemoglobin: Hemoglobin is the part of the red blood cell that carries oxygen. During the life span of a red blood cell, glucose in the blood binds to hemoglobin A, the major form of hemoglobin in the red blood cell. When glucose binds to hemoglobin A, the hemoglobin is said to be glycosylated. Glycosylated hemoglobin values reflect average blood glucose levels during the past six to 12 weeks, and they are a useful indicator of how well a client is controlling his/her blood glucose level. Normal values for the laboratory used by your institution should be consulted.
- Body weight.

Follow-up is needed at least every six to 12 months for adults and every three to six months for children to assure good control of blood sugar, to evaluate any changes or complications, and to reinforce education.

MEDICAL NUTRITION THERAPY OF OVERWEIGHT AND OBESITY

Americans trying to lose weight have plenty of company. Tens of millions of Americans are dieting at any given time, spending billions of dollars every year on weight-reduction products, such as diet foods and drinks. Overweight and obesity are among the most prevalent health problems in the US today.

Obesity is a medical affliction, not a moral failing. According to the Institute of Medicine, obesity is a disease involving genetic, environmental, psychological, and other factors. There is no single cause for obesity, and therefore no single cure. It occurs when energy intake exceeds the amount of energy expended over time. Over time, every 3,500 excess calories become one extra pound of body weight. Only in a small minority of cases is obesity caused by illness, such as hypothyroidism, or by medications, such as steroid hormones, which cause weight gain.

Chapter 8 provides more detail about evaluating body weight and determining what is ideal for a given individual. Research suggests that the location of body fat also is an important factor in health risks for adults. Excess fat in the abdomen (stomach area) is a greater health risk than excess fat in the hips and thighs. Extra fat in the abdomen is linked to high blood pressure, diabetes, early heart disease, and certain types of cancer. Smoking and too much alcohol increase abdominal fat and the risk for diseases related to obesity. Vigorous exercise helps to reduce abdominal fat and decrease the risk for these diseases. Waist-to-hip ratio can be calculated by dividing the number of inches around the waistline by the circumference of the hips. For example, someone who has a 27-inch waist and 38-inch hips would have a ratio of 0.71. A woman whose ratio is 0.8 or higher would be at high risk of weight-related health problems (such as heart disease, hypertension, and diabetes), as would a man whose ratio is 0.95 or above.

Overweight individuals who lose even relatively small amounts of weight are likely to:

- Lower their blood pressure
- Reduce abnormally high levels of blood glucose
- Bring blood levels of cholesterol and triglycerides down to more desirable levels
- Reduce sleep apnea, or irregular breathing during sleep
- Decrease the risk of osteoarthritis
- Decrease depression
- Improve appearance and self-esteem

Treatment of Obesity

Obesity has been and continues to be resistant to treatment. The prospect of attaining and maintaining normal weight is very low—about 5%. Preventing obesity is a preferable approach to reversing it. Because many factors affect how much or how little food a person eats and how that food is used, losing weight is not simple. A comprehensive approach to treating obesity focuses on the whole person, rather than just the extra weight that needs to be shed. Treatment success is measured not only by the number of pounds lost, but also by other factors, such as improved self-image. Components of this approach typically include nutrition education, exercise, behavior modification, attitude modification, social support, and maintenance support.

More and more health professionals are adopting a non-dieting approach to obesity. This approach steers clear of dieting and emphasizes helping clients adopt a healthier lifestyle. In many cases, diets simply don't work. By restricting food intake, diets can lead to unmanageable hunger and obsession with food, which may lead to binge eating. Those who follow extremely low-calorie regimens essentially starve their bodies. The body may also respond by reducing basal energy expenditure as a response to perceived starvation. The result is

Figure 6.12

CALORIES AND EXERCISE

ACTIVITY	CALORIES BURNED PER HOUR	ACTIVITY	CALORIES BURNED PER HOUR
Bicycling, 6 mph	240	Swimming, 25 yards/minute	275
Bicycling, 12 mph	410	Swimming, 50 yards/minute	500
Jogging, 5½ mph	740	Tennis, singles	400
Jogging, 7 mph	920	Walking, 2 mph	240
Jumping rope	750	Walking, 3 mph	320
Running in place	650	Walking, 4½ mph	440
Running, 10 mph	1,280		

These are calories expended by a 150-pound person. For a 100-pound person, reduce the calories by ⅓; for a 200-pound person, multiply by 1⅓.

Source: National Heart, Lung, and Blood Institute

that the body begins to require fewer calories. Anyone who follows an extremely restrictive diet or a low carbohydrate diet is likely to lose lean body mass (e.g. muscle) as well as fluid. This may look great on the scales, but it doesn't last, and isn't a healthy condition. A realistic weight loss plan avoids this yo-yo syndrome by targeting one to two pounds of weight loss per week. Knowing that 3,500 calories equal about one pound of fat, we can calculate that a daily change in energy balance of 500 calories totals to one pound of weight loss over one week. In other words, eating 500 calories less than usual each day through moderate food choices will result in a pound of fat lost after a week. An even better way to make this 500-calorie per day adjustment is to "burn" about 100 calories per day in additional exercise (see Figure 6.12) and eat 400 fewer calories. Eating fewer fat calories and exercising can help many obese people to lose some weight—and keep it off, too.

Nutrition Education

Anyone who wants to lose weight needs to understand several basic concepts of nutrition before planning a diet:

Calories should not be overly restricted during dieting because this practice decreases the likelihood of success. A progressive weight loss of one to two pounds a week is considered safe. For many dieters, the emphasis will be on decreasing fat calories and including nutrient-dense foods.

No foods should be forbidden, as that only makes them more attractive.

Eating regularly (not skipping meals) is crucial to minimize the possibility of getting overly hungry. People tend to overeat when hungry.

Portion control is vital. Measuring and weighing foods is helpful because "eyeballing" is not always accurate.

Variety, balance, and moderation are key to satisfying all nutrient needs.

Weighing oneself is important but should not be done every day because minor weight gains and losses can occur on a daily basis due to fluid shifts. Weekly weigh-ins are more meaningful and less likely to cause disappointment.

Exercise

Exercise is a vital component of any weight loss program. It may be more effective in reducing fat stores than dieting alone, and can result in significant weight loss even without eating less. Regular physical activity:

- Burns off calories to help lose extra pounds or maintain desirable weight
- Tones muscles
- Helps control appetite
- Helps in coping with stress
- Improves self-image
- Increases resistance to fatigue; energizes
- Helps counter anxiety and depression
- Promotes relaxation

Besides burning calories, an added bonus of a regular exercise regimen is that it helps shift the body's balance to include proportionally more muscle and less fat. In turn, this change in body composition increases the basal energy expenditure. Even at rest, a person with more muscle needs more calories. In short, exercise can help an overweight person feel and look better.

Behavior Modification

Behavior modification deals with identifying and changing behaviors that affect weight gain. Keeping a food diary helps to identify eating habits. A food diary is a daily record of types and amounts of foods and beverages consumed, as well as time and place of eating, with whom a person eats a meal, mood at the time, and degree of hunger. A diary can increase awareness about how and why a person eats. Once harmful patterns that encourage overeating are identified, the behavior can be changed to become more positive.

For example, overeating may occur in reaction to stressful situations, emotions, or cravings. A client can learn to handle these situations in new ways. Solutions may include exercising or using relaxation techniques to relieve stress; or switching to a new activity—such as taking a walk, knitting, or reading. Delay can also be effective. A client simply decides to wait five minutes before eating. A craving may dissipate during this time. Positive self-talk is important for good control. Instead of saying to oneself, "I cannot resist that cookie," a client can say, "I will resist that cookie." An understanding of causes of unhealthy eating, if applicable, forms a crucial basis for long-term weight management. Clients can use behavior modification to make long-lasting lifestyle changes.

Attitude Modification

The most common attitude problem obese people have is thinking they are either on or off a diet. Being "on a diet" implies that at some point the diet will be over, resulting in weight gain if old habits are resumed. Dieting should not be so restrictive and with such unrealistic goals that the person cannot wait to get "off the diet." When combined with exercise, behavior and attitude modification, social support, and a maintenance plan, dieting is really a plan of sensible eating that allows for periodic indulgences.

Setting realistic goals, followed by monitoring and self-reward when appropriate, is critical to the success of any weight loss program. Through goal setting, goals involving complex behavior changes can be broken down into a series of small, successive steps. Goals need to be reasonable and stated in a positive, behavioral manner. For example, if a problem behavior is buying a chocolate bar every afternoon at work, a goal may be to bring an appropriate afternoon snack in from home. If this goal is not truly attainable, perhaps one chocolate bar per week should be allowed and worked into the diet.

Even with reasonable goals, occasional lapses in behavior occur. A constructive attitude is critical. After eating and drinking too much at a party one night, for example, feelings of guilt and failure are not uncommon. The solution is to accept the situation and simply continue as planned.

Two other attitudes concern hunger and foods that are "bad for you." Hunger is a physiological need for food, whereas appetite is a psychological need. Eating should be in response to hunger, not to appetite. Obese people frequently think certain foods are good for them and certain foods are bad. No food is inherently good or bad. Some foods do contain more nutrients per calorie, and some are empty calories with few nutrients. However, no food is so bad that is can never be eaten.

Social Support

In general, obese people are more likely to lose weight when their families and friends are supportive and involved in their weight loss plans. When possible, clients need to enlist the help of someone who is easy to talk to, understanding, and genuinely interested in helping. Partners can model good eating habits and give praise and encouragement. The client needs to tell the partner exactly how to be supportive by, for example, not offering high calorie snacks. Requests of the partner need to be specific and positive. For their help, partners should be rewarded.

Drugs and Surgery

In some situations, obesity becomes so severe that it threatens health, even in the immediate short-term. Or, it may be so difficult to manage that a physician feels more aggressive treatment is in order. These may be among the reasons that a physician will decide to prescribe drugs for weight loss. Fervent research continues on the mechanisms that cause obesity. Based on findings, which are plentiful and complex, researchers have developed some drugs that may alter appetite, feelings of fullness, and body metabolism. So far, experts agree there is no perfect diet drug. One drug currently approved by the FDA is Orlistat, which cuts down on the action of lipase. Lipase is an enzyme that helps the body digest fat. Reduced action from lipase results in less fat absorption. It's a way to change the bioavailability of fat in the diet. Other drugs include Sibutramine and Fenfluramine. Both of these affect body chemicals in the brain, such as one called serotonin, to regulate appetite. Over-the-counter drugs and herbal supplements also exist for weight loss. One over-the-counter drug, phenylpropanolamine, can cause serious side effects and stroke. The FDA issued a public health advisory about this drug in 2000, and a ban may be forthcoming. Some consumers turn to herbal products for help, mistakenly assuming they are entirely safe. One herb that has caused heart palpitations, heart attacks, seizures, psychiatric crises, and even death is ephedra, also known as Ma Huang. The FDA has has banned this supplement from use.

Surgery for obesity is an extreme measure. One technique, *gastric bypass surgery*, actually reduces the size of the stomach. It makes eating very much food at one time difficult, because the smaller stomach becomes full easily. About 80% of patients lose weight following gastric bypass, but only 30% attain a desirable weight. Over time, many patients re-gain weight. This dramatic procedure requires long-term behavior change, as does any approach to weight management.

Menu Planning for Weight Loss and Maintenance

Without drugs, surgery, or non-existent miracle cures, an individual who wishes to lose weight is back to commonsense nutrition. While it's not as exciting—or expensive—as many approaches in the marketplace, a gradual approach to dietary change can have lasting effects on weight control. This is a big advantage over dramatic treatments, many of which tend to produce only temporary results. A commonsense approach combines regular exercise with reduced caloric intake to shift the balance of calories and achieve weight loss. One tool for nutritional planning is the weight loss pyramid described in Chapter 3 (Figure 3.10). The following advice can be useful:

- Eat a variety of foods that are low in calories and high in nutrients.
- Eat less fat and fewer high fat foods.
- Eat smaller portions and limit second helpings of foods high in fat and calories.

- Eat more vegetables and fruits without fats and sugars added in preparation or at the table.
- Eat pasta, rice, breads, and cereals without fats and sugars added in preparation or at the table.
- Eat less sugar and fewer sweets (like candy, cookies, cake, soda).
- Drink less or no alcohol.

Maintenance Support

Only recently has weight maintenance started to receive the attention it deserves as a crucial component of a weight loss program. Unfortunately, little is known about factors associated with weight maintenance success or what support is needed during the first few months of weight maintenance, when a majority of dieters begin to relapse. Being at a normal, or more normal, weight can bring about stress, as adjustments are needed. Food is no longer a focal point, and old friends and activities may not fit very well into the new lifestyle. Support and encouragement from significant others may diminish. A formal maintenance program can help deal with those issues as well as others.

GASTROINTESTINAL PROGRESSION DIETS

Often, surrounding surgery, testing, or various stresses and disorders affecting the gastrointestinal system, physicians will prescribe special diets such as a clear liquid diet, a full liquid diet, or a soft diet. Typically, these therapeutic diets are used temporarily.

Clear Liquid Diet

The clear liquid diet allows foods that are clear liquid foods or become clear liquid at room temperatures. Figure 6.13 lists foods included in a clear liquid diet, and Figure 6.14 shows a sample menu. The clear liquid diet may be used:

- After surgery (Usually it's the first diet because it is easily digested and absorbed.)
- Before surgery (Note that starting about eight hours before surgery, the clear liquid diet may end. At this time, all foods and fluids are usually withheld. This is to prevent vomiting while under anesthesia, which could lead to aspiration—when food, vomit, or other foreign substances accidentally enter the lungs.)
- Before various diagnostic tests (such as tests involving the intestinal tract, because the clear liquid diet helps keep the intestines clear)
- Following periods of vomiting, diarrhea, or other upset of the digestive tract
- In the acute stages of many illnesses, such as fever, when only the clear liquid diet may be tolerated
- To test the ability to tolerate oral feedings

Figure 6.13

FOODS INCLUDED IN A CLEAR LIQUID DIET

- Apple, grape, cranberry, or cranapple juice
- Strained orange or grapefruit juice
- Fruit punch, lemonade, limeade
- Carbonated beverages
- Clear broth, bouillon, consommé

- Flavored gelatin
- Fruit ice, popsicle
- Tea and coffee
- Sugar and salt

Figure 6.14

SAMPLE MENU FOR A CLEAR LIQUID DIET

BREAKFAST	LUNCH	DINNER
1 cup strained orange juice	1 cup apple juice	1 cup cranberry juice
½ cup gelatin	¾ cup clear broth	¾ cup consommé
2 tsp sugar	½ cup fruit ice	½ cup gelatin
1 cup coffee	2 tsp sugar	1 cup tea
12 oz ginger ale	1 cup tea	12 oz Sprite
	12 oz 7-up	

The clear liquid diet is intended to provide fluids, electrolytes, and some energy, with minimal stimulation of the digestive tract and minimal development of fecal material (also called residue). It is useful in preventing dehydration and relieving thirst. This diet is inadequate in all nutrients except vitamin C and should not be used for more than three days without supplementation.

Full Liquid Diet

The full liquid diet contains foods that are either liquid at room temperature or become liquid at room temperature. It differs from the clear liquid diet mostly by the addition of cereals and milk products. Figure 6.15 lists foods included in a full liquid diet, and Figure 6.16 shows a sample menu.

The full liquid diet is indicated in postoperative situations when the client has not fully recovered the ability to consume and tolerate solid food. In this case, a full liquid diet often acts as a transition between a clear liquid and soft or regular diet. It may also be indicated for clients who have esophageal or stomach disorders that interfere with the normal handling of solid foods.

The full liquid diet is adequate in calories, protein, vitamin C, calcium, sodium, and potassium. It is inadequate in iron, niacin, and folacin, and other nutrients. However, due to the limited selection of foods, a multivitamin and mineral

Figure 6.15

FOODS INCLUDED IN A FULL LIQUID DIET

- Carbonated beverages, coffee and tea (regular & decaffeinated), fruit drinks
- Milk and milk drinks, yogurt without seeds or nuts
- Pureed meat added to broth or cream soup
- Custard, gelatin desserts, smooth ice cream, sherbet, puddings, popsicle
- Cooked, refined cereal; mashed potatoes in cream soup
- All vegetable juices, pureed vegetables in soup

- All fruit juices
- Sugar, honey, syrup, clear hard candy
- Butter, margarine, cream, vegetable oils
- Consomme, broth, bouillon, strained soup made from allowed foods
- Salt
- Commercial liquid formulas that are nutritionally complete

Figure 6.16

SAMPLE MENU FOR A FULL LIQUID DIET

BREAKFAST
1 cup whole milk

1 cup eggnog

1 cup orange juice

½ cup cooked strained oatmeal

nondairy creamer

2 tsp sugar

1 T honey

salt

coffee

LUNCH
1 cup whole milk

1 cup vanilla milkshake

1 cup apple juice

nondairy creamer

¾ cup strained cream of potato soup

1 tsp sugar

½ cup sherbet

salt, pepper

tea

DINNER
1 cup whole milk

1 cup chocolate milkshake

½ cup egg custard

1 cup cranberry juice

nondairy creamer

¾ cup strained vegetable beef soup

1 tsp sugar

salt, pepper

tea

supplement may be necessary if this diet is to be used for more than two weeks and a commercial liquid formula is not used.

Soft Diet (or "GI Soft Diet")

The soft diet is designed for use during transition from liquid to regular diet after surgery. It provides a modified consistency, but is also intended to be easy on the gastrointestinal tract during a sensitive time. Foods in a soft diet are:

- Soft in consistency (but not ground or chopped)
- Mildly spiced
- Moderately low in fiber content

Cooked vegetables and fruits without seeds or peels are allowed. Raw vegetables, highly seasoned or fried foods, and nuts and seeds are not allowed. This diet must be individualized to each client.

MODIFIED CONSISTENCY DIETS

Some clients have difficulty chewing or swallowing due to surgery, loosely-fitting dentures, missing teeth, inadequate saliva production (this commonly occurs in aging), mouth injury or infection, surgery of the head and neck, or stroke. Depending on the nature and severity of the problem, any of the following diets that are modified in consistency may be needed: full liquid diet (as described above), puree diet, mechanical soft diet, or dysphagia diet. Each is described below.

Puree Diet

The puree diet includes foods that require very little, if any, chewing. It may be recommended for alert clients with impaired ability to chew or swallow. Because pureed foods do not look very appetizing, many hospital and nursing home cooks and managers are making efforts to improve the appearance of pureed diets. For example, some cooks use thickeners to make pureed foods cohesive and then shape them to look like the original foods. Although there are several commercial thickeners available, some cooks use thickeners such as cornstarch or instant mashed potato flakes. Many of the commercial food thickeners are powdered and can be mixed directly with liquids and pureed foods.

Mechanical Soft Diet

The mechanical soft diet is a modification of the regular diet, and consists of foods that are easy to chew. Figure 6.17 lists guidelines for a mechanical soft diet. It includes many of the foods on the regular diet, simply modified for consistency. Because each client's need for chopped or ground foods will vary, this diet must be individualized to each client.

Dysphagia Diets

Dysphagia means difficulty swallowing. A number of signs may suggest a problem with dysphagia:

- Oral leaking or drooling
- Choking or gagging
- Pocketing food (capturing it in the cheeks)
- Taking longer than two to 10 seconds to swallow
- Weakness, poor motivation
- Poor chewing ability, which may lead to choking on food

If any of these signs occurs, the client may need further evaluation to avoid severe choking or aspiration. This information should be referred to the dietitian or nursing supervisor so the speech pathologist can be notified. In all, up

GUIDELINES FOR A MECHANICAL SOFT DIET

▶ Meat and poultry must be ground, chopped, or moist and tender. Ground meats can be used in soups, stews, and casseroles. Cooked dried beans and peas, soft cheeses, and eggs are additional softer protein sources. Fish must be flaked.

▶ Cook vegetables thoroughly, without skins, and dice or chop by hand if necessary before or after cooking.

▶ Serve mashed potatoes or rice with gravy if desired.

▶ Salads are possible if chopped.

▶ Soft fruits such as fresh bananas, berries, or melon; and canned peaches, pears, or applesauce are some possible choices.

▶ Soft breads can be made even softer by removing the crust.

▶ Puddings and custard are good dessert choices.

▶ Many foods that are not soft can be easily chopped by hand or blended in a blender or food processor to allow a wider variety of foods.

▶ No nuts or seeds are allowed, as they are hard to chew.

to 14% of hospitalized patients and up to 50% of residents in nursing homes may be experiencing a form of dysphagia. Dysphagia may be caused by stroke, neurological disease, dementia, or other factors. It poses the danger of aspiration and choking, while also increasing the likelihood of dehydration and malnutrition over time. There are many variations of dysphagia; it's a very individualized condition. A speech pathologist can perform an in-depth evaluation of swallowing, and recommend the type of dietary treatment required.

There is no universal diet for clients with dysphagia. One misconception about dysphagia clients is that foods need to be thin and liquid in order to be swallowed. On the contrary, liquids (especially thin liquids) are usually harder to swallow than solid foods. As needed, liquids can be thickened to nectar, honey, or pudding consistency. Pre-thickened liquids or thickening products on the market can help in providing appropriate foods.

The **National Dysphagia Diet (NDD)**, now the national standard for dietary treatment of dysphagia, accounts for modifications in food textures, as well as liquids. Based on evaluation, a customized dysphagia diet recommendation contains two specifications: one for food texture, and a second one for liquids. Thus, a dysphagia diet may be specified as: NDD 3 or Dysphagia Advanced with thin liquids, or NDD Level 1 or Dysphagia Pureed with honey-like liquids. Figure 6.18 describes NDD guidelines.

When clients have swallowing problems, the speech pathologist may encourage special positioning and other suggestions to help ease swallowing during

Figure 6.18

NATIONAL DYSPHAGIA DIET

NDD Food Texture Levels: NDD Level 1 • Dysphagia Pureed
Smooth pureed, homogenous, very cohesive, pudding-like foods that require very little chewing ability.

GENERAL GUIDELINES:

1. Bread should be pre-gelled through the entire thickness, pureed or pureed into other foods in accordance with recipes.

2. Fruits and vegetables should be pureed with no pulp, seeds or chunks.

3. Mashed potatoes should be served with gravy, sauce, butter or margarine to moisten.

4. Soups should be pureed smooth.

5. Avoid scrambled, fried or hard-boiled eggs. Souffles are allowed.

6. Avoid fruited yogurt, un-blenderized cottage cheese, peanut butter, and any food with lumps, including soups and hot cereal.

NDD Food Texture Levels: NDD Level 2 • Dysphagia Mechanically-Altered
Cohesive, moist, semisolid foods that require some chewing ability. Included in this level are fork-mashable fruits and vegetables. Excluded are most bread products, crackers, and other dry foods.

GENERAL GUIDELINES:

1. Bread should be pre-gelled through the entire thickness or pureed according to recipe.

2. Fruits should be soft, canned or cooked. Soft, ripe bananas are allowed. Avoid canned pineapple.

3. Vegetables should be soft, well cooked, easily mashed with a fork, and in pieces smaller than ½ inch.

4. Meat should be tender and moist, ground, or cubed smaller than ¼ inch. Moisten with gravy.

5. Avoid dry whole grain cereal with nuts, seeds and coconut.

6. Avoid items that are difficult to chew, including large chunks or nuts.

NDD Food Texture Levels: NDD Level 3 • Dysphagia Advanced
Soft-solid foods which require more chewing ability. This level is nearly regular textures. Included are easy-to-cut whole meats, fruits, and vegetables. Excluded are hard, crunchy fruits and vegetables, sticky foods, and very dry foods.

GENERAL GUIDELINES:

1. Breads and cereals should be well moistened.

2. Fruits such as bananas or soft, peeled fruits such as peaches, berries, nectarines, kiwi or melon without seeds may be tolerated.

3. Avoid potato skins, corn, and raw vegetables.

4. Meat must be very tender, small pieces, or ground, and well moistened.

5. Avoid items that are difficult to chew: nuts, seeds, popcorn, potato chips, coconut, etc.

NDD Food Texture Levels: NDD Level 4 • Regular
Any solid food texture

NATIONAL DYSPHAGIA DIET, *CONTINUED*

NDD Liquid Levels: Thin
Thin liquids include clear liquids, milk, commercial nutritional supplements, water, tea, coffee, soda, beer, wine, broth, and clear juice. Individuals tolerating thin liquids will also be able to tolerate foods containing thin liquids, such as watermelon, grapefruit or oranges. Foods like ice cream, frozen yogurt, or plain gelatin which turn to liquid in the mouth are also considered thin liquids.

NDD Liquid Levels: Nectar-like
Medium thickness liquids include nectars, vegetable juices, and handmade milkshakes or shakes made with thickeners. Thin liquids can be thickened with commercial thickeners or purchased pre-thickened to nectar-like thickness.

NDD Liquid Levels: Honey-like
Honey-like is thicker than the nectar-like level and resembles the consistency of honey at room temperature. Commercial thickeners can be added using package instructions to bring any liquids to this level of thickness or purchased commercially pre-thickened to honey-like thickness.

NDD Liquid Levels: Spoon-thick
This includes high viscosity liquids too thick for a straw. Commercial thickeners can be added to any beverage to obtain this level of thickness or purchased commercially pre-thickened to spoon-thick.

Reprinted from Dining with Dysphagia, by Carlene Russell, MS, RD, LD, FADA. The Master Track Series, Dietary Managers Association, 2003.

meals. In general, positioning residents as close to a 90-degree angle as possible makes swallowing easier and safer. If clients are in bed, you may need to support their heads, backs, necks, and sides. It may also be helpful to wait for the client to swallow prior to placing any more food in the mouth, and alternate solids and liquids.

Finger Food Diet
The Finger Food Diet has existed for many years. However, the increased attention to this diet is due to the emphasis on maintaining quality of life by providing additional rehabilitation services. Finger foods are useful for residents with physical or functional impairments who have lost their ability to eat with utensils. They allow a resident to maintain independent eating ability, e.g. in the case of Alzheimer's disease.

The biggest obstacle with this diet may be family members who feel it is socially unacceptable to eat with fingers and beneath the dignity of the resident. If the family is not aware of the need to maintain independence in eating, they may believe it is more acceptable to eat with a spoon and/or be fed by staff. A team effort among the resident, family, dietary staff, speech therapy, and nursing will help make this diet a successful intervention.

The characteristics of finger foods include:

▶ Bite size pieces—not too large or too small
▶ Not too soft, squishy, slippery, or crumbly
▶ No thick, gooey sauces or gravy poured on the food

A finger food diet may include foods such as: pudding in an ice cream cone, chicken nuggets, sandwiches cut into quarters, cold cereals formed in large pieces, bar cookies, donuts, turnovers, peanut butter on crackers, tater tots or baked potatoes cut into pieces, batter-dipped vegetables, corn on the cob, thin soup served in a mug, popcorn, bite-sized fruit or vegetable pieces.

LACTOSE INTOLERANCE

Lactose intolerance is a condition caused by inadequate amounts of lactase in the body. *Lactase* is an enzyme needed by the intestine to digest lactose, the form of sugar that appears in milk and other dairy products. **Food intolerance** is an important term that describes unfavorable reactions to foods. Often, these reactions are uncomfortable but not dangerous. Symptoms of lactose intolerance include abdominal cramps, bloating, and diarrhea, which can start about 30 minutes to two hours after ingesting milk products. Symptoms stem from the activity of intestinal bacteria that digest the lactose and produce gas and acid. The symptoms normally clear up within two to five hours.

Certain groups of people are more susceptible to lactose intolerance than others, e.g. Asian Americans, Native Americans, Latinos, and African Americans. Individuals suffering from lactose intolerance vary tremendously as to severity of symptoms. Most can drink small amounts of milk without any symptoms, especially if eaten with other foods. Chocolate milk and whole milk are sometimes better tolerated than skim or 2% milk, due to variations in fat content and the presence of other sugars which may delay emptying of the stomach. Lactose-reduced milk and other modified dairy products are available, as is the enzyme lactase, which can be added to milk to reduce the lactose content. Eight fluid ounces of lactose-reduced milk contain only three grams of lactose, compared with 12 grams in regular milk. Lactase enzyme is available at pharmacies and many supermarkets.

Although most dairy foods (such as milk, ice cream, cottage cheese, eggnog, and cream) contain much lactose, some contain less. Yogurt is often well tolerated because it is cultured with live bacteria that digest lactose. This is not always the case with frozen yogurt, because most of it does not contain nearly the number of bacteria that are found in fresh yogurt. Also, some yogurts have milk solids added to them that can cause problems. Hard cheeses contain very little lactose and usually do not cause symptoms because most of the lactose is removed during processing, or is digested by the bacteria used in making certain cheeses. Anyone who suffers lactose intolerance may be at risk for consuming inadequate calcium, as milk and dairy products are the chief sources in most diets. Without a comfortable alternative, many lactose-intolerant individuals may need to take calcium supplements.

Lactose intolerance is not an allergy. A **food allergy** is an immune system response to specific proteins in foods, and it can be life-threatening. True milk allergy is less common than lactose intolerance. For more information about food allergy, see *Nutrition in the News* (Food Allergy) at the end of this chapter.

Gastroesophageal Reflux Disease (GERD)

Gastroesophageal reflux disease (GERD) or reflux esophagitis is the medical term for what many people call acid indigestion or heartburn. As described in Chapter 4, a muscle called the lower esophageal sphincter relaxes to let food into the stomach, and then closes immediately so the acidic stomach contents won't go back up the esophagus. When this muscle doesn't close tightly, the acidic stomach contents splash up into the esophagus, causing irritation. This irritation is described as acid indigestion or heartburn. Reflux esophagitis frequently develops due to aging. It can also be caused by a condition called a hiatal hernia. Normally the lower esophageal sphincter sits right in the diaphragm, a strong muscle that separates the abdominal cavity from the chest cavity. The esophagus is above the diaphragm and the stomach is below it. In the case of a hiatal hernia, part of the stomach extends up through the diaphragm into the chest cavity. Because the diaphragm no longer reinforces the esophageal sphincter, stomach contents reflux into the esophagus.

Unfortunately, reflux esophagitis can do much more harm than just causing a burning sensation. Chronic heartburn can result in inflamed and scarred tissue in the esophagus, which can reduce its inner diameter. This is known as esophageal stricture. Cells that line the esophagus can eventually become cancerous.

Nutritional care goals include reducing gastric acidity and preventing esophageal reflux. Treatment for reflux esophagitis often includes the following:

- Avoid/limit foods that irritate the esophagus: citrus fruits and juice, tomatoes, spicy foods (especially chili powder and black pepper), and coffee.
- Avoid/limit foods that decrease pressure: alcohol; caffeine-containing drinks such as coffee, tea, and cola soft drinks; chocolate, peppermint, spearmint, and fat.
- Eat smaller amounts of food at meals. Drink most fluids between meals.
- Reduce fat intake. High-fat meals empty from the stomach slowly.
- Wait two to three hours after eating a meal to lie down or exercise.

▶ Wear clothing that does not constrict the waist or abdomen, so as not to increase the upward pressure on the lower esophageal sphincter.

▶ Refrain from stooping over; instead bend from the knees.

▶ Elevate the head of the bed.

▶ Reduce weight if overweight because obesity increases pressure within the stomach.

▶ Avoid smoking.

In addition, physicians may prescribe any of a variety of medications to help control GERD, including antacids and drugs that prevent acid production in the stomach.

GASTRITIS AND PEPTIC ULCER DISEASE

Gastritis is a painful inflammation of the mucosal lining of the stomach. The top layer of cells lining the stomach, called the mucosa, protects the stomach lining from the acidic gastric juices. Gastritis symptoms may include nausea, vomiting, anorexia, pain, bleeding, and belching.

Gastritis may be either acute (meaning it has a relatively short duration) or chronic (meaning it lasts a long time). Food allergies, overeating, chronic doses of aspirin or nonsteroidal anti-inflammatory drugs (such as ibuprofen), radiation therapy, stress, and/or infections can cause acute gastritis. Nutritional care generally includes withholding food for one to two days to let the stomach rest and heal.

Chronic gastritis is often seen in elderly populations. As this type of gastritis progresses, stomach cells become smaller in size, stomach secretions decrease, and production of intrinsic factor (needed for vitamin B12 absorption) falls. Nutritional care for chronic gastritis involves an individualized diet that avoids foods causing discomfort.

Ulcers affect more than 25 million Americans at some point in their lives, according to the National Institutes of Health. Ulcer sufferers describe an ulcer as a burning, cramping, gnawing, or aching in the abdomen that comes in waves, for three to four days at a time, but may subside completely for weeks or months. Pain is worst before meals and at bedtime, when the stomach is usually empty.

Mention "ulcer" and most people envision a stressed-out, workaholic, junk food-gobbling worrier. But that image is substantially incorrect. Now, the medical community views painful ulcers in a new light—as an easily treatable bacterial infection. The name of the bacteria is Helicobacter pylori. The ulcer itself in an open sore in the lining of the stomach (called a gastric ulcer) or in the first few centimeters of the duodenum (called a duodenal ulcer). The mucosa is eroded away, exposing the underlying submucosa, which is rich in nerves and blood vessels. Ulcers therefore cause pain and possibly bleeding. Both types of ulcers are termed *peptic ulcer disease (PUD)*, which means chronic inflammation of the stomach and duodenum.

Treatment for peptic ulcers generally includes anti-secretory drugs (drugs that reduce the amount of acid secreted in the stomach), antibiotics, antacids, and nutritional care. Examples of anti-secretory drugs used in peptic ulcer disease include Tagamet (cimetidine), Pepcid (famotidine), and Zantac (ranitidine hydrochloride). The use of antibiotics to remove Helicobacter pylori prevents most peptic ulcers from recurring.

The nutritional care goals for PUD revolve around reducing and neutralizing stomach acid secretion and limiting discomfort. These goals can be met by:

- Avoiding any foods or beverages that cause indigestion (in medical terms, indigestion is called *dyspepsia*)
- Eating small, frequent meals and avoiding large meals that cause stomach distention
- Following a bland diet

The foods allowed on the bland diet have changed over the years, and now the diet is much more liberal. Because of the success of drugs and antacids in reducing gastric acid levels, this diet is not recommended often, and may be nearly obsolete. A bland diet usually excludes the following gastric stimulants:

- Alcohol
- Regular and decaffeinated coffee
- Red and black pepper

Like many other diets, the bland diet needs to be individualized to meet each client's needs.

CONSTIPATION

Constipation is among the most common gastrointestinal problems in the US, and it accounts for 2 million visits to the doctor every year, according to the National Institutes of Health. **Constipation** is passage of small amounts of hard, dry bowel movements, usually fewer than three times a week. Bowel movements may be difficult and/or painful. Some people also experience a feeling of being bloated.

Because the gastrointestinal system tends to slow down with aging, occurrence of constipation is common in older Americans. It is also more common among individuals who have limited mobility, as imposed by an injury, disability, or medical condition. Constipation can be an after effect of stroke, or a side effect of various neurological disorders. It may also occur in certain hormonal disorders, gastrointestinal disorders, and other conditions. In addition, lifestyle habits can influence constipation. Infrequent exercise, low intake of dietary fiber, high intake of fat, and low intake of fluids can all contribute to constipation. Laxative abuse can also trigger constipation. Laxatives are considered habit-forming, and can damage nerve cells in the colon and interfere with the colon's natural ability to contract. Likewise, frequent use of enemas can diminish normal bowel functioning. Furthermore, many medications can cause constipation; it's a common side effect of drugs such as narcotics, antacids, antidepressants, blood pressure medications, antispasmodics, and even dietary iron supplements. Individuals who change the consistency of their diets because of chewing or swallowing problems may inadvertently reduce dietary fiber intake, too.

Treatments for constipation include diet, laxatives, stool softeners, and drugs that stimulate bowel contractions, such as Correctol, Dulcolax, Purge, and Senokot. Exercise may also be a component of treatment. A diet that helps to correct constipation includes 20-35 grams of fiber daily and adequate fluid intake.

NAUSEA AND VOMITING

Nausea is an unpleasant feeling in the stomach, accompanied by an urge to vomit. A number of medical conditions and medications can prompt nausea. Because nauseous clients do not feel like eating, nausea that lasts for more than a few days can create nutritional concerns. Figure 6.19 lists suggestions to combat nausea.

Whereas a muscular process called peristalsis normally moves foods down the gastrointestinal tract, vomiting occurs when the waves of peristalsis reverse direction. Vomiting is often seen as a symptom of a disease or of the body's equilibrium being upset, such as on a ship. Vomiting is the body's way to get rid of an irritating substance, and is not dangerous unless large amounts of

---

Figure 6.19

SUGGESTIONS FOR DEALING WITH NAUSEA AND VOMITING

- Smaller meals seem to work. They are easier to digest and get through the stomach faster.
- Eat more frequently.
- Avoid liquids at mealtimes. Take them between meals.
- Clear, cool beverages are recommended. Sip liquids slowly. Enjoy a popsicle or ice cubes made of any kind of favorite liquid.
- Dry carbohydrate foods, such as toast or crackers, are helpful after getting up in the morning.
- Do not lie down flat for at least two hours after eating.
- Loose clothing and fresh air can help.

fluids are lost. The best advice for simple cases of vomiting includes at least four hours of no food or water, followed by drinking small amounts of fluid as tolerated and resting. When vomiting is more prolonged and therefore serious, medical care to replace lost fluids and restore electrolyte balance is essential.

INFLAMMATORY BOWEL DISEASE

Inflammatory bowel disease (IBD) includes two conditions with similar symptoms and clinical management: Crohn's disease and ulcerative colitis. The causes for either disease are not known, and there is no cure. They often first show up between 15 and 30 years of age, but may continue for a lifetime.

Crohn's disease, also called regional enteritis, is characterized by long-term, progressive inflammation of sections of the intestinal tract and lesions in the mucosal wall of the small intestine, large intestine, and/or rectum. The lesions often go through the entire intestinal wall. Chronic inflammation can cause fistulas (abnormal passages from an internal organ to a body surface or to another internal organ), abscesses (localized inflammation), and obstruction. Symptoms include persistent diarrhea, abdominal pain, fatigue, malabsorption, weight loss, anemia, fever, and anorexia.

During acute phases of Crohn's disease, enteral and parenteral nutrition may be used particularly if the client has part of the intestines surgically removed. Once the acute phase closes, medical nutrition therapy often includes a diet high in protein (due to the protein losses from the mucosal lesions and poor dietary intake) and calories (due to weight loss commonly seen). Fiber is generally limited if intestines are inflamed, and fat is limited if it is not being absorbed properly. Any other offending foods, such as milk in the case of lactose intolerance, should be omitted. Supplemental vitamins and minerals are often used.

Ulcerative colitis is a disease that causes inflammation and sores, called ulcers, in the lining of the large intestine. Ulcerative colitis usually affects the lower part of the colon. Inflammation destroys intestinal cells, resulting in ulcers. Intestinal mucosa become so fragile that they bleed easily. Symptoms include painful diarrhea (often bloody), rectal bleeding, dehydration, anorexia, and malnutrition.

During active phases of ulcerative colitis, bowel rest is often necessary, meaning the client cannot eat or drink anything by mouth. Once the client resumes eating, the same guidelines are used for ulcerative colitis as for Crohn's disease.

A high protein diet is one in which high protein snacks or supplements, such as from the dairy and meat groups, are given in addition to the regular diet. The diet consists of approximately 1.5 grams of protein/kilogram of body weight per day for an adult. An effective diet is also high in calories.

DIVERTICULAR DISEASE

Diverticulosis is a disease of the intestine in which the intestinal walls become weakened and bulge out into pockets called *diverticula*. (A single one of these pockets is called a *diverticulum*.) About 10% of Americans over 40, and half of Americans over 60 have diverticula. Most don't know it. There are no symptoms unless these pouches become infected or inflamed due to fecal matter collecting in the pockets. This condition develops in about 1 or 2 out of every 10 people who have diverticula, and is called diverticulitis. If the terminology seems confusing, consider this rule of medical terminology:

The word ending *osis* or *asis* means "presence of"
Diverticulosis means "presence of diverticula"

The word ending *itis* means "inflammation of"
Diverticulitis means "inflammation of diverticula"

This trick can help you understand and remember many other medical terms, such as gastritis (inflammation of the stomach), arthritis (inflammation of the joints), and others.

A low fiber diet, along with decreased strength of intestinal muscle walls that occurs during aging, probably explain why diverticula develop. Increased fiber is recommended to decrease the pressure in the intestine that causes the pockets to form. A high fiber diet (20-35 grams per day) is often prescribed.

While an individual with diverticulosis will benefit from a high fiber diet, this is not true for the acute, temporary condition of diverticulitis. Dietary treatment of diverticulitis often restricts fiber so that it doesn't add to the inflammation. Typically, this diet eliminates most fresh fruit (except ripe bananas) and raisins, substituting canned or cooked fruits without seeds. Fruit juices are allowed. Nuts, crunchy peanut butter, popcorn, wild rice, bran, whole grains, coconut, and other foods with small particles that could become trapped in diverticula are also omitted. Cooked or canned vegetables without skins or seeds are permitted. Dried beans (legumes), peas, sauerkraut, and winter squash are not. During this treatment, a patient may receive antibiotics. When the problem has resolved, an individual can usually return to a high fiber diet.

DIARRHEA AND IRRITABLE BOWEL SYNDROME

Diarrhea, frequent watery bowel movements, may be the result of emotional upset, food allergies, lactose intolerance, foodborne illness, gastrointestinal disease, medications, radiation therapy, or other conditions. Prolonged diarrhea can be serious, causing dehydration, weight loss, and malnutrition.

Diarrhea is often treated with a mixture of water, salts, and sugar, called *oral rehydration therapy (ORT)*. In serious cases of diarrhea, bowel rest may be necessary. This allows the gastrointestinal tract to heal. Fluid and electrolytes are given intravenously in these cases. After adequate bowel rest, the client may start on a clear liquid diet and slowly progress back to a regular diet. Lactose and any irritating foods are omitted from the diet.

Diarrhea alternating with constipation may be a sign of *irritable bowel syndrome (IBS)*, a condition of unknown cause that first presents itself around age 20. Other symptoms of irritable bowel syndrome are abdominal pain, bloating, gas, indigestion, nausea, and rectal pain. According to the National Institute of Diabetes & Digestive & Kidney Diseases, a whopping one-in-five adults suffers from irritable bowel syndrome. The good news, though, is that this condition does not lead to any serious harm. It really describes a cluster of gastrointestinal symptoms that are, unfortunately, common.

The National Institute of Diabetes & Digestive & Kidney Diseases says that the following have been associated with a worsening of IBS symptoms:

- Large meals
- Bloating from gas in the colon
- Medicines
- Wheat, rye, barley, chocolate, milk products, or alcohol
- Drinks with caffeine, such as coffee, tea, or colas
- Stress, conflict, or emotional upsets

Symptoms may respond to stress, and for women—to phases in the menstrual cycle. Dietary recommendations include a high fiber diet (unless diarrhea is present), adequate fluid intake, and smaller meals.

MALABSORPTION

Malabsorption describes a condition in which nutrients are not absorbed properly. We have already seen malabsorption of some nutrients in Crohn's disease and ulcerative colitis. Another disease associated with malabsorption is gluten-sensitive enteropathy.

Gluten-Sensitive Enteropathy (GSE)

Gluten-sensitive enteropathy (GSE) is also known as celiac disease or celiac sprue. Gluten is a protein present in wheat and some other grains. Gluten has two components: gliadin and glutenin. It is the gliadin fraction that causes serious damage to intestinal mucosa, causing malabsorption of many nutrients to occur. As the disease progresses, the villi of the intestinal mucosa are damaged. The end result of this damage is that the surface area for absorption of nutrients decreases by as much as 95%. Symptoms include diarrhea, weight loss, anemia, and other nutrient deficiencies.

The primary treatment for GSE is a gluten-free diet. A gluten-free diet often brings quick, dramatic results within days, followed by weight gain in about one week. Abnormal stools may take several weeks and abdominal distention even longer to disappear. It will take two to three months before the intestine regains its normal appearance.

This diet eliminates foods prepared with the grains wheat, rye, oats, and barley, buckwheat (also called kasha), quinoa, and millet—and flours made from any of the grains wheat, rye, oats, or barley. Arrowroot, corn, potato, rice, soybean, and low-gluten wheat starch flour may be used instead. When foods are selected properly, it is expected that the diet will be adequate in nutrients. Compliance with the gluten-restricted diet may decrease the risk of malignancy of the small intestine, which is a risk. A caregiver also needs to check labels for the following, and avoid these food ingredients:

- Graham
- Bulgur
- Triticale
- Malt and malt flavoring (unless made from corn)
- Starch (unless it is cornstarch)
- Modified food starch (unless it is made from arrowroot, corn, potato, tapioca, maize, or rice)
- Vegetable gums (unless carob or locust bean gum, cellulose or sugar gum, gum acacia, gum Arabic, gum tragacanth, xanthan gum, guar gum)
- Soy sauce and soy sauce solids unless made without wheat
- Hydrolyzed or texturized vegetable protein (allowed if made from corn or soy)
- Monosodium glutamate (MSG)

Nutrition counseling is the cornerstone of treatment for clients with GSE. The gluten-restricted diet is a difficult diet to follow, and requires intensive education and support.

TOOTH DECAY

The major health problems caused by eating sugary foods, and also starchy foods, are tooth decay and cavities (*dental caries*). The more often these foods—even small amounts—are eaten and the longer they are in the mouth before teeth are brushed, the greater the risk for tooth decay. This is because every time we eat something containing sugar or starch, the bacteria that naturally live on teeth produce acid for 20 to 30 minutes. This acid eats away at the teeth, and cavities may eventually develop. Eating sugary or starchy foods as frequent between-meal snacks may be more harmful to teeth than having them at meals. Foods such as dried fruits, candies, soda pop, breads, cereals, cookies, and crackers increase chances of dental caries when eaten frequently. Fruit chews and chewy candies are particularly troublesome. Foods that do not seem to cause cavities include some vegetables, meats, fish, aged cheeses, and nuts. To prevent cavities, it is important to brush teeth frequently and thoroughly, floss daily, and avoid chewy sweets.

FATTY LIVER, HEPATITIS, AND CIRRHOSIS

The liver, the largest organ in the body, has many important roles. Following are some of its functions:

- The liver converts blood glucose to fat and glycogen. The liver can also make glucose. The liver has an important role in regulating blood glucose levels.
- The liver makes triglycerides and cholesterol. It also excretes cholesterol in bile.
- The liver makes many of the proteins found in the blood, such as the proteins necessary for blood to clot after an injury.
- The liver removes drugs, hormones, and other molecules by excreting them in the bile.

Fatty liver, a condition in which triglycerides build up in the liver and cause it to swell, is often an early sign of more liver problems to come. Fatty liver most often occurs due to excessive alcohol intake, infection, or malignant disease. It can also be caused by certain drugs or by extremely low protein intake (to the point of protein malnutrition). Treatment for fatty liver centers on removing its cause, whether it be alcohol, drugs, or a poor diet. The effects of fatty liver can be reversed when the cause is eliminated.

Hepatitis is more serious than fatty liver, and refers to inflammation of the liver due to alcohol, viruses, drugs, toxins, or viral infection. Symptoms include low fever, fatigue, nausea, anorexia, vomiting, constipation or diarrhea. Symptoms cause malnutrition in some instances, particularly in cases of alcohol abuse. A high calorie, high protein diet is appropriate for malnourished clients, and fat soluble vitamins in water soluble form are often prescribed.

Cirrhosis is a term used for advanced stages of liver disease that occurs when fatty liver or hepatitis are not reversed. At this point, liver cells harden and die. The damage can't be reversed. The liver shrinks and is not able to complete all of its vital functions. Cirrhosis due to alcohol abuse is called Laennec's cirrhosis. It is the most common type of cirrhosis.

Symptoms of cirrhosis include nausea, anorexia, weight loss, weakness, iron-deficiency anemia, stomach pain, esophageal varices (blood vessels that project into the esophagus), steatorrhea (fat is malabsorbed and is found in the stool), and ascites. *Ascites* is the abnormal accumulation of fluid in the abdomen. The level of ammonia in the blood, which is toxic to the brain and nervous system, also increases.

When cirrhosis progresses to the point where the liver function has decreased to 25% or less, hepatic failure occurs. Liver failure is characterized by *jaundice*, a yellowing of the skin. Over time, liver failure results in *portal systemic encephalopathy (PSE)*, which affects the brain and is a life-threatening complication of liver failure. Symptoms range from confusion and poor coordination to flapping of the hands (called *asterixis*), and finally to loss of consciousness and coma.

Several laboratory tests help in evaluation of liver function. Elevated liver enzymes mean the liver cells are being destroyed and the enzymes are released into the blood. This suggests liver failure. Blood ammonia tests are also used as a measurement of the degree of liver failure. The liver converts proteins into amino acids. Ammonia is a byproduct. The liver converts ammonia into urea. Urea is excreted by the kidneys. When the liver is failing, it cannot convert ammonia to urea. Thus, high blood ammonia level is an early sign of liver failure. It may be accompanied by symptoms of confusion. A low protein diet may be part of the therapy at this point, because this minimizes the production of ammonia. In cases of hepatic coma, hepatic formulas that are low in a type of amino acid called aromatic amino acids, and high in branched-chain amino acids may be used.

Medical nutrition therapy for cirrhosis includes the following:

1. High calories (about 35 to 45 calories per kilogram body weight) due to frequent weight loss and increased energy needs due to disease.

2. High protein (1.0 to 1.5 grams of protein per kilogram body weight) due in part to protein being broken down for energy and a poor diet. Protein is restricted to 40 to 60 grams per day or less when the client is in, or close to being in, hepatic coma, because dietary protein adds to the ammonia level of the blood.

3. Moderate fat due to client's decreased ability to metabolize triglycerides. Fat is restricted when steatorrhea is present. Clients with steatorrhea are often given medium-chain triglyceride (MCT) oil. MCT oil is a readily absorbed form of fat.

4. Vitamin and mineral supplementation are almost always necessary due to malnutrition.

5. Fluid and sodium restrictions if ascites and edema are present. **Edema** is unhealthy water retention.

Gallbladder Disease

The liver also makes and secretes bile, a substance that aids in the digestion and absorption of fats. Bile is carried by ducts from the liver to the gallbladder. The gallbladder stores and concentrates bile until food is in the stomach and duodenum. Then the gallbladder contracts and bile travels to the duodenum.

There are various diseases of the gallbladder, such as gallstones (*cholelithiasis*), or inflammation of the gallbladder (*cholecystitis*), which is usually caused by gallstones. A low fat diet, usually interpreted to mean 40 grams of fat per day, may be used to treat these diseases in the hospital. Clients with chronic cholecystitis may need a long-term diet with 25 to 30% of calories from fat. Less fat in the diet results in fewer gallbladder contractions and less pain. Figure 6.20 outlines a fat-restricted diet. A client who has the gallbladder removed can progress as tolerated to a regular diet.

PANCREATITIS

Pancreatitis is an inflammation of the pancreas in which pancreatic enzymes are blocked from emptying, causing some of these strong enzymes to digest the pancreas itself. Pancreatitis can be either acute or chronic. Gallstones are the most common cause of acute pancreatitis, while alcohol abuse is a common cause of chronic pancreatitis. Symptoms include tender abdomen, nausea, vomiting, fever, and rapid pulse. Pancreatitis causes fat malabsorption and steatorrhea. When fat is lost in the stool, so are calories and fat-soluble vitamins.

During acute pancreatitis, oral feedings are usually withheld until the acute phase subsides to give the pancreas a rest, at which time the client may slowly progress as tolerated to a low fat diet. For clients with chronic pancreatitis, dietary treatment includes pancreatic enzyme replacements (taken orally with meals), a low fat diet, vitamin and mineral supplements, and MCT oil if steatorrhea is present.

RENAL DISEASE

The kidneys perform the vital function of maintaining the proper balance of water, electrolytes (sodium, potassium, and chloride), and acids in body fluids. This is done by secreting some substances into the urine and holding back others in the bloodstream for use in the body. In addition to forming urine, the kidneys also have an endocrine function, meaning they produce hormones. The kidneys secrete rennin (a substance that is important in maintaining normal blood pressure), erythropoietin (a hormone that regulates the production of red blood cells), and a form of vitamin D.

Certain conditions damage the cells of the kidneys, making it difficult for the kidneys to perform their jobs. **Renal failure** occurs when the kidneys fail to maintain normal fluid and electrolyte balance and to excrete waste products within normal limits. It may strike at any age, due to a variety of causes. Renal failure may occur over a period of time (chronic renal failure) or suddenly (acute renal failure). Acute renal failure may result from shock, burns, or severe injuries. It is often reversible.

Chronic renal failure (CRF) is not reversible, due to the progressive destruction of kidney tissue. Many diseases can damage the kidneys, such as *nephritis* (inflammation of the kidneys), high blood pressure, and complications of

Figure 6.20

FAT-RESTRICTED DIET FOR GALLBLADDER DISEASE

Type of Food	Include	Avoid
BEVERAGES	Skim milk or buttermilk made with skim milk, 1% milk, coffee, tea, fruit juice, soft drinks, cocoa made with cocoa powder and skim milk	Whole milk, evaporated and condensed milk, buttermilk made with whole milk, 2% milk, chocolate milk, cream (in excess of amounts allowed under fats)
CHEESES	¼ cup of low fat cottage cheese may be substituted for 1 oz of meat; low fat cheeses containing less than 5 g of fat/oz may be substituted for part of the meat allowance	Whole milk cheeses
EGGS	3 per week (prepared without fat), egg whites; as desired, low fat egg substitutes (1 egg equals 1 meat equivalent)	More than 1 per day (unless substituted for part of meat allowed)
MEAT, MEAT SUBSTITUTES	A 20 g fat diet will be limited to 3 lean meat equivalents/day; a 40 g fat diet will be limited to 5 lean meat equivalents/day; poultry without skin, fish (¼ cup water-packed tuna or salmon equals 1 equivalent), veal (all cuts), liver, lean beef, pork, and lamb (1 oz cooked weight equals 1 equivalent; remove all visible fat)	Fried or fatty meats, sausage, scrapple, frankfurters, poultry skins, stewing hens, spareribs, salt pork, beef (unless lean), duck, goose, ham hocks, pig's feet, luncheon meats, gravies (unless fat free), tuna and salmon packed in oil, peanut butter
BREADS, CEREALS, STARCHES	Plain, nonfat cereals, spaghetti, noodles, rice, macaroni, plain whole grain or enriched bread	Biscuits, quick breads, cheese bread, pancakes, waffles, sweet rolls, doughnuts, fritters, chips, snack foods and popcorn prepared with fat, muffins, natural cereals and breads to which extra fat is added
VEGETABLES	All prepared without fat	Avocado in excess of amount allowed on fat list
FRUITS	All	None
DESSERTS	Sherbet made with skim milk, fruit ice, gelatin, rice, bread, cornstarch, tapioca or junket pudding made with skim milk, fruit whips with gelatin, sugar, and egg white; fruit, angel food cake, meringues	Cake, pie, pastry, ice cream; doughnuts, cookies, or any dessert containing shortening, chocolate, or fats of any kind, unless especially prepared using part of fat allowance

FAT-RESTRICTED DIET FOR GALLBLADDER DISEASE, *CONTINUED*

Type of Food	Include	Avoid
SWEETS	Jelly, jam, marmalade, honey, syrup, molasses, sugar, hard candies, fondant, gumdrops, jelly beans, marshmallows	Any candy made with chocolate, nuts, butter, cream, or fat of any kind
FATS	A 20 g fat diet is limited to 1 serving of fat/day; a 40 g fat diet will be limited to 3 servings of fat/day; choose up to the limit allowed on diet from the following (1 serving in the amount listed equals 1 fat choice): 1 tsp butter or fortified margarine, 1 tsp shortening or oil, 1 tsp mayonnaise, 1 T Italian or French dressing, 1 strip crisp bacon, ¼ avocado (4" diameter), 2 T light cream, 1 T heavy cream, 6 small nuts, 5 small olives	Any in excess of amount prescribed on diet, all others
SOUPS	Bouillon, clear broth, fat free vegetable soup, cream soup made with skimmed milk, packaged dehydrated soups	All others
SEASONINGS	As desired	None

Source: Shands Hospital at the University of Florida

diabetes. Clients who suffer from chronic renal failure may eventually require dialysis, in which waste materials such as urea (a byproduct of protein metabolism that can be toxic at high levels) are separated from the bloodstream. *Dialysis* removes excess wastes and fluids but can't perform any of the hormonal functions of the kidney. When the client is to the point of requiring dialysis or a kidney transplant, the disease is referred to as *end-stage renal disease (ESRD)*.

Part of the treatment for ESRD may be dialysis, a mechanical process that removes wastes. There are two types of dialysis: *hemodialysis* and *peritoneal dialysis*. In hemodialysis, the client's blood is routed through a dialysis machine, which performs many of the kidney's functions. Then, the blood is returned to the body. In peritoneal dialysis, fluid is introduced into the abdominal cavity by a catheter or tube permanently placed into the abdomen.

The goals of the renal diet are as follows:

- To provide normal growth in children.
- To achieve and maintain an optimal nutritional status through adequate protein, energy, vitamin, and mineral intake.
- To attain and maintain a desirable body weight.
- To lighten the work of a diseased kidney by reducing the amount of waste products, such as urea made from protein, that have to be excreted.
- To control edema and electrolyte imbalance by controlling sodium, potassium, and fluid intake.
- To replace proteins that are lost in hemodialysis.
- To prevent or slow down the development of bone disease (called renal osteodystrophy) by controlling phosphorus (the blood level of which increases during renal failure, leading to bone disease) and increasing calcium intake.
- To provide a palatable diet.

Of all the modified diets, the renal diet is probably the most complex. The intake of protein, sodium, potassium, phosphorus, and fluid are carefully regulated from day to day. Actual nutrient restrictions vary based on many factors, such as:

- Degree of kidney failure
- Age of the client
- Mode of treatment and/or dialysis
- Need to maintain or achieve an ideal or desired weight
- Other medical conditions: diabetes, high blood pressure, hyperlipidemia, or malnutrition

General diet recommendations for renal clients are listed in Figure 6.21.

The National Renal Diet, using food exchanges much like the diabetic diet, provides a guide for renal diet planning. The exchange lists are customized for each of these situations, which have different nutritional concerns:

- Pre-end-stage renal disease
- Pre-end-stage renal disease and diabetes
- Hemodialysis
- Hemodialysis and diabetes
- Peritoneal dialysis
- Peritoneal dialysis and diabetes

RENAL DIET RECOMMENDATIONS

TREATMENT	PRE-ESRD	HEMODIALYSIS	PERITONEAL DIALYSIS
Protein (g/kg IBW)	0.6-0.8*	1.1-1.4	1.2-1.5
Nephrotic syndrome	0.8-1.0		
Energy (cal/kg IBW)	35-40	30-35	25-35
Phosphorous (mg/kg IBW)	8-12	17	17
Sodium (mg/d)	1000-3000 if necessary	2000-3000	2000-4000
Potassium (mg/kg IBW)	Typically unrestricted	Approximately 40	Typically unrestricted
Fluid (ml/d)	Typically unrestricted	500-700 + daily urine output *or* 1000 ml if anuric	2000+
Calcium (mg/d)	1200-1600	Depends on serum level	Depends on serum level

*The upper end of this range is preferred for diabetes and malnourished patients.

© 1993, American Dietetic Association, "A Healthy Food Guide for Hemodialysis". Used with permission.

Below is a description of the food lists.

Milk choices. Because milk is high in phosphorus, potassium, and protein, the portion size is one-half cup, and a typical renal diet plan limits milk to one half-cup serving per day.

Nondairy milk substitute choices. This group includes substitutes, such as nondairy frozen topping, that are much lower in phosphorus, potassium, and protein than regular milk choices.

Meat choices. Each serving on this list is equal to one ounce of meat. A typical renal diet plan might limit meat to a total of about 5 oz. per day.

Starch choices. This group include breads, rolls, cereals, grains, starchy vegetables, crackers, snack foods such as pretzels, and some desserts. Dried beans, peas, and lentils are not included because they are high in potassium and phosphorus. Whole grains and bran are discouraged because they are high in phosphorus.

Vegetable choices. For clients on dialysis, this list is further divided into low, medium, and high potassium groups. High potassium vegetables and fruits are sharply limited.

Figure 6.22

SAMPLE RENAL DIET MEAL PLAN

	Sample	Exchanges	Protein (grams)	Sodium (milligrams)	Potassium (milligrams)	Phosphorus (milligrams)
BREAKFAST						
Fruit, low	½ cup apple juice	1	0.5	tr	70	15
Fruit, med						
Fruit, high						
Meat	1 small egg	1	7	25	100	65
Starch	1 toast ½ cup grits	2	4	160	70	70
Milk	½ cup milk	1	4	80	185	110
Fat	2+ tsp margarine	2+	0	100	20	10
LUNCH						
Meat	2 oz chicken	2	14	50	200	130
Starch	½ cup rice	2	4	160	70	70
Veg, low						
Veg, med	½ cup steamed broccoli	1	1	15	150	20
Veg, high						
Fruit, low	baked apple	1	0.5	tr	70	15
Fruit, med						
Fruit, high						
Fat	1+ tsp margarine	1+	0	55	10	5
SUPPER						
Meat	2 oz meat balls	2	14	50	200	130
Starch	1 cup spaghetti and 1 slice Italian bread	3	6	240	105	105
Veg, low						
Veg, med	free salad with Italian dressing					
Veg, high	½ cup tomato sauce	1	1	15	270	20
Fruit, low						
Fruit, med						
Fat		1+	0	55	10	5
HS SNACK						
Milk	½ cup vanilla sugar-free pudding	1	4	80	185	110
			60	1100*	2000	900
Fruit, high	½ banana sliced	1	0.5	tr	270	15

Source: Smathers, J. 1995 Practical Application of the National Renal Diet. Dietary Manager Magazine March/April, p.11.

Fruit choices. Again, for clients on dialysis, this list is divided by potassium level. Fruit choices such as sweetened fruits are not allowed for diabetics, so the average calories per serving from this group is lower for them.

Fat choices. Nuts and seeds are not allowed on the renal diet because of their phosphorus, potassium, and low-quality protein content.

High calorie choices. This list includes high carbohydrate, and low protein foods such as lemonade and jam, that can add calories, but little protein, to the diet.

Salt choices. Salt, and other high sodium condiments appear on this list, and these are limited.

Beverage choices. This list is used only for clients on hemodialysis and some clients on peritoneal dialysis, because fluid intake is limited. Certain beverages, such as coffee, may be restricted due to potassium content.

A sample meal plan using these food lists is displayed in Figure 6.22. The detailed food lists appear in Appendix E.

CANCER

Cancer is a disease characterized by unrestricted and excessive multiplication of body cells. *Tumors* are growths of cancerous cells and may be either *malignant* (meaning cancerous growth is continuing and may be life-threatening) or *benign* (meaning not cancerous). Cancerous cells can also leave their original site of growth and travel through the blood and lymph to spread throughout the body, referred to as *metastasis*.

Sometimes the first signs of cancer are weight loss and anorexia. Cancer cells require calories and nutrients to grow, and basal energy use is increased in cancer clients. This helps explain part of the weight loss. Cancer clients may need 35 to 50 calories per kilogram of body weight simply to maintain their current weight. To complicate matters more, cancer clients often have little interest in eating. They experience nausea and vomiting, feel full quickly, and do not taste many foods normally. These symptoms may be caused by the cancer or by the treatment, which may include radiation, chemotherapy, and surgery. Good nutritional status is important to withstand the effects of treatment.

The traditional cancer therapies, radiation therapy and chemotherapy, interfere with nutritional status. In radiation therapy, high-energy rays are used to destroy cancerous tissues and stop the growth of cancer cells. Chemotherapy is the treatment of cancer with drugs. Some effects of radiation therapy and chemotherapy include nausea, vomiting, taste alterations, diarrhea, malabsorption, and reduced salivary secretions in the case of radiation treatment of the head and neck. The result can be *cancer cachexia* (malnutrition).

Surgery is another major approach to treating cancer. Surgery removes cancerous tissue. In these situations, providing proper nutrition will require dietary modifications such as small, frequent meals for clients who have had part of the stomach removed. About half of cancer clients experience an extreme state of malnutrition and wasting of the body called *cancer cachexia*. Symptoms include significant weight loss, loss of appetite, feeling full early, abnormal taste and smell abilities, anemia, and other nutritional deficiencies.

Following are approaches to overcome some of the nutritional problems that present in cancer clients.

Loss of Appetite

Causes of anorexia and weight loss include emotional stress and depression, chemotherapy, radiation treatment, and the cancer itself, especially if it is in the gastrointestinal tract. These strategies may help stimulate appetite:

- Ask the physician and nursing staff about effective medications to control nausea and pain. Give these one hour before meals to promote better intake.
- Large amounts of food tend to overwhelm a reluctant eater. Try smaller portions of nutrient-dense food.
- Update food preferences and dislikes often, since these may change during the course of the illness.
- Cater to special requests, even if this means purchasing food not normally stockcd.
- Offer high calorie, high protein foods (described in Chapter 19).

Even though many high calorie foods are high in fat, and in some cases also saturated fat, keep in mind that there are situations where taking in adequate calories is more important than worrying about fat content.

Early Satiety

Feeling full midway through the meal is a common occurrence. These tips may be useful:

- Encourage five or six mini-meals throughout the day.
- Serve a well balanced, nutrient-dense breakfast since many clients feel good in the morning.
- Instruct the client to save high fat foods until the end of the meal because these promote satiety.
- Have high calorie snacks available at the bedside.

Nausea and Vomiting

In addition to medications, the following tactics may help control nausea and vomiting:

- Allow the client to eat when less nauseated; be flexible with mealtimes.
- Encourage nutrient-dense fluids between meals to prevent dehydration. Use fruit juice, milkshakes, and liquid medical nutritional products.
- Avoid food with strong odors and flavors if these are offensive.
- Offer cold meals rather than hot foods, as this minimizes aromas.
- Bland or dry food like toast or crackers may be well tolerated.

Dry or Sore Mouth

Changes in saliva make the client more prone to dental problems. Encourage good oral hygiene and frequent saline (saltwater) rinses. These nutrition tips will help bring relief during meals:

- Use sugarless gum to stimulate salivation.
- Analgesics may relieve pain while eating.
- Avoid crisp and raw food, which may scratch the mouth and throat causing discomfort. Also, acidic and salty food may irritate these areas.
- Soft foods are better tolerated; a pureed texture may be needed temporarily.
- Add liquid, gravy, and sauces to moisten food.

Swallowing Difficulties

Swallowing problems occur when the esophagus is exposed to radiation, usually two to three weeks after treatment begins.

- Soft and pureed consistencies are better tolerated.
- Serve food at room temperature or very cold.
- Liquids may be easier to manage; consider liquid medical nutritional products.
- Request an evaluation from the speech pathologist.

Changes in Taste and Smell

Sensations may be decreased or may just be different from normal. Check with the client often to inquire about food aversions, and then make appropriate substitutions for the offending foods.

- Highly seasoned food may be appreciated.
- Meat may be better accepted cold.
- Try soybean-based tofu and dairy products as protein alternatives if meats are refused.
- Pay particular attention to the presentation of food on the plate and to mealtime ambiance.

Diarrhea

A temporary lactose intolerance may develop, causing diarrhea. Eliminate milk and milk products to determine whether the diarrhea is from lactose intolerance.

- Try low lactose milk or a lactose-free medical nutritional product.
- Encourage potassium rich food to replace losses. Good sources are bananas, apricots, raisins, citrus fruits, and potatoes.
- Avoid high fat food, which may aggravate the situation.

AIDS

Acquired Immunodeficiency Syndrome (AIDS) is a serious illness that affects the body's ability to fight infection. The human immunodeficiency virus (HIV) causes AIDS. HIV is spread primarily through sexual intercourse with an HIV-infected person, contaminated needles or blood, or from mother to infant during pregnancy or lactation. When first infected with HIV, a client generally has no symptoms. As time progresses, symptoms appear and often include exhaustion, fever, diarrhea, weight loss, muscle pain, and mouth infections. AIDS actually refers to the final stage of HIV infection, when health problems such as recurrent pneumonia, cancers, severe diarrhea, and malabsorption are the most serious.

The wasting and malnutrition just discussed with regard to cancer cachexia are commonly seen in HIV-infected clients. There are many possible reasons for this, such as anorexia, inadequate diet, increased metabolic rate, GI tract infections, drugs, reduced gastric acid secretion, diarrhea, and malabsorption.

As you can imagine, early nutrition support is important to build up nutrient stores and body weight. As long as possible, an oral diet is generally preferable, using high protein, high calorie foods and supplements as necessary. A concern for HIV-infected and AIDS clients is making sure food is safe to eat. The body ordinarily is well-equipped to deal with bacteria that cause food-borne illness, but these clients are at far greater risk of serious illness. Because of weakened immune systems, these individuals are more susceptible to contracting a foodborne illness. Once contracted, these infections, with their severe vomiting and diarrhea, can be difficult to treat and they can come back again and again. This can further weaken the immune system and hasten the progression of HIV infection, and be fatal for persons with AIDS.

Individuals with AIDS may lose up to 34% of their ideal body weight in the 4-5 months before death. They have inadequate nutrient intakes for reasons similar to those of people with cancer—altered perceptions, drug therapy, dry mouth, lack of energy to eat, depression, nausea/vomiting, etc. Accelerated nutrient losses may occur because of diarrhea, drug therapy, infections, or malabsorption. Sound nutritional status may improve a person's response to drug therapy, reduce duration of hospital stays, and promote physical independence. Dietary considerations include:

- Aim to maintain body weight at 95-100% of usual body weight.
- Provide small, frequent meals (6-9 per day) for better tolerance and reduced mealtime fatigue.
- Provide adequate fluid and potassium.
- Provide 20-30 cal/kg actual body weight with 1.5 gm protein/kg actual body weight.
- A general multivitamin-mineral supplement may be needed. Two to five times the RDA of all water-soluble vitamins may be useful. Maintain fat-soluble vitamins at regular levels.

ALZHEIMER'S DISEASE

Alzheimer's Disease is the most common form of dementia (impairment of mental functioning). It proceeds in stages over months or years and gradually destroys memory, reason, judgment, language, and eventually the ability to carry out even simple tasks. About half of individuals over age 85 have Alzheimer's Disease, but it can also appear as early as middle age. It accounts for 60% of admissions to nursing homes. Managing the nutritional well-being of a resident with Alzheimer's disease is challenging and ever-changing, as no two individuals' needs and abilities are the same. Techniques that successfully maintain food intake and weight in some residents may not work for others. Nutrition management of a resident with Alzheimer's must be individualized according to the person's ability and current stage of the disease.

Understanding the progression of the disease is the first step toward nutrition management. There are basically three stages of Alzheimer's:

Early Stage. This stage is characterized by forgetfulness, a tendency to misplace things, and some withdrawal from usual interests. Individuals may have trouble finding the right words to communicate their thoughts. Initially, they may not have problems eating their meals, but environmental surroundings may cause a problem. They may not want to eat in public or in a noisy environment. This stage of Alzheimer's may go unnoticed.

Intermediate Stage. Persons with Alzheimer's usually cannot initiate a specific movement or course of action without assistance during this stage. There is confusion and difficulty carrying out usual routines. Individuals may begin to need re-direction at mealtime as they forget how to use flatware or are unaware of what to do with the food in front of them. Some individuals also wander at mealtimes and therefore require constant supervision. Partial to total feeding is usually required. At times, they may refuse to open their mouths, making the dining experience a conflict situation between resident and caregiver. Situations like this can promote violent behavior in some individuals. Also, patients become disoriented with respect to their surroundings, time, and place. This may explain why they become lost walking to the dining room or forget if they have eaten meals. Losing the ability to remember whether they have eaten not only can lead to weight loss, but also to weight gain.

Late Stage. At this stage, the person's motor skills deteriorate. Patients lose the ability to chew and swallow, and often to speak. Their sensitivity to seizures, aspiration, and pneumonia increases, making it difficult for caregivers to provide them with fluids and food orally. Food and fluid textures have to be modified to promote oral intake as long as possible. Correct feeding and positioning techniques must be exhibited by the caregiver during mealtimes. Decisions by families and medical staff must be made regarding enteral nutrition support.

Compiling a comprehensive nutrition assessment upon admission of each resident with Alzheimer's is a key aspect in nutritional management. Continuous assessment is necessary due to the disease progression. During the initial three to five days after admission, the resident must be closely monitored at mealtimes for changes in eating/feeding ability. Depending on the severity of the eating skill deficiency, close monitoring should be done weekly to monthly.

Nutritional care strategies must be individualized to patients and their current stages of the disease. All techniques do not work for all residents with Alzheimer's. The old saying, "If at first you don't succeed, try, try again," is never more true than for this population. Nutritional management of persons with Alzheimer's requires implementing techniques appropriate for specific problems, as outlined below.

To maintain weight and appetite:

- Serve the larger meals at breakfast when the resident is more alert and his or her appetite is larger. Even residents with good appetites will consume smaller evening meals due in part to the "sundowning" effect (increased restlessness and anxiety as evening approaches).

- Provide nutrient-dense foods routinely in the diet, such as whole milk with meals, fortified cereal at breakfast, and additional juices and whole grain breads.
- Offer nutritious snacks between meals, such as juice and graham crackers, sandwich halves, fruit, and cheese.
- Implement a weekly weight program for all residents. Close monitoring is a must.
- Involve all facility staff during mealtimes to assist residents in the dining rooms and those who receive room service.

Observe for changes in a resident's eating habits, such as decreased use of utensils, playing with food, or using fingers. If observed, make appropriate changes in meal service to maintain their independence. To maintain feeding independence:

- If there is a decreased use of utensils: offer utensils only as needed, use "hand-over-hand" techniques in promoting self-feeding, and provide verbal cues for resident, e.g., "Mrs. Jones, pick up your fork".
- If the client is playing with or mixing food: offer one food at a time, place foods in individual bowls, put condiments on food before serving, and have staff provide constant redirection and verbal cues at mealtimes.
- If the client is using fingers to eat, maximize the situation. Offer finger foods to allow resident to maintain independence, yet eat in a dignified manner.

If the client experiences confusion at meal times:

- Offer meals at the same, time, same place, and same seating arrangement every day.
- Serve the meal immediately after the resident is in the dining room.
- Allow adequate time for meals.
- Make the physical environment pleasant and calming.
- Limit the use of intercoms.
- Play soft background music.
- Seat residents in groups of four to six.
- Use square rather than round tables.
- Set the table with solid, contrasting colors between the china and the tablecloth.
- Limit the centerpieces at mealtimes.
- Maintain a high staff-to-resident ratio at mealtime.

If the client has difficulty chewing and/or swallowing:

- Check fit of dentures, if applicable.
- Position the resident correctly (at 90-degree angle) in chair, wheelchair, or bed.
- Provide verbal cues in a soft, gentle manner to remind residents to chew food, eat slowly, and swallow.
- Evaluate for need of a texture-modified diet. Offer soft or ground meat first, then go to soft scoop pureed consistency.
- Use gravies and sauces to moisten food.
- Ensure that food temperatures are safe.
- Avoid offering a food with a combination of textures, e.g. vegetable soup.
- Consult a speech therapist for swallowing evaluation.
- Learn techniques to overcome problems of refusing to open mouth or of pocketing food.

IMMOBILIZATION

Long periods of immobilization, such as following an injury or simply being bedridden, can result in development of pressure ulcers. **Pressure ulcers**, or pressure sores, are lesions caused by unrelieved pressure resulting in damage to underlying tissue. Over one million patients in hospitals and nursing homes suffer from pressure ulcers. The first preventive step is to identify clients at high risk for pressure ulcers, explained in Figure 6.23. Clients with pressure ulcers need to be followed closely, using a staging system (Figure 6.24).

Figure 6.23

RISK FACTORS FOR PRESSURE ULCERS

- Impaired transfer or bed mobility
- Bedridden, hemiplegia, quadriplegia
- Loss of bowel or bladder control
- Peripheral vascular disease
- Diabetes mellitus
- Hip fracture
- Weight loss/poor nutrition
- Pressure ulcer history
- Impaired tactile sensory perception
- Medications

- Restraints
- Severe chronic pulmonary obstructive disease
- Sepsis
- Terminal cancer
- Chronic or end-stage renal, liver, and/or heart disease
- Disease or drug related immunosuppression
- Full body cast
- Steroid, radiation or chemotherapy
- Renal dialysis
- Head of bed elevated the majority of the day

Figure 6.24

PRESSURE ULCER STAGING & NUTRITIONAL NEEDS

A staging system describes the extent of tissue damage in pressure ulcers. Stages also influence nutritional recommendations. The stages and related nutritional advice are as follows:

Stage	Needs:	Calories	Protein	Fluid
STAGE I: A persistent area of skin redness (without a break in the skin) that does not disappear within 30 minutes when pressure is relieved.		30 cal/kg	1.0-1.1 gm/kg	30 ml/kg
STAGE II: A partial thickness of skin is lost that presents clinically as an abrasion, blister, or shallow crater.		30	1.2	30
STAGE III: A full thickness of skin is lost, exposing tissues below the skin, presents as a deep crater with or without undermining adjacent tissue.		35	1.3-1.4	30-35
STAGE IV: A full thickness of skin and subcutaneous tissue is lost, exposing muscle and/or bone.		35	1.5-1.6	35

Nutrition plays a vital role in preventing and treating pressure ulcers. Clients who are malnourished and/or eating and drinking poorly have a greater chance of developing pressure ulcers. Medical nutrition therapy for this condition commonly includes a high calorie, high protein diet along with adequate fluids.

The nutritional needs for calories, protein, and fluid increase with the stage of the ulcer, as shown in Figure 6.24. Multivitamin/mineral supplements are frequently given for Stages II-IV. Additional vitamin C and zinc are given for Stage IV. More aggressive calorie, protein, and vitamin/mineral supplementation is needed for a client with multiple pressure ulcers.

DEVELOPMENTALLY DISABLED AND HANDICAPPED CLIENTS

The term *developmental disability* refers to a severe, chronic disability that:

- ▶ Is attributable to a mental or physical impairment, or a combination of mental and physical impairments.
- ▶ Is manifested before the person reaches the age of 22 years.
- ▶ Is likely to continue indefinitely.
- ▶ Results in substantial functional limitations in three or more of the following areas of major life activity: self-care, receptive and expressive language, learning, mobility, self-direction, capacity for independent living, and economic self-sufficiency.

▶ Reflects the person's need for a combination and sequence of special interdisciplinary or generic care, treatment, or other services that are lifelong or of extended duration and individually planned and coordinated (Developmental Disabilities Assistance and Bill of Rights Act, 1978).

Examples of developmental disabilities are mental retardation, cerebral palsy (partial paralysis and lack of muscular coordination), muscular dystrophy (progressive weakness and deterioration of muscles), epilepsy (sudden, passing disturbances of brain function), and autism (withdrawal and lack of responsiveness to others). Developmentally disabled children are at high risk for nutritional problems and deficiencies. Frequent nutrition-related problems that contribute to nutritional risk include the following:

Feeding problems. There may be either physical or psychological factors that cause feeding problems. For example, in children with cerebral palsy, the muscles involved in chewing and swallowing may not function normally. In children with autism, eating becomes very much of a ritual that is hard to change.

Drug-nutrient interactions. Many individuals with developmental disabilities are on long-term medications to treat chronic problems such as epilepsy and infections. Nutrition counseling may be needed as well as vitamin or mineral supplements.

Obesity. Some of the developmentally disabled are more prone to obesity due to limited activity, poor muscle tone, small stature, and/or overeating. Nutrition counseling and exercise may be useful.

Constipation. Constipation is common due to decreased activity and certain medications.

Dehydration. Some developmentally disabled individuals are not able to feel or express thirst. Others need extra fluids because of drooling or to prevent frequent urinary infections. Fluid intake should be encouraged and individuals assisted when necessary.

Nutrition intervention is more effective with an interdisciplinary team approach that includes other professionals such as nurses, occupational therapists, physical therapists, social workers, and dentists. Nutrition intervention is also more effective when the traditional nutrition assessment process has been modified for this population. For example, it is necessary to overcome difficulties in weighing and measuring clients and in selecting appropriate standards (such as weight) for comparison. Nutrition programs for the developmentally disabled can greatly benefit these individuals by improving their health and their capacity to socialize and function in an educational, work, or home environment.

Figure 6.25

FEEDING PROBLEMS AND ADAPTATIONS

PROBLEM/CHALLENGE	POSSIBLE ADAPTATION
One handedness; difficulty cutting meat	Rocker knife or roller knife
Poor hand coordination	Weighted utensils, scoop dish, plate guard, covered cups with slotted opening
Hand deformity, difficulty grasping	Built-up handles on eating utensils
Limited neck motion—unable to tilt head back	Cut-out plastic cup (nose cup)
Muscle weakness	Utensil holder, two-handled cups, clamp-on handles
Visual problems	Clock method for locating food on tray, plate guard, scoop dish
Shakiness	Sippy cup, swivel utensils

Source: Becky Dorner. 1996. Dignity in dining: feeding techniques for elderly and disabled clients.
Dietary Manager Magazine.

A physical handicap can be caused by a variety of illnesses or accidents. Some of the common causes are arthritis, amputations, spinal cord injuries, stroke, Parkinson's disease, or multiple sclerosis. These illnesses can result in feeding problems for either emotional or physical reasons. Depression, which can occur with any illness, can result in a loss of appetite leading to weight loss, or in increased consumption of high calorie, easily consumed foods, leading to obesity. Depressed clients may be extremely demanding and very selective in their food preferences. Demands requiring many substitutions can be very frustrating to the dietary staff. Tremors or paralysis may make it difficult for a client to use utensils. Dysphagia may make eating certain consistencies of food difficult. Figure 6.25 addresses feeding problems and adaptations.

DIET MANUALS

A **diet manual** specifies therapeutic diets and their application. Usually, a diet manual takes the form of a reference book. The manual standardizes names for diets, which is important. When a physician orders a diet, standard terminology allows communication among the physician, dietary caregivers, and the entire healthcare team. For example, if a physician were to order a "Diabetic Diet," what would you do to implement this order? Now that you know the range of dietary interventions for diabetes, you know that this term doesn't specify enough. But perhaps your institution develops a diet for diabetes centered on the Food Guide Pyramid. Then perhaps, your diet manual will describe a diet named something like: "Diabetes Pyramid Diet." Your diet manual will outline the detail about how each food group is used in developing menus and serving meals. For some diets, the manual may specify foods to be used and foods to omit. In some ways, a diet manual may resemble an expanded version of this chapter, minus the background on medical conditions. It will also give more information about how to dictate an order. A carbohydrate counting diet, for instance, must include a level of carbohydrate or daily goal. It may read: "Carbohydrate Counting—210 grams per day". This form of control is helpful so that a physician's intent and the actual result coincide.

Most healthcare institutions adopt or adapt a diet manual from an outside source. The American Dietetic Association, as well as many state and local chapters of dietitians, develop diet manuals and offer them in the professional marketplace. Usually, very large healthcare institutions develop their own manuals—a massive undertaking. Whatever your source, as a dietary manager in healthcare, you will need to identify this standard for dietary planning. Deciding on a diet manual and nutritional care specifications is done in communication with physicians and other members of the healthcare team. In a large institution, a formal approval process may be required. In a small institution, the medical director alone may approve the diet manual. A diet manual should be readily available for reference by all caregivers, and should form the basis for menu planning and meal service. The diet manual also dictates what information must be relayed in nutrition education.

LIBERALIZING MODIFIED DIETS

From the information in this chapter, it is apparent that therapeutic diets can become quite complex, and can limit food offerings. Sometimes, adherence to a modified diet can do more harm than good. When has a modified diet gone too far? Often, the answer is: when it limits food intake and compromises overall nutrition status, or when it reduces enjoyment and the quality of life. This is of special concern among elderly individuals, as well as anyone suffering from a terminal illness. In longterm care facilities, federal regulations emphasize respect for residents' rights. A resident must enjoy informed choice in many matters, including diet. The American Dietetic Association supports liberalizing therapeutic diets as follows:

> "It is the position of the American Dietetic Association (ADA) that the quality of life and nutritional status of older residents in long-term care facilities may be enhanced by a liberalized diet. The Association advocates the use of qualified dietetics professionals to assess and evaluate the need for medical nutrition therapy according to each person's individual medical condition, needs, desires, and rights. One of the major determinants among the predictive factors of successful aging is nutrition. Long-term care includes a continuum of health services ranging from rehabilitation to supportive care. Nutrition care for older adults in long-term settings must meet two goals: maintenance of health through medical care and maintenance of quality of life. However, these goals often seem to compete, resulting in the need for a unique approach to medical nutrition therapy (MNT). Typically, MNT includes assessment of nutritional status and

development of an individualized nutrition intervention plan that frequently features a theraperutic diet appropriate for managing a disease or condition. MNT must always address medical needs and individual desires, yet for older adults in long-term care this balance is especially critical because of the focus on maintaining quality of life. Dietetics professionals must help residents and health care team members assess the risks versus the benefits of therapeutic diets. For frail older adults, overall health goals may not warrant the use of a therapeutic diet because of its possible negative effect on quality of life. A diet that is not palatable or acceptable to the individual can lead to poor food and fluid intake, which results in weight loss and undernutrition, followed by a spiral of negative health effects. Often, a more liberalized nutrition intervention that allows an older adult to participate in his or her diet-related decisions can provide for the person's nutrient needs and allow alterations contingent on medical conditions while simultaneously increasing the desire to eat and enjoyment of food. This ultimately decreases the risks of weight loss, undernutrition, and other potential negative effects of poor nutrition and hydration."

(excerpted from the Journal of the American Dietetic Association, Liberalized Diets for Older Adults in Long-Term Care, 2002)

According to the ADA, benefits of liberalizing diets in longterm care may include:

- Improved dietary compliance
- Improved psychosocial status of residents
- Improved appearance and flavor of food
- Enhanced calorie and nutrient intake
- Increased accuracy and efficiency of trayline
- Improvement of fasting blood glucose levels
- Improvement in ability to maintain acceptable weight and nutritional parameters for residents
- Decreased labor and food costs
- Improved surveys due to reduced chance of error
- Improved quality of life for residents
- Happy, healthy, and satisfied residents

How may a diet be liberalized? The ADA emphasizes the importance of individuals receiving a less restricted diet of regular foods. This may include a carbohydrate controlled diet instead of a calorie controlled diabetic diet, in tandem with blood glucose monitoring. It may involve a no added salt diet instead of a 2 gm sodium diet. The appropriateness of low cholesterol diets for older adults in longterm care facilities is questioned since epidemiologic evidence indicates that after age 65, the importance of elevated serum cholesterol levels as a risk factor for coronary heart disease virtually disappears. Dietary caregivers must carefully weigh health-related priorities and use sound judgment to tailor nutritional care for each resident.

UNDERSTANDING FOOD ALLERGY

Allergies affect the lives of millions of people around the world. Fresh spring flowers, a friend's cat or dog, even the presence of dust can make people itch, sneeze and scratch almost uncontrollably. But what about that seemingly innocent peanut butter sandwich, glass of milk or fish fillet?

Almost 2% of American adults have an allergy to these or other foods. Food allergies can be life threatening. Knowledge about food allergies can help save a life.

What is a food allergy?

Food allergy is a reaction of the body's immune system to something in a food or an ingredient in a food—usually a protein. It can be a serious condition and should be diagnosed by a board-certified allergist. A true food allergy (also called "food hypersensitivity") and its symptoms can take many forms.

Which foods cause food allergy?

The eight most common food allergens—milk, eggs, peanuts, tree nuts, soy, wheat, fish and shellfish—cause more than 90% of all food allergic reactions. However, many other foods have been identified as allergens for some people.

What are the symptoms of food allergy?

Symptoms of food allergy differ greatly among individuals. They can also differ in the same person during different exposures. Allergic reactions to food can vary in severity and time of onset, and may be affected by when the food was eaten.

Common symptoms of food allergy include skin irritations such as rashes, hives and eczema, and gastrointestinal symptoms such as nausea, diarrhea and vomiting. Sneezing, runny nose and shortness of breath can also result from food allergy. Some individuals may experience a more severe reaction called anaphylaxis.

What is anaphylaxis?

Anaphylaxis is a rare but potentially fatal condition in which several different parts of the body experience allergic reactions. These may include itching, hives, swelling of the throat, difficulty breathing, lower blood pressure and unconsciousness.

Symptoms usually appear rapidly, sometimes within minutes of exposure to the allergen, and can be life threatening. Immediate medical attention is necessary when anaphylaxis occurs. Standard emergency treatment often includes an injection of epinephrine (adrenaline) to open up the airway and blood vessels.

Do I have a food allergy?

Of all the individuals who have any type of food sensitivity, most have food intolerances. Fewer people have true food allergy involving the immune system. According to the National Institutes of Health, approximately 5 million Americans, (5 to 8% of children and 1 to 2% of adults) have a true food allergy.

What are other reactions or sensitivities to foods called?

Other reactions to foods are called food intolerance and food idiosyncrasy. Food intolerance and food idiosyncrasy reactions are generally localized, temporary, and rarely life threatening, whereas food allergy can cause life threatening reactions.

Food intolerance is an adverse reaction to a food substance or additive that involves digestion or metabolism (breakdown of food by the body) but does not involve the immune system. Lactose intolerance is an example of food intolerance. It occurs when a person lacks an enzyme needed to digest milk sugar. If a person who is lactose intolerant eats milk products, they may experience symptoms such as gas, bloating and abdominal pain.

Food idiosyncrasy is an abnormal response to a food or food substance. The reaction can resemble or differ from symptoms of true food allergy. Idiosyncratic reactions to food do not involve the immune system. Sulfite sensitivity or sulfite-induced asthma is an example of a food idiosyncrasy that affects small numbers of people in the population. However, sulfite-induced asthma can be potentially life-threatening.

Other suspected adverse reactions to foods such as to corn, high fructose corn syrup and sugar have rarely been demonstrated as true food allergies. Some foods contain a variety of either naturally occurring or added components that can cause a chemical, or drug-like reaction. The "burning" sensation when eating foods like chili peppers is an example of a chemical food reaction.

What should I do if I believe I have an adverse reaction to a certain food?

You should see a board-certified allergist to get a diagnosis. An allergist and dietitian can best help the food-allergic patient manage diet issues with little sacrifice to nutrition or the pleasure of eating. Making a diagnosis may include:

- A thorough medical history;
- The analysis of a food diary; and
- Several tests including skin-prick tests, RAST tests (blood tests), and food challenges (using different foods to test for allergic reactions).

Once a diagnosis is complete, an allergist will help set up a response plan to manage allergic reactions that may occur. A response plan may include taking medication by injection to control allergic reactions.

Am I allergic to food additives?

Probably not. Misconceptions abound regarding allergy to food additives and preservatives. Although some food components have been shown to trigger asthma or hives in certain people, these reactions are not the same as those observed with food.

Many of these additives, including aspartame, monosodium glutamate and several food dyes have been studied extensively. Scientific evidence shows that they do not cause allergic reactions.

© International Food Information Council (IFIC) Foundation. Reprinted with permission.

- Medical nutrition therapy is an integral component of healthcare. It involves nutritional assessment and treatment of medical conditions, illnesses, or injuries, and can improve health.

- Dietary treatment for high blood cholesterol aims to reduce LDL and increase HDL.

- A dietary plan for reducing risk of cardiovascular disease limits total fat to 30% of calories (with saturated fat as 7-10%), and dietary cholesterol to 300 mg/day.

- Limiting intake of meat (especially fatty meats) and dairy fat while increasing plant foods in the diet can help with compliance.

- The DASH diet is designed to improve hypertension. The DASH diet limits sodium to 2400 mg/day or less, while boosting potassium and calcium intake and limiting alcohol.

- Most dietary sodium comes from processed foods, rather than the salt shaker. High sodium foods include processed and cured meats, salty snack foods, canned soups and vegetables, many convenience food mixes, many condiments, and some cheeses.

- Diabetes is a condition in which glucose in the blood does not enter body cells efficiently. Glucose builds up in the blood, causing risks and complications.

- Type 1 diabetes results from inadequate insulin production, and treatment typically requires insulin injection.

- Type 2 diabetes usually strikes adults, and is often controlled with oral hypoglycemic drugs.

- Both types of diabetes require medical nutrition therapy to stabilize blood glucose levels from day to day. Nutrition therapy may take the form of a modified Food Guide Pyramid, an exchange system diet, or carbohydrate counting.

- Causes of obesity are not well understood, and it can be difficult to control over the long term.

- Weight management can be achieved through a combination of exercise and moderately reduced caloric intake to tip the calorie balance.

- Commonsense dietary guidance for weight management includes eating a variety of foods, eating smaller portions, eating less fat, and limiting foods at the top of the Food Guide Pyramid. Plant foods, fruits, and vegetables can help fill the gaps.

- Behavior modification, attitude modification, and social support all play important roles in weight management.

- After surgery a patient may temporarily follow a clear liquid diet, which may progress to a full liquid diet, and then a soft diet. The first two of these are generally nutritionally inadequate.

- An individual who has difficulty chewing may require a pureed or mechanical soft diet.

- Swallowing disorders (dysphagia) are very individual, and must be evaluated by a speech therapist.

- A diet for dysphagia has two parts: one specifying food texture, and one specifying the type of liquid recommended.

- A finger food diet for adults can help an individual with physical impairments or dementia and allow for eating independence.

- Diets for gastroesophageal reflux disease and peptic ulcer disease use small meals and limit any foods that irritate the gastrointestinal system.

- Dietary treatment for constipation includes plenty of fiber and fluids.

- Over time, inflammatory bowel disease (Crohn's disease and ulcerative colitis) may lead to malabsorption and malnutrition and require nutritional intervention.

- Many people have diverticula, pouches in the intestines. Prevention includes a high fiber diet.

- When diverticula become inflamed (diverticulitis), dietary fiber is limited, and nuts and seeds are avoided.

- Irritable bowel syndrome, a very common complaint, may be indicated by alternating diarrhea and constipation. Often, a high fiber diet (except during diarrhea), and smaller meals may help.

- Individuals with gluten-sensitive enteropathy must avoid grains and read food labels carefully.

- Lactose intolerance is a limited ability to digest lactose (milk sugar) due to a deficiency of lactase (an enzyme). Tolerance varies. Individuals with lactose intolerance may need to avoid or limit most dairy products, or use special products.

- During hepatitis, an inflammation of the liver, individuals may need a high calorie, high protein diet and supplementation of fat-soluble vitamins.

- During advanced cirrhosis and portal system encephalopathy, brain functioning is impaired. Dietary intervention may include a low protein diet, branched chain amino acid formulas, fluid and sodium restrictions, and fat in the form of MCT oil.

- During cholecystitis (inflammation of the gallbladder), a very low fat diet of about 40 grams per day may be required.

- Renal failure occurs when the kidneys cannot adequately remove waste and fluid from the body. A diet for advanced renal failure usually follows an exchange system to track restrictions in intake of protein, sodium, potassium, phosphorous, and fluid. Special care is essential to achieve an adequate calorie intake and maintain nutritional status.

- Due to the condition and/or treatments, cancer patients may experience loss of appetite, early satiety, nausea and vomiting, dry or sore mouth, swallowing difficulties, changes in taste or smell, and/or diarrhea. Each requires individualized nutritional care.

- AIDS patients may need extra calories and protein, adequate fluid, and special attention to food sanitation.

◗ Nutritional care for an individual with Alzheimer's disease addresses needs such as orientation and assistance with feeding, modifications in food consistency, and maintaining nutritional status.

◗ Adequate nutrition can help prevent and/or speed the healing of pressure ulcers, which may occur when a person is immobilized for extended periods of time. A high protein, high calorie diet, adequate fluids, and sometimes vitamin and mineral supplementation play important roles in treatment.

◗ Developmental disability or handicap can bring about many types of nutritional problems. Each requires intervention.

◗ A diet manual specifies therapeutic diets and their application.

◗ In longterm care, dietary caregivers must weigh nutritional and health priorities, and make commonsense judgments to tailor nutritional care to residents. The American Dietetic Association supports liberalizing therapeutic diets in this environment.

Key Terms

Alzheimer's Disease: a common, progressive form of dementia (impairment of mental functioning)

Atherosclerosis: A process in which deposits of cholesterol and other substances accumulate on the inside of arteries. Atherosclerosis is also called hardening of the arteries.

Cancer: a disease characterized by unrestricted and excessive multiplication of body cells

Chronic obstructive pulmonary disease (COPD): a group of diseases that includes chronic bronchitis, emphysema and asthmatic bronchitis

Congestive heart failure (CHF): a condition in which the heart becomes weak, beats faster, and enlarges

Constipation: passage of small amounts of hard, dry bowel movements, usually fewer than three times a week

DASH Diet: Developed by the National High Blood Pressure Education Program of the National Institutes of Health to treat hypertension. DASH stands for Dietary Approaches to Stop Hypertension.

Diabetes mellitus: a metabolic disorder in which the body cannot use glucose properly

Diet Manual: a reference book approved by the institution; specifies diets and their application

Dysphagia: difficulty swallowing

Edema: unhealthy water retention

Exchange lists: a meal planning system in which foods within a group can be exchanged for others

Food allergy: an immune system response to specific proteins in foods, which can be life-threatening

Food intolerance: describes unfavorable reactions to foods

Gestational diabetes: a condition characterized by abnormal glucose tolerance during pregnancy

Glycosuria: a condition caused when the kidneys remove extra glucose from the blood and dump it into the urine

High-Density Lipoproteins (HDL): "good cholesterol"; carries cholesterol away

Hyperglycemia: high blood glucose levels

Hypoglycemia: low blood glucose levels

Hypertension: a medical condition involving chronic high blood pressure

Inflammatory bowel disease (IBD): includes two conditions with similar symptoms and clinical management, Crohn's disease and ulcerative colitis

Low-Density Lipoproteins (LDL): "bad cholesterol"; source of blockage in arteries

Malabsorption: a condition in which nutrients are not absorbed properly

Medical nutrition therapy: the nutritional assessment and treatment of a condition, illness, or injury that places an individual at risk

National Dysphagia Diet (NDD): the national standard for dietary treatment of dysphagia; specifies modifications in food textures as well as liquids

Pressure ulcers: lesions caused by unrelieved pressure resulting in damage to underlying tissue, also known as pressure sores

Renal failure: occurs when the kidneys fail to maintain normal fluid and electrolyte balance and to excrete waste products within normal limits

Stroke: Occurs when blood vessels bringing oxygen to the brain burst or become clogged. The interruption of blood flow to the brain interrupts body functions and damages nerve cells.

Type 1 diabetes: occurs when a group of cells in the pancreas, called the beta cells, is unable to make insulin

Type 2 diabetes: occurs when an individual's pancreas makes insulin but the cells are not as sensitive to it

1. Which of the following is NOT a risk factor for atherosclerosis?
   A. High LDL
   B. High HDL
   C. Obesity
   D. A sedentary lifestyle

2. Which of the following advice would help a person reduce intake of saturated fat and cholesterol?
   A. Avoid beans
   B. Eat more whole eggs
   C. Eat more fruits and vegetables
   D. Avoid fiber

3. Most sodium in the average diet comes from:
   A. Processed foods
   B. Table salt
   C. Milk
   D. Canned fruit

4. Which of the following is good advice for implementing a DASH diet?
   A. Eat high amounts of meat
   B. Avoid starchy foods
   C. Limit intake of high potassium fruits, such as oranges
   D. Eat plenty of fruits, vegetables, and fat free dairy products

5. In the exchange system, which of the following is true?
   A. An individual should limit intake of foods to one serving from each group at each meal.
   B. One item in a food group can be exchanged for another for roughly equal value of protein, carbohydrate, fat, and calories.
   C. Combination foods, such as casseroles and sandwiches, are not allowed.
   D. A client should focus on just one item in each group and avoid variety.

6. In a carbohydrate counting system, which of the following is true?
   A. An individual tracks the grams of carbohydrate consumed to meet a specified daily level.
   B. Refined sugars are not permitted.
   C. Carbohydrate is limited to less than 10% of calories.
   D. An individual is encouraged to consume most of the daily carbohydrate at breakfast.

7. Which of the following is sound advice for a person who wishes to lose weight?

    A. Avoid exercise until you meet your weight goal.
    B. Avoid carbohydrate rich foods such as breads, cereals, and potatoes.
    C. Limit intake of high fat foods such as excessive meat, whole milk, regular salad dressing, and fried foods.
    D. Set a weight loss goal of 3-6 pounds per week.

8. Which of the following foods is NOT allowed on a clear liquid diet?

    A. Flavored gelatin
    B. Ginger ale
    C. Popsicle
    D. Skim milk

9. Which of the following is appropriate on a mechanical soft diet?

    A. Mixed nuts
    B. Flaked fish
    C. Fresh apple
    D. Celery sticks

10. Which of the following items would be appropriate to include on a dysphagia diet specified as: dysphagia mechanically-altered with nectar-like liquids?

    A. Dry Cheerios and apple juice
    B. Sliced roast beef and 2% milk
    C. Sloppy Joe meat and milkshake with thickener
    D. Canned pineapple and frozen yogurt

Alternative therapies often come up during the provision of nutritional care. A dietary manager needs to understand alternative therapies and know how to assess them to promote optimum nutrition for clients.

After completing this chapter, you should be able to:

- Define the terms *conventional medicine, complementary medicine, alternative medicine,* and *integrative medicine.*
- Name types of complementary and alternative medicine, and list examples of each.
- Identify the potential risks of using dietary supplements without being well-informed.
- List questions to ask in evaluating dietary supplements and other complementary and alternative treatments.
- Identify the role of basic nutrition concepts in assessment and implementation of complementary and alternative therapies.
- Identify the role of a dietary manager in assisting healthcare clients who use or wish to use alternative therapies.

Alternative practices often come up during the provision of nutritional care. A dietary manager needs to understand complementary and alternative approaches to medical care and know how to assess them in order to promote optimum nutrition for clients. What do these terms mean? Both terms describe practices that fall outside of conventional medicine in the US. They may describe practices that healthcare professionals have not learned to use in treating various health conditions.

The National Center for Complementary and Alternative Medicine (NCCAM) of the National Institutes of Health provides this definition:

> *Complementary and alternative medicine is a group of diverse medical and healthcare systems, practices, and products that are not presently considered to be part of conventional medicine.*

What do we mean by **conventional medicine**? This is the science used by physicians (Medical Doctors—MDs and Doctors of Osteopathy—DOs), as well as allied health professionals, as they are trained in the US. Sometimes, conventional medicine is also called mainstream medicine, orthodox medicine, biomedicine, or allopathy.

Anything that does not fall within this broadly accepted group of practices is Complementary and Alternative Medicine (CAM). **Complementary medicine** is an unconventional medical practice that is used to complement or *add to* conventional medical practice. **Alternative medicine** is an unconventional medical practice that is used *instead of* conventional medicine. CAM therapies may also be called unconventional medicine, simply meaning they are not part of the routine therapeutic approach to treatment.

Integrative medicine is medical practice that combines conventional practice with CAM practices. For example, a physician treating anxiety who prescribes both a drug regimen and meditation is practicing integrative medicine.

NCCAM explains: "While some scientific evidence exists regarding some CAM therapies, for most there are key questions that are yet to be answered through well-designed scientific studies—questions such as whether they are safe and whether they work for the diseases or medical conditions for which they are used.

"The list of what is considered to be CAM changes continually, as those therapies that are proven to be safe and effective become adopted into conventional healthcare and as new approaches to healthcare merge."

TYPES OF CAM

NCCAM identifies five types of CAM: alternative medical systems, mind-body interventions, biologically based therapies, manipulative and body-based methods, and energy therapies. Figure 7.1 shows some common terms. Here is a closer look at types of CAM:

Alternative Medical Systems

These represent complete and separate systems for understanding health and illness. One example is Ayurveda, which emphasizes the use of body, mind, and spirit in disease prevention. Ayurveda strives to bring three types of energies into balance. Ayurvedic treatment may include exercise, diet, and herbal remedies.

Another example is homeopathic medicine or homeopathy, which focuses on the idea that "like cures like". Practitioners of homeopathic medicine believe that a substance that can cause an illness can also cure it. The cure, however, is a small, highly diluted quantity. Based on symptoms, a homeopathic practitioner selects a medicine and gives it in very weak doses. These principles contradict conventional medical science.

Yet another alternative medical system is naturopathic medicine, in which practitioners work with natural healing forces within the body, with a goal of helping the body recover from disease and attain better health. Naturopathic therapies may include dietary modifications, massage, exercise, and acupuncture.

Mind-Body Interventions

These therapies use the influence of the mind on the body. One example of mind-body influence that is part of mainstream medicine today is biofeedback. In biofeedback, a trained technician attaches sensors to various parts of the

Figure 7.1

Common Terms: Complementary and Alternative Medicine

Aromatherapy ("ah-roam-uh-THER-ah-py") involves the use of essential oils (extracts or essences) from flowers, herbs, and trees to promote health and well-being.

Ayurveda ("ah-yur-VAY-dah") is a CAM alternative medical system that has been practiced primarily in the Indian sub-continent for 5,000 years. Ayurveda includes diet and herbal remedies and emphasizes the use of body, mind, and spirit in disease prevention and treatment.

Chiropractic ("ki-roh-PRAC-tic") is a CAM alternative medical system. It focuses on the relationship between bodily structure (primarily that of the spine) and function, and how that relationship affects the preservation and restoration of health. Chiropractors use manipulative therapy as an integral treatment tool.

Electromagnetic fields (EMFs, also called electric and magnetic fields) are invisible lines of force that surround all electrical devices. The earth also produces EMFs; electric fields are produced when there is thunderstorm activity, and magnetic fields are believed to be produced by electric currents flowing at the earth's core.

Homeopathic ("home-ee-oh-PATH-ic") medicine is a CAM alternative medical system. In homeopathic medicine, there is a belief that "like cures like" meaning that small, highly diluted quantities of medicinal substances are given to cure symptoms, when the same substances given at higher or more concentrated doses would actually cause those symptoms.

Massage ("muh-SAHJ") therapists manipulate muscle and connective tissue to enhance function of those tissues and promote relaxation and well-being.

Naturopathic ("nay-chur-o-PATH-ic") medicine is a CAM alternative medical system in which practitioners work with natural healing forces within the body, with a goal of helping the body recover from disease and attain better health. Practices may include dietary modifications, massage, exercise, acupuncture, minor surgery, and various other interventions.

Osteopathic ("ahs-tee-oh-PATH-ic") medicine is a form of conventional medicine that, in part, emphasizes diseases arising in the musculoskeletal system. There is an underlying belief that all of the body's systems work together, and disturbances in one system may affect function elsewhere in the body. Some osteopathic physicians practice osteopathic manipulation, a full-body system of hands-on techniques to alleviate pain, restore function, and promote health and well-being.

Qi gong ("chee-GUNG") is a component of traditional Chinese medicine that combines movement, meditation, and regulation of breathing to enhance the flow of qi (an ancient term given to what is believed to be vital energy) in the body, improve blood circulation, and enhance immune function.

Reiki ("RAY-kee") is a Japanese word meaning Universal Life Energy. Reiki is based on the belief that when spiritual energy is channeled through a Reiki practitioner, the patient's spirit is healed, which in turn heals the physical body.

Therapeutic Touch is derived from an ancient technique called laying-on of hands. It is based on the premise that it is the healing force of the therapist that affects the patient's recovery; healing is promoted when the body's energies are in balance; and, by passing their hands over the patient, healers can identify energy imbalances.

Source: National Center for Complementary and Alternative Medicine (NCCAM), National Institutes of Health

body. The technician gives a patient feedback as the patient focuses to relax, reduce blood pressure, reduce the heart rate, or control pain. This procedure helps to train a patient in using the mind to produce positive effects. Other examples of mind-body interventions are meditation, hypnosis, prayer, mental healing, and creative endeavors, such as art or music therapy.

Biologically Based Therapies

These approaches use biological agents, such as herbs, special foods, or nutritional supplements to produce therapeutic results. An example is using shark cartilage to cure cancer. This is an example of a CAM therapy whose effectiveness is not proven.

Manipulative and Body-Based Methods

Manipulative therapies involve moving or manipulating parts of the body to promote healing. Massage is a familiar example. In addition, osteopathic medicine, which is well recognized as conventional medicine, bases treatment on the idea that disturbances in bones, spinal alignment, and muscle can create other medical problems. An osteopathic physician (DO), who receives the same training as an MD, may use hands-on techniques to alleviate pain, restore function, and promote health and well-being. Chiropractors also use body manipulation. Their medical training, however, is more limited, compared with osteopathic physicians. While chiropractors often use nutrition therapies as well, their training does not include extensive nutrition science.

Energy Therapies

These therapies use energy fields believed to surround and penetrate the body. This is a concept that has not been identified by conventional science. Examples of energy therapies include Reiki, qi gong, therapeutic touch, and electromagnetic treatments.

BACKGROUND

Complementary and alternative medicines are becoming prevalent in the US today. Why? For many people, they represent a way to take control of personal health. The *Journal of the American Medical Association* has reported that from 1990-97, healthcare consumers made more visits to CAM practitioners than they did to primary care physicians. The strength of consumer motivation becomes apparent when we note that medical insurance typically does not cover CAM. Most consumers pay for these services out-of-pocket, with no reimbursement.

In addition to personal control, CAM offers some individuals beliefs that they can treat themselves in a "natural" way, or that they may not risk side effects that can accompany conventional treatments. In addition, use of technology in medicine today is distressing to some individuals, who may choose CAM as a low-technology alternative. Sometimes, a CAM therapy is easy to use. Taking a dietary supplement, for example, may seem easier than going to a hospital for chemotherapy.

Furthermore, some CAM practices have ancient roots, and this inspires confidence for many patients. Acupuncture, for example, is thousands of years old. Use of herbal remedies began long before today's pharmaceutical industry developed. For some consumers, cultural tradition inspires trust and confidence. Interestingly, many observers think that some CAM therapies are effective simply because of consumer confidence. Belief in a cure can produce a

placebo effect. This means a patient's condition improves not because of the treatment itself, but because of the belief that the treatment works.

Is CAM really safer than conventional medicine? The answer can vary. What is important in evaluating any medical treatment is whether it is safe, and whether it is effective. Confidence in treatment stems from well-controlled research. In many cases, CAM treatments simply have not undergone adequate research for medical scientists to draw conclusions. This is changing, however. Research about CAM therapies is increasing. Some have been found to be safe and

COMMON CAM THERAPIES

THERAPY	USED FOR	SAFE?	EFFECTIVE?
Chiropractic manipulation	Back pain	Probably	Yes, according to some research
Massage	Relaxation; muscle soreness	Yes, with precautions (e.g. not over an open wound, or with phlebitis)	Yes, but additional therapies may be required
Glucosamine and chondroitin supplements	Osteoarthritis	Probably	Maybe; is under further study
Ephedra herbal supplement	Weight loss	No, can cause heart palpitations and death, especially if combined with other stimulants; banned in 2004	Yes, for short-term weight loss
Garlic supplements	Preventing heart attack	Generally, yes	Inconclusive
St. John's Wort herbal supplement	Depression	Yes, but can cause problem drug interactions	May be effective for mild depression
Coenzyme Q10	Parkinson's Disease	Poses drug interaction concerns	Yes, slows progression of the disease
Plant estrogens /soy products	Menopause symptoms	Probably	Inconclusive
Laetrile	Cancer treatment	No, can cause cyanide poisoning	No
Kava herbal supplement	Anxiety, insomnia	No, can damage the liver	Inconclusive
Wearable magnets	Arthritis pain	Probably, except if close to a pacemaker	Possibly
Acupuncture	Pain management	Can cause nerve damage if technique is poor or hepatitis B under unsanitary conditions	Inconclusive

Source: National Center for Complementary and Alternative Medicine

Figure 7.2

effective. Others have been found to pose serious risks. Figure 7.2 provides examples of common CAM therapies, with information about safety and effectiveness.

HERBS AND DIETARY SUPPLEMENTS

Herbs, large doses of vitamins and minerals, and other food components are common forms of CAM. In fact, sales of dietary supplements total more than $15 billion per year, according to the Food and Nutrition Board of the Institute of Medicine. As the role of nutrition in health gains increasing attention from the scientific community, it is easy to believe there is a dietary solution to nearly every condition. This is not exactly true. Dietary practices can become an important component of overall healthcare, however.

When it comes to herbs and other nutritional supplements, it's important to understand that "natural" does not necessarily mean "safe". Many of nature's poisons are entirely natural—but deadly. Arsenic is an example. Meanwhile, some of today's drug therapies have been derived from plants. An example is digitalis, a medicine for regulating heartbeat. Thus, the key point is that any chemical compound that has biological activity—whether derived from natural sources or created in a laboratory—must be evaluated scientifically. It needs to be proven safe and effective. In addition, the manufacture and dosage need to be controlled.

According to the FDA, a **dietary supplement**:

- is a product (other than tobacco) that is intended to supplement the diet that bears or contains one or more of the following dietary ingredients: a vitamin, a mineral, an herb or other botanical, an amino acid, a dietary substance for use by man to supplement the diet by increasing the total daily intake, or a concentrate, metabolite, constituent, extract, or combination of these ingredients.
- is intended for ingestion in pill, capsule, tablet, or liquid form.
- is not represented for use as a conventional food or as the sole item of a meal or diet.
- is labeled as a "dietary supplement."

Under the Dietary Supplement Health and Education Act passed by Congress in 1994, dietary supplements are considered foods, not drugs. It is a manufacturer's responsibility to ensure that its products are safe and properly labeled prior to marketing. This means that dietary supplements are not subject to the same controls as prescription and over-the-counter drugs. For a drug to reach the market, its manufacturer must first prove safety and effectiveness to the FDA. Dietary supplements, in contrast, must be proven unsafe by the FDA to be removed from the market.

In addition, the regulation prohibits dietary supplement manufacturers from making health claims on product labels. For example, a label cannot state that this supplement will "cure cancer" or "treat arthritis". However, manufacturers are allowed to describe the supplement's effects on "structure or function" of the body or "well-being". To use these claims, manufacturers must have substantiation that the statements are truthful and not misleading. A product label must bear the note: "This statement has not been evaluated by the Food and Drug Administration. This product is not intended to diagnose, treat, cure, or prevent any disease." A dietary supplement must have a label identifying its ingredients and must provide nutrition labeling.

Clearly, a dietary supplement package can imply health benefits that may not be well substantiated. What else is not regulated? Controls on product composition, purity and quality, and quantities are minimal. In 2003, the FDA proposed a new rule to control these issues. In short, the contents of a dietary supplement preparation may not be exactly what a consumer thinks. For example, the FDA evaluated a group of soy products on the market and found that some contained as little as half the amount of isoflavones (active ingredients) claimed. Another review found that a supplement of folic acid contained only 35% of its declared dose. Conversely, a supplement may contain much larger doses of active ingredients than the label indicates. This can pose risks related to overdosage. In addition, a dietary supplement may contain contaminants such as lead, pesticides, bacteria, or undeclared ingredients. Among other things, the proposed new rule would establish good manufacturing practices for dietary supplements.

Meanwhile, in 2001, the US Pharmacopeia (USP), which is a research group that is not a part of the government, announced a certification program for dietary supplements. Based on testing, a supplement can contain a USP certification mark to indicate that ingredients are as claimed. Of course, this mark does not verify that the supplements are effective treatments for specific health conditions.

It's important to note that safe and effective dosages for herbs and other dietary supplements may not be well established. At least for recognized vitamins and minerals, we have reference standards. Thus, even for an herb that may have beneficial effects, a consumer might not take a dosage that proves beneficial. Or, a consumer may easily overdose. Meanwhile consumers may mistakenly assume that "more is better" when it comes to supplementation. This can be dangerous. Even a vitamin or mineral known to be essential for life can become toxic in excessive doses. Figure 7.3 identifies overdose risks of several dietary supplements.

To avoid overdose of vitamins and minerals, it's helpful to return to basic nutrition science. The body has basic requirements for nutrients. Excesses of many of the water-soluble vitamins are simply excreted in urine. Fat-soluble vitamins

Figure 7.3

RISKS OF OVERDOSE

DIETARY SUPPLEMENT	EFFECTS OF OVERDOSE
Vitamin B6 > 100 mg/day	Neurological toxicity, nerve injury
Niacin > 500 mg/day	Gastrointestinal distress, liver damage, very low blood pressure, occasionally life-threatening conditions
Vitamin A > 25,000 International Units (IU)/day	Liver damage, birth defects, damage to bones and cartilage
Selenium > 800 micrograms/day	Tissue damage
Germander	Liver disease
Comfrey	Liver damage/cirrhosis, sometimes life-threatening
Chaparral	Liver damage

and minerals can, in some cases, accumulate in the body. Generally, nutritionists recommend that supplementation of vitamins and minerals be used to correct deficiencies, based on an assessment of nutritional status and nutritional needs. As explained in Chapter 3, a tolerable upper intake level (UL) is the highest level of daily nutrient intake that is likely to pose no risk of adverse health effects for most people. This is different from a recommended level of intake. It provides a reference for evaluating the safety of supplementation. Tolerable upper intake levels appear in the CD-ROM that accompanies this book.

Drug Interactions

Among the risks of using dietary supplements can be the interactions they present. Herbs, for example, may interact with each other to cause dangerous effects. Herbs may also interact with conventional drugs to modify their action. For instance, the herbal supplement ginko has many potential drug interactions. Gingko can increase blood levels of antidepressant drugs, accidentally building high drug levels. Used with an antipsychotic medication, gingko can cause seizures. Both gingko and coenzyme Q10 are supplements that can interfere with the action of anticoagulant medications, such as warfarin or coumadin. The result can be excessive bleeding. Both ginseng and coenzyme Q10 can enhance the action of a drug designed to lower blood sugar. The result can be a crisis with hypoglycemia (very low blood sugar). St. John's Wort may eliminate a number of drugs from the body very quickly. There is concern that taking this supplement may reduce the effectiveness of oral contraceptives. It can also interact with antidepressant drugs to cause headache, upset stomach, and restlessness. Before surgery, it can be dangerous to take certain herbal supplements, including ginseng or goldenseal, which may raise blood pressure. Other herbs can slow down blood clotting and increase the risk of excessive bleeding. These include garlic, ginger, gingko, and feverfew.

Because many consumers use dietary supplements as complementary or alternative therapies, they may not choose to discuss these therapies with physicians. Typically, an individual using dietary supplements considers this treatment "separate" from a physician's care. However, it is actually important for a physician to know the complete picture. A dietary manager can facilitate this process by asking patients questions about what dietary supplements they use, reporting this information in the diet history, and discussing it with other members of the healthcare team.

EVALUATING CAM THERAPIES

The following questions can help you evaluate any type of medical therapy.

- What research supports the safety of this treatment?
- What are the possible risks and side effects?
- What research indicates this treatment is effective?
- Has research been published in a medical journal that is reviewed by trained medical scientists?
- Has the research been well-controlled, or is the therapy based on anecdotal reports?
- What will the treatment involve?
- What will it cost?
- Is this treatment intended to complement other therapies or replace them (alternative medicine)?
- Has this treatment been discussed with a physician?
- What are the other options, and how does this treatment compare?

Figure 7.4 identifies red flags that may indicate fad or fraud in proposed treatments. In addition, the FDA notes that four key assumptions often come into play when consumers are making decisions about therapies. These appear in Figure 7.5.

HEALTHCARE POLICY

In 2003, the White House Commission on CAM Policy issued policy suggestions for the healthcare industry. They recommended 10 principles for healthcare policy:

1. **A wholeness orientation in healthcare delivery.** Health involves all aspects of life—mind, body, spirit, environment—and high-quality healthcare must support care of the whole person.

2. **Evidence of safety and efficacy.** The Commission is committed to promoting the use of science and appropriate scientific methods to help identify safe and effective CAM services and products and to generate evidence that will protect and promote the public health.

Figure 7.4

FADS, FRAUDS, AND QUACKERY

The following claims are cause for caution. Each is a red flag suggesting that the scientific basis for safety and effectiveness may be missing. Based on these red flags, a treatment could be a fad, fraud, or form of quackery. **Quackery** is medical treatment that does not perform as claimed and is offered by an untrained or uninformed individual.

Miracle cure: The treatment is described as a miracle, breakthrough, or cure-all. Few treatments are actually this effective!

Anecdotal evidence: Descriptions of the treatment use stories about individual success, rather than citing controlled medical research.

Shaky terminology: Some unfounded treatments may claim to purify, energize, or detoxify the body. These terms have little scientific meaning.

Too good to be true: A claim tells only the good, without identifying possible risks or side effects.

Source: FDA

Figure 7.5

FOUR QUESTIONABLE ASSUMPTIONS

Check assumptions about the following:

QUESTIONABLE ASSUMPTION #1
"Even if a product may not help me, at least it won't hurt me." It's best not to assume that this will always be true. When consumed in high enough amounts, for a long enough time, or in combination with certain other substances, all chemicals can be toxic, including nutrients, plant components, and other biologically active ingredients.

QUESTIONABLE ASSUMPTION #2
"When I see the term 'natural,' it means that a product is healthful and safe." Consumers can be misled if they assume this term assures wholesomeness, or that these food-like substances necessarily have milder effects, which makes them safer to use than drugs. The term "natural" on labels is not well defined and is sometimes used ambiguously to imply unsubstantiated benefits or safety. For example, many weight-loss products claim to be "natural" or "herbal" but this doesn't necessarily make them safe. Their ingredients may interact with drugs or may be dangerous for people with certain medical conditions.

QUESTIONABLE ASSUMPTION #3
"A product is safe when there is no cautionary information on the product label." Dietary supplement manufacturers may not necessarily include warnings about potential adverse effects on the labels of their products. If consumers want to know about the safety of a specific dietary supplement, they should contact the manufacturer of that brand directly. It is the manufacturer's responsibility to determine that the supplement it produces or distributes is safe and that there is substantiated evidence that the label claims are truthful and not misleading.

QUESTIONABLE ASSUMPTION #4
"A recall of a harmful product guarantees that all such harmful products will be immediately and completely removed from the marketplace." A product recall of a dietary supplement is voluntary and while many manufacturers do their best, a recall does not necessarily remove all harmful products from the marketplace.

Source: FDA

3. **The healing capacity of the person.** The person has a remarkable capacity for recovery and self-healing, and a major focus of healthcare is to support and promote this capacity.

4. **Respect for individuality.** Every person is unique and has the right to healthcare that is appropriately responsive to him or her, respecting preferences and preserving dignity.

5. **The right to choose treatment.** Every person has the right to choose freely among safe and effective care or approaches, as well as among qualified practitioners who are accountable for their claims and actions and responsive to the person's needs.

6. **An emphasis on health promotion and self-care.** Good healthcare emphasizes self-care and early intervention for maintaining and promoting health.

7. **Partnerships as essential for integrated healthcare.** Good healthcare requires teamwork among patients, healthcare practitioners (conventional and CAM), and researchers committed to creating optimal healing environments and to respecting the diversity of all healthcare traditions.

8. **Education as a fundamental healthcare service.** Education about prevention, healthful lifestyles, and the power of self-healing should be made an integral part of the curricula of all healthcare professionals and should be made available to the public.

9. **Dissemination of comprehensive and timely information.** The quality of healthcare can be enhanced by promoting efforts that thoroughly and thoughtfully examine the evidence on which CAM systems, practices, and products are based and making this evidence widely, rapidly, and easily available.

10. **Integral public involvement.** The input of informed consumers and other members of the public must be incorporated in setting priorities for healthcare, healthcare research, and in reaching policy decisions, including those related to CAM, within the public and private sectors.

In its report, the White House Commission on CAM Policy also offered more perspective that is helpful to dietary managers in evaluating CAM: "Although most CAM modalities have not yet been proven to be safe and effective, it is likely that some of them eventually will be proven to be safe and effective, whereas others will not...."

"The question is not, *Should Americans be using complementary and alternative medicine modalities?* as many—perhaps most—already are doing so. For the most part, however, they are making these choices in the absence of valid scientific information to guide them in making informed and intelligent choices.

"Many of the commissioners agree with the editors of *The New England Journal of Medicine* who stated in 1998: 'There cannot be two kinds of medicine—conventional and alternative. There is only medicine that has been adequately tested and medicine that has not, medicine that works and medicine that may or may not work. Once a treatment has been tested rigorously, it no longer matters whether it was considered alternative at the outset. If it is found to be reasonably safe and effective, it will be accepted.'"

A Dietary Manager's Role

In line with recommended healthcare policy and the state of knowledge on CAM therapies today, dietary managers and others involved in providing healthcare can take several approaches to CAM:

- Recognize the individual rights of healthcare consumers to choose their own care.
- Respect individual preferences.
- Facilitate communications with patients about CAM therapies, particularly use of dietary supplements.
- Help communicate information about individuals' CAM therapy choices to the entire healthcare team.
- Inform patients of possible risks; help to educate.
- Keep an open mind, and continue to keep abreast of new findings in this fast-growing area of medical science.

Key Points

- Complementary and alternative medicine is a group of diverse medical and healthcare systems, practices, and products that are not presently considered to be part of conventional medicine.

- Types of CAM include: alternative medical systems, mind-body interventions, biologically based therapies, manipulative and body-based methods, and energy therapies.

- Many consumers choose CAM therapies to take control of personal health, often perceiving CAM therapies as more "natural" than conventional medicine.

- When it comes to herbs and other nutritional supplements, "natural" does not necessarily mean "safe".

- Some dietary supplements can have dangerous effects if taken in excessive amounts.

- Some herbal supplements may interfere with drug treatments, so physicians should know about dietary supplements a patient uses.

▶ The public can be deceived or misled. Possible signs of fraud include claims for a miracle cure, use of anecdotal evidence ("stories"), shaky terminology, and claims that sound too good to be true.

▶ The two key questions for evaluating CAM are: Is the treatment safe? Is the treatment effective?

▶ Recommended healthcare policy about CAM includes applying a wholeness orientation to healthcare delivery, and using science and appropriate scientific methods to help identify safe and effective CAM therapies.

▶ In providing dietary care, a dietary manager can promote respect for individual choices and facilitate communication about CAM treatments.

Key Terms

Alternative medicine: an unconventional medical practice that is used instead of conventional medicine

CAM: Complementary and Alternative Medicine, a group of diverse medical and healthcare systems, practices, and products that are not presently considered to be part of conventional medicine

Complementary medicine: an unconventional medical practice that is used to complement or add to conventional medical practice

Conventional medicine: the science used by physicians and allied health professionals, as they are trained in the US. Sometimes, conventional medicine is also called mainstream medicine, orthodox medicine, biomedicine, or allopathy.

Dietary supplement: a product that is intended to supplement the diet that bears or contains one or more of the following dietary ingredients: a vitamin, a mineral, an herb or other botanical, an amino acid, a dietary substance for use to supplement the diet by increasing the total daily intake, or a concentrate, metabolite, constituent, extract, or combination of these ingredients

Integrative medicine: a medical practice that combines conventional practice with CAM practices

Placebo effect: improvement in a patient's condition because of the belief that the treatment works

Quackery: medical treatment that does not perform as claimed and is offered by an untrained or uninformed individual

1. The difference between complementary medicine and alternative medicine is that:
   A. Complementary medicine adds to conventional treatment, while alternative medicine replaces conventional treatment.
   B. Complementary medicine is safe, while alternative medicine is dangerous.
   C. Complementary medicine is dangerous, while alternative medicine is safe.
   D. Complementary medicine involves herbs, while alternative medicine involves acupuncture.

2. Which of the following is an example of a manipulative therapy?
   A. Biofeedback
   B. Goldenseal herbal supplement
   C. Massage
   D. Ayurveda

3. Reiki, qi gong, therapeutic touch, and electromagnetic treatments are examples of what type of CAM?
   A. Energy therapies
   B. Alternative medical systems
   C. Mind-body interventions
   D. Biologically based therapies

4. The placebo effect occurs when someone uses a treatment and then:
   A. Feels better because of the belief that the treatment works
   B. Experiences no side effects
   C. Experiences serious side effects
   D. Feels better due to drug interactions

5. Liver damage, birth defects, and damage to bones and cartilage may be adverse effects of taking too much:
   A. Iron
   B. Vitamin A
   C. Kava root
   D. Insulin

6. Concerns about dietary supplement composition include all of the following EXCEPT:
   A. Uncertainty about the quality of ingredients
   B. Possible contamination with other ingredients
   C. Uncertainty about the quantity of active ingredients
   D. Whether the herb is named on the label

7. A patient is taking gingko supplements with the hopes of improving memory, and is also taking antipsychotic medication. A dietary manager who knows this should:

    A. Tell the patient gingko appears to be effective for memory.

    B. Alert the physician, in order to manage a potential herb-drug interaction.

    C. Suggest the patient take extra doses of garlic supplements instead.

    D. Look the other way, because this is the patient's choice.

8. A key concern about taking ginseng before surgery is that:

    A. It may raise blood pressure and cause problems.

    B. It may prevent a patient from relaxing.

    C. It has been prohibited from the market by the FDA.

    D. It may cause an offensive off-odor.

9. According to current regulations for dietary supplements:

    A. A manufacturer can make any health claim desired on a product label.

    B. It is the manufacturer's responsibility to determine that the supplement it produces or distributes is safe, and FDA's responsibility to prove a product unsafe.

    C. Manufacturers do not have to provide nutrition facts labeling when relevant.

    D. Herbal products in pills or capsules are subject to regulation, but herbal teas are not.

10. A positive aspect of the CAM movement is:

    A. It has brought scientific research on CAM therapies to a halt.

    B. It encourages patients to become involved in their own healthcare and take responsibility for wellness.

    C. It eliminates the need for nutrition practitioners in healthcare.

    D. It replaces the need for trained medical professionals in many healthcare institutions.

Nutrition screening helps a dietary manager identify healthcare clients in need of nutrition intervention. It is also required for compliance with regulations and standards.

After completing this chapter, you should be able to:

- Identify the goal of nutrition screening.
- Explain the difference between nutrition screening and nutrition assessment.
- Identify sources for nutrition screening standards and tools.
- Relate the rationale for developing a policy and procedure for performing nutrition screening.
- List factors a dietary manager may check during nutrition screening.
- Explain the term body mass index (BMI).
- Calculate *ideal body weight (IBW).*
- Give examples of common food-drug interactions.
- Name some components of a diet history.
- Define *basal energy expenditure (BEE).*
- Calculate BEE and total energy needs.

As explained in Chapter 6, nutrition can have a dramatic effect on the overall wellness of many individuals—especially those who are at risk for nutrition problems. Healthcare institutions as well as legislators recognize the benefits of providing appropriate medical nutrition therapy to many patients in hospitals and residents in longterm care facilities. The natural question is: How do we know who is at risk and may need nutrition therapy? And next: How do we know what intervention a person may need?

NUTRITION SCREENING

The answers come in stages, as shown in Figure 8.1. We know who may need nutrition therapy by performing nutrition screening. In a healthcare institution such as a nursing home or hospital, every individual who is admitted should undergo nutrition screening as a routine. In other types of healthcare settings—such as an outpatient WIC (Women, Infants, and Children) Program, a renal dialysis program, or many others—nutrition screening is part of a standard outpatient procedure as new clients enter the service. **Nutrition screening** is a systematic method for identifying individuals at risk for nutrition problems. It is a process applied to an entire group, in order to select members of that group who are candidates for further intervention.

Clients whose nutrition screening suggests concerns move to the next step in the nutrition care process—**nutrition assessment**. This is an in-depth evaluation of a client's nutritional well-being. The person who conducts nutrition

Figure 8.1

MEDICAL NUTRITION THERAPY: THE NUTRITION CARE PROCESS

1. Screen patients for nutrition risk

⬇

2. Assess each patient identified by the screening process as being at risk

⬇

3. Develop a nutrition care plan for each patient

⬇

4. Document, communicate, and implement the plan

⬇

5. Re-assess the patient at defined intervals ⬅

⬇

6. As appropriate, revise the plan ──

screening may be a dietary manager, dietetic technician, or other caregiver as dictated by institutional policy. Ordinarily, the person who performs a nutrition assessment is a registered dietitian (RD). The RD uses interviews, laboratory data, clinical information, body measurements, information gathered from healthcare team members, and other tools to develop an assessment. In some institutions, other members of the healthcare team may help to gather information for the nutrition assessment. In these situations, it is typically the responsibility of the dietitian to make a final evaluation of the complete set of information. The nutrition assessment forms a basis for developing a personalized nutrition care plan. Chapter 13 addresses nutrition care planning, and Chapter 14 explains some of the follow-up required to assure effectiveness of a nutrition care plan. In this chapter, we will focus on Step 1 of the nutrition care process.

One of the responsibilities of many dietary managers who happen to work in healthcare institutions is to conduct routine nutrition screening. Screening is typically a fairly simple process, based on indicators. **Indicators** are pieces of information that might suggest a concern or risk. Many are numbers or measurements. They are built upon statistics. For example, we might discover that many individuals found to be less than 90% of their ideal body weight turn out to have significantly higher rates of complications from surgery. Based on that, we might set an indicator for nutrition screening as: less than 90% of ideal body weight. In fact, there is a huge body of research on this idea. Through research, experts have been able to identity findings and figures that can help to predict the level of nutrition risk. Other indicators might be based on diagnosis, or usual food intake, or laboratory data.

If we determine that some of the indicators for risk are present, what happens next? There are several approaches to determining the level of risk based on indicators. One method is simply to count the risk factors. A screening policy may specify something like this: *If three or more indicators of nutrition risk are present, this patient will be flagged for a complete nutrition assessment.*

In another scheme, each risk factor receives a point value. Factors judged to heighten nutrition risk the most receive the most points. In a **nutrition risk scoring system**, each risk indicator has a point value, and the total point value identifies the level of nutrition risk. Some systems even define risk levels based on the score. One system may have two levels of risk, such as: moderate risk and high risk. Another may have three levels, or even five.

Figure 8.2 provides a sample nutrition screening tool (nutrition risk assessment tool) developed by The American Dietetic Association Consulting Dietitians practice group. Figure 8.3 provides a nutrition screening and assessment tool from Nestle Clinical Nutrition. Note that both of these examples use scoring systems. In the ADA example, more points equal greater risk. In the Nestle example, fewer points mean greater risk. Whether to use high scores or low scores for expressing a risk is not important. However, it is important to understand any tool you happen to be applying in your place of employment, and to use and interpret it accurately.

Even a nutrition risk scoring system may incorporate certain overrides or automatic flags. Let's say you work with a system that specifies 20 points or higher as indicating risk. The system might also say that any individual who has been diagnosed with a pressure ulcer is automatically classified as being at nutrition risk. Even a resident who scores only 16 on the nutrition risk score would be "flagged" for nutrition assessment based on the presence of a pressure ulcer. Overrides or automatic flags can be helpful to be certain that individuals who might benefit from medical nutrition therapy receive appropriate assessment.

Also note that the example in Figure 8.3 combines screening and assessment into one document. This can be a simple method of keeping important information together. A nutrition screening result usually becomes part of a permanent medical record. Screening information is thus available to other caregivers. For example, a dietary manager may complete a nutrition screening and place it into the formal record. In follow-up, a registered dietitian may gather and evaluate more information to develop a nutrition assessment.

SOURCES FOR NUTRITION SCREENING TOOLS

As you have already noticed, many sources and standards exist for nutrition screening. Tools vary from one institution to another. If you join the staff of a healthcare institution, you will most likely find that there is a tool in place. Your job, then, will be to become familiar with the tool and to apply it. Often, a registered dietitian or clinical nutrition manager will help to locate and/or develop

Figure 8.2

SAMPLE NUTRITION SCREENING TOOL (ADA CONSULTING DIETITIANS)

Instructional Guide for Nutrition Risk Assessment

Nutrition risk is determined by the presence of characteristics that are associated with an increased likelihood of poor nutritional status. This includes various non-acute or chronic diseases and conditions, unintended weight change, inadequate or inappropriate food/fluid intake, dependency, disability, chronic medication use, and abnormal lab values. The Nutrition Risk Assessment form is designed for use in nursing facilities and can be used as the assessment form.

Frequency: The Nutrition Risk Assessment form should be completed on the same cycle as the Minimum Data Set (MDS) as follows:

(I) Initial, upon admission as part of nutrition assessment

(Q) Quarterly, with each care plan review if nutrition changes are identified in the MDS

(SC) With each significant change in condition, if nutrition-related

(R) Readmission

(A) Annual review

Data collection: The Nutrition Risk Assessment data will be collected by a registered dietitian (RD); dietetic technician, registered (DTR); or as appropriate, the certified dietary manager (CDM).

Form completion: The Nutrition Risk Assessment form will be completed, signed, and dated by a qualified dietetic professional (i.e., RD, DTR).

Procedures:

1. Complete the top of the form as indicated. The 'assessment type' is determined by the frequency (see Frequency above).

2. After reviewing the resident's medical record, interviewing the resident and/or family, monitoring the resident's actual dining performance (e.g. intake, positioning), and discussing with pertinent staff members, evaluate each resident for individual risk factors. Circle the description/terms that apply to the resident. Use the comment column to specify details of the assessment.

3. Record the appropriate number in the point column for each risk factor. The total for each risk factor cannot exceed three points.

4. If the resident falls into more than one category within a risk factor, assign the points for the most severe level. For example, if DM is controlled, but the resident receives dialysis, assign 3 points.

5. Total the number of points, determine the resident's Overall Risk Category, and record on the bottom of the form.
   0-2 points = No/Low Risk
   3-7 points = Moderate Risk
   ≥8 points = High Risk

6. If the resident is identified to be at Moderate or High Risk for *any* risk factor, follow the appropriate Strategies/Interventions and document in nutrition progress notes and care plan.

7. The nutrition professional must communicate with the interdisciplinary team to coordinate care for residents at risk.

8. File the Nutrition Risk Assessment form in the Nutrition Section of the clinical record or in the appropriate section identified by the facility and communicate recommendations to approriate team members.

9. Do not count vitamin and mineral supplements as medications. Use progress notes to document needs.

10. Document lab values obtained within the past quarter.

Nutrition Risk Assessment

Name_____ Adm date_____ Rm_____ Asess type_____

DOB_____ Age_____ Sex: M F Advance directive_____ Physician_____

Diagnosis_____

Ht (in)_____ Wt (lb)_____ Wt (kg)_____ Usual body wt range_____ BMI_____

BEE_____ Activity factor_____ Injury factor_____ Total cal_____ Total protein_____g (____g/kg)

Total fluids_____cc (_____cc/kg) Fluid restriction_____

Diet order_____ Food allergies/sensitivities_____

Supplement/snacks_____ Cultural/religious preferences_____

Risk Factor	No/Low Risk (0 pts)	Moderate Risk (1 pt)	High Risk (3 pts)	MDS Ref	Pts	Comments
Weight status; loss or gain	BMI 19-27 No weight change	<5% wt change in 30 days <7.5% within 90 days; or <10% within 6 mo	BMI <19 or >27 ≥5% wt change in 30 days; ≥7.5% in 90 days; or ≥10% within 6 mo	J,K, E		
Oral/nutrition intake; food	Intake meets 76-100% of estimated needs	Intake meets 26-75% of estimated needs	Intake meets ≤25% of estimated needs	AC, J, K		
Oral/nutrition intake; fluids	Consumes 1,500-2,000 cc/day	Consumes 1,000-1,499 cc/day	Consumes <1,000 cc/day	AC, J, K		
Medications; nutrition-related	0-1 drugs/day	2-4 drugs/day	5 or more drugs/day	O		
Relevant conditions and diagnoses	HTN, DM, heart disease or other controlled diseases/conditions	Anemia, infection, CVA (recent), fracture, UTI, alcohol abuse, drug abuse COPD, edema, surgery (recent), osteoporosis, hx of GI bleed, food intolerances and allergies, poor circulation, constipation, diarrhea, GERD, anorexia, Parkinson's	Cancer (advanced), septicemia, liver failure dialysis, ESRD, Alzheimer's, dementia, depression, dehydration, dysphagia, radiation/chemo, active GI bleed, chronic nausea, vomiting, ostomy, gastrectomy, fecal impaction, uncontrolled diseases or conditions	E, H, I, J, M, P		
Physical and mental functioning	Ambulatory, alert, able to feed self, no chewing or swallowing problems	Out of bed w/assistance, motor agitation (tremors, wandering), limited feeding assistance, supervision while eating, chewing or swallowing problems, teeth in poor repair, ill-fitting dentures or refusal to wear dentures, edentulous, taste and sensory changes, unable to communicate needs	Bedridden, inactive, total dependence, extensive or total assistance or dependence while eating, aspirates, tube feeding, TPN, mouth pain	A, B, E, G, L, P		
Lab values	Albumin and other nutrition-related lab values WNL	Albumin 3.0-3.4 g/dl, 1-2 other nutrition-related labs abnormal	Albumin less than 3.0 g/dl, 3-5 other nutrition-related labs abnormal	P		
Skin conditions	Skin intact	Stage I/II pressure ulcers or skin tears not healing, hx of pressure ulcers, stasis ulcer, fecal incontinence	Stage III/IV pressure ulcers or multiple impaired areas	M		

Figure 8.3

NUTRITION SCREENING AND ASSESSMENT TOOL (NESTLE CLINICAL NUTRITION)

NESTLÉ NUTRITION SERVICES

Mini Nutritional Assessment
MNA®

Last name:	First name:	Sex:	Date:

Age:	Weight, kg:	Height, cm:	I.D. Number:

Complete the screen by filling in the boxes with the appropriate numbers.
Add the numbers for the screen. If score is 11 or less, continue with the assessment to gain a Malnutrition Indicator Score.

Screening

A Has food intake declined over the past 3 months
due to loss of appetite, digestive problems,
chewing or swallowing difficulties?
0 = severe loss of appetite
1 = moderate loss of appetite
2 = no loss of appetite ☐

B Weight loss during last months
0 = weight loss greater than 3 kg (6.6 lbs)
1 = does not know
2 = weight loss between 1 and 3 kg (2.2 and 6.6 lbs)
3 = no weight loss ☐

C Mobility
0 = bed or chair bound
1 = able to get out of bed/chair but does not go out
2 = goes out ☐

D Has suffered psychological stress or acute
disease in the past 3 months
0 = yes   2 = no ☐

E Neuropsychological problems
0 = severe dementia or depression
1 = mild dementia
2 = no psychological problems ☐

F Body Mass Index (BMI) (weight in kg) / (height in m)²
0 = BMI less than 19
1 = BMI 19 to less than 21
2 = BMI 21 to less than 23
3 = BMI 23 or greater ☐

Screening score (subtotal max. 14 points) ☐ ☐

12 points or greater   Normal – not at risk –
no need to complete assessment

11 points or below   Possible malnutrition – continue assessment

Assessment

G Lives independently (not in a nursing home or hospital)
0 = no   1 = yes ☐

H Takes more than 3 prescription drugs per day
0 = yes   1 = no ☐

I Pressure sores or skin ulcers
0 = yes   1 = no ☐

J How many full meals does the patient eat daily?
0 = 1 meal
1 = 2 meals
2 = 3 meals ☐

K Selected consumption markers for protein intake
• At least one serving of dairy products
(milk, cheese, yogurt) per day?   yes ☐ no ☐
• Two or more serving of legumes
or eggs per week?   yes ☐ no ☐
• Meat, fish or poultry every day   yes ☐ no ☐
0.0 = if 0 or 1 yes
0.5 = if 2 yes
1.0 = if 3 yes   ☐ . ☐

L Consumes two or more servings
of fruits or vegetables per day?
0 = no   1 = yes ☐

M How much fluid (water, juice, coffee, tea, milk…)
is consumed per day?
0.0 = less than 3 cups
0.5 = 3 to 5 cups
1.0 = more than 5 cups   ☐ . ☐

N Mode of feeding
0 = unable to eat without assistance
1 = self-fed with some difficulty
2 = self-fed without any problem ☐

O Self view of nutritional status
0 = view self as being malnourished
1 = is uncertain of nutritional state
2 = views self as having no nutritional problem ☐

P In comparison with other people of the same age,
how do they consider their health status?
0.0 = not as good
0.5 = does not know
1.0 = as good
2.0 = better   ☐ . ☐

Q Mid-arm circumference (MAC) in cm
0.0 = MAC less than 21
0.5 = MAC 21 to 22
1.0 = MAC 22 or greater   ☐ . ☐

R Calf circumference (CC) in cm
0 = CC less than 31   1 = CC 31 or greater ☐

Assessment (max. 16 points) ☐ ☐ . ☐

Screening score ☐ ☐

Total Assessment (max. 30 points) ☐ ☐ . ☐

Malnutrition Indicator Score

17 to 23.5 points   at risk of malnutrition ☐

Less than 17 points   malnourished ☐

Ref.: Guigoz Y, Vellas B and Garry P.J. 1994. Mini Nutritional Assessment: A practical assessment tool for grading the nutritional state of elderly patients. *Facts and Research in Gerontology.* Supplement #2:15-59.
Rubenstein LZ, Harker J, Guigoz Y and Vellas B. Comprehensive Geriatric Assessment (CGA) and the MNA: An Overview of CGA, Nutritional Assessment, and Development of a Shortened Version of the MNA. In: "Mini Nutritional Assessment (MNA): Research and Practice in the Elderly". Vellas B, Garry PJ and Guigoz Y., editors. Nestlé Nutrition Workshop Series. Clinical & Performance Programme, vol. 1. Karger, Bâle, in press.

® Société des Produits Nestlé S.A., Vevey, Switzerland, Trademark Owners

0698 USA

a screening tool. Some institutions develop nutrition screening tools in-house, drawing on the expertise of dietitians and healthcare team members. On the other hand, a screening tool may come from professional organizations, such as The American Dietetic Association or other dietetics group. It may come from researchers or educational institutions. It may come from a provider of products to support medical nutrition therapy. Nutrition screening standards and forms are sometimes components of diet manuals. Finally, nutrition screening may be built into a clinical nutrition management software package. Software-based systems may have default screening criteria and scoring values built-in. Typically, however, a dietitian can select indicators and thresholds in the software in order to customize scoring to institutional policies and procedures. Another advantage of using software support in the screening process is that most programs can then generate a report or list for follow-up assessment. If a priority system is used (e.g. Level 1 Risk, Level 2 Risk, etc.), software may sort the list by priority level. Software also automates the calculations involved in nutrition screening.

Regardless of the choice of tools, an effective nutrition screening process:

- Uses meaningful screening criteria, as identified by a qualified individual (e.g. dietitian)
- Sets meaningful thresholds that correspond to known risks
- Is applied to every client
- Is implemented quickly upon admission
- Is implemented uniformly and consistently

The screening process is implemented uniformly and consistently through the use of standardized forms, such as the examples in Figures 8.2 and 8.3. Using a form ensures that as you screen, you review the same key indicators among all clients, without overlooking any piece of the screening standard. It's like a shopping list; it ensures you won't forget anything! A software program accomplishes the same objective, but through an electronic process. By following a methodical process for nutrition screening, you can be reasonably confident that you are finding the clients whose personal health may benefit from medical nutrition therapy. You can ensure that each of these clients receives a nutrition assessment.

Furthermore, nutrition screening is generally dictated by relevant healthcare regulations, both federal and state. Guidelines from the Joint Commission on Accreditation of Healthcare Organizations (JCAHO) also apply to most healthcare institutions. Standards may require that nutrition screening be conducted within a given timeframe after admission, and again at prescribed intervals. Based on regulations, the role of a dietary manager in screening may vary from one institution to another. Likewise, the method of documenting screening activities may also vary. Thus, it is imperative to become familiar with all relevant regulations and standards at any place of employment, and to follow them. Each healthcare institution needs to develop a policy and procedure for nutrition screening that achieves the objective of identifying clients at risk and stipulates a mechanism for assuring regulatory compliance and documentation.

NUTRITION SCREENING INDICATORS

There are many factors that may suggest nutrition risk. By no means is it necessary to use all possible criteria to identify risk. Criteria used in screening are usually representative of a cluster of related findings. In other words, a key indicator used for nutrition screening may represent the tip of an iceberg. If this factor exists, we consider it likely that other risk factors exist along with it. Indicators used in screening (and in nutrition assessment) fall into four basic categories, which some people think of as A-B-C-D:

- Anthropometric measurements
- Biochemical tests
- Clinical information
- Diet history

Clearly, there are many types of information that can suggest nutritional risk. A nutrition screening process will use only a few pieces of information as indicators or predictors. However, a nutrition assessment uses most or all of the relevant information available.

Nutritional status is a person's state of nutritional health. We focus the most attention on information that reflects overall nutritional status, or *protein-calorie status*. Basically, this is a measurement of status for the macronutrients. If a person is in negative energy balance, losing weight rapidly, we assume some protein has been lost from the body. Weight loss and protein loss are associated with negative health outcomes. If we examine whether a person is in a deficiency state for iron, we are looking at *iron status*. Nutritional status can describe any nutrient or groups of nutrients. Most screening focuses on calories and protein in the body. In some environments, a dietary manager may assist in screening, and/or in gathering some of the nutrition-related information. Here is a closer look at the information involved:

Anthropometric Measurements

Anthropometric measurements are measurements of the human body. The most common examples are height and weight. These two figures are actually very useful, provided that accurate measurements are made. Adults should be weighed on a beam balance scale that is calibrated regularly to ensure accuracy. The best time to weigh a client is in the morning before breakfast and after the bladder has been emptied. For consistency, clients should always be weighed at the same time of day, and on the same scale, wearing the same amount of clothing. This makes comparisons of weights from one date to another most meaningful. There are specialized scales available for clients who are unable to stand. Even when weights are taken correctly, factors such as fluid retention, adaptive equipment on wheelchairs, and wedges or pillows may adversely affect a weight reading. It is important to obtain a weight upon admission and regularly thereafter. Do not simply rely on a weight recorded at a different facility.

An accurate measurement of height is also important. Relying upon the client's self-reported height or a visual estimate is not adequate. Whenever possible, height should be measured with the client standing straight against a measuring tape or stick on a vertical wall or instrument. If this is not possible, using a tape measure to check height from feet to head is an option. Another alternative is to measure the distance from the fingertip to the midpoint of the chest, and then double that number. Usually, this gives a reasonable estimate of actual height. However, it is not highly accurate.

There are many guidelines and standards that may be used for evaluating body weight. Standards are generally based on height. In general, a good standard also accounts for differences between males and females, as well as differences in body frame size. For example, a person with a small frame (small bones) should ideally weigh less than a person of the same height who has a larger frame size. Weight alone doesn't tell all, however. Another consideration is what that weight is made of. A person who exercises a great deal, and in particular someone who does strength training, may accumulate a great deal of muscle mass. This may translate into a high body weight, but it may be a healthy condition. Some experts use various methods to evaluate percent body fat.

Using weight and height, we can determine ideal body weight. **Ideal body weight (IBW)** is an estimate of what would be a healthy weight for an individual. It is based on height, sex, and frame size. **Frame size** refers to the thickness of bones, or underlying body build. You may check reference tables to determine ideal body weight, or use a simple formula (Figure 8.4) to calculate it. Here is an example for a 5 foot, 11-inch male with a large frame:

106 pounds + (11 x 6) = 172 pounds
172 pounds x 0.10 = 17 pounds
172 pounds + 17 pounds = 189 pounds IBW

Figure 8.4

How to Calculate Ideal Body Weight (IBW)

WOMEN
IBW = 100 lbs + 5 x (number of inches over 5 feet)

MEN
IBW = 106 lbs + 6 x (number of inches over 5 feet)

FRAME ADJUSTMENTS (MEN AND WOMEN)
For a small frame, subtract 10% of the total

For a large frame, add 10% to the total

Figure 8.5

How to Calculate Percent of IBW

Percent of IBW = (Actual weight ÷ IBW) x 100

Figure 8.6

How to Calculate Percent Weight Change

Percent weight change = [(Usual weight - Actual weight) ÷ usual weight] x 100

Once we know a person's ideal body weight, we can compare this with actual weight. **Actual weight** is what a person weighs right now. When we compare the two figures, we examine percent of IBW. **Percent of IBW** describes how closely a person's actual weight resembles the ideal. Figure 8.5 shows how to calculate percent of IBW. Here are two examples:

Marla weighs 156 lbs. Her IBW is 115 lbs.
Percent of IBW = (156 lbs ÷ 115 lbs) x 100
$$= 1.36 \text{ x } 100$$
$$= 136$$
Marla is at 136% of her IBW.

Jacob weighs 137 lbs. His IBW is 148 lbs.
Percent of IBW = (137 lbs ÷ 148 lbs) x 100
$$= 0.93 \text{ x } 100$$
$$= 93$$
Jacob is at 93% of his IBW.

Note that in these examples, we are rounding calculations to the nearest whole number. IBW and related calculations are only estimates, so it is not necessary to extend decimal places. Roughly speaking, percent of ideal body weight gives an indication of whether a person is potentially undernourished or overweight. For example, one rule of thumb says that a person at or below 90% of IBW may be a nutritional risk. However, this measurement alone does not tell all. Imagine Jacob from the example above. Currently, he is below his IBW. To better understand his nutritional state, what we really need to know is what the recent trend has been. Jacob weighs 137 lbs. right now. We have to wonder: Has he always been a thin man? If so, maybe there is not a concern here. On the other hand, what if Jacob weighed 159 lbs. just six months ago, and is now down to this weight? This should concern us greatly, because it indicates a severe downward trend in his weight. We can guess his weight will continue to fall without intervention. This rapid weight loss may be due to health conditions, such as cancer, or dysphagia, or depression. Furthermore, if he is losing weight at a rapid clip, he may be losing some of his lean body mass. **Lean body mass** describes the weight of all parts of the body that are NOT fat, e.g. muscle, bones, and organs. If Jacob is losing lean body mass, his body systems may not be functioning at their best. He is likely at risk.

How can we determine what is really going on here? The answer is: by calculating percent weight change. **Percent weight change** indicates by what proportion the body weight has changed over a certain period of time. Figure 8.6 shows the calculation. Here is an example:

Jacob weighs 137 lbs. now. He weighed 159 lbs. six months ago.

$$
\begin{aligned}
\text{Percent weight change} &= [(159 \text{ lbs} - 137 \text{ lbs}) \div \text{usual weight}] \times 100 \\
&= [22 \div \text{usual weight}] \times 100 \\
&= [22 \div 159] \times 100 \\
&= 0.14 \times 100 \\
&= 14\%
\end{aligned}
$$

Jacob has experienced a 14% weight change over six months. Another way to say this is: He has lost 14% of his body weight over the past six months.

To calculate percent weight change, it's important to find the most reliable weight information possible for past data. Sources may include: a medical record, the report from the client, or a report from a family member. Unfortunately, it is not always possible to obtain highly reliable information about past weights. Also, there is no specific time frame for a percent weight loss calculation. Common standards suggest that the following percent weight changes indicate nutrition risk:

▶ a weight loss of 5% over the past one month,

▶ a weight loss of 7.5% over the past 90 days, or

▶ a weight loss of 10% over the past six months.

Another method for comparing weight with height to gauge overweight or underweight is the **body mass index (BMI)**. This formula simply describes weight proportionately to height. Figure 8.7 shows a reference table for determining BMI. The BMI associated with the lowest health risk is between 20 to 25. Usually, underweight is defined as a BMI of less than 18. Overweight corresponds to a BMI of 25-29.9, and obesity >30.

A final way to measure body mass is to examine the percentage of body weight that is fat. For men, a desirable percentage of body fat is 13 to 25%, and for

Figure 8.7

BODY MASS INDEX TABLE

To use the table, find the appropriate height in the left-hand column labeled Height. Move across to a given weight (in pounds). The number at the top of the column is the BMI at that height and weight.

BMI→	19	20	21	22	23	24	25	26	27	28	29	30	31	32	33	34	35	36	37	38	39	40
Height (Inches)																						
58	91	96	100	105	110	115	119	124	129	134	138	143	148	153	158	162	167	172	177	181	186	191
59	94	99	104	109	114	119	124	128	133	138	143	148	153	158	163	168	173	178	183	188	193	198
60	97	102	107	112	118	123	128	133	138	143	148	153	158	163	168	174	179	184	189	194	199	204
61	100	106	111	116	122	127	132	137	143	148	153	158	164	169	174	180	185	190	195	201	206	211
62	104	109	115	120	126	131	136	142	147	153	158	164	169	175	180	186	191	196	202	207	213	218
63	107	113	118	124	130	135	141	146	152	158	163	169	175	180	186	191	197	203	208	214	220	225
64	110	116	122	128	134	140	145	151	157	163	169	174	180	186	192	197	204	209	215	221	227	232
65	114	120	126	132	138	144	150	156	162	168	174	180	186	192	198	204	210	216	222	228	234	240
66	118	124	130	136	142	148	155	161	167	173	179	186	192	198	204	210	216	223	229	235	241	247
67	121	127	134	140	146	153	159	166	172	178	185	191	198	204	211	217	223	230	236	242	249	255
68	125	131	138	144	151	158	164	171	177	184	190	197	204	210	216	223	230	236	243	249	256	262
69	128	135	142	149	155	162	169	176	182	189	196	203	210	216	223	230	236	243	250	257	263	270
70	132	139	146	153	160	167	174	181	188	195	202	209	216	222	229	236	243	250	257	264	271	278
71	136	143	150	157	165	172	179	186	193	200	208	215	222	229	236	243	250	257	265	272	279	286
72	140	147	154	162	169	177	184	191	199	206	213	221	228	235	242	250	258	265	272	279	287	294
73	144	151	159	166	174	182	189	197	204	212	219	227	235	242	250	257	265	272	280	288	295	302
74	148	155	163	171	179	186	194	202	210	218	225	233	241	249	256	264	272	280	287	295	303	311
75	152	160	168	176	184	192	200	208	216	224	232	240	248	256	264	272	279	287	295	303	311	319
76	156	164	172	180	189	197	205	213	221	230	238	246	254	263	271	279	287	295	304	312	320	328

Source: National Institutes of Health

women, about 17 to 29%. When a man's body fat exceeds 25% (or a woman's exceeds 30%), health risks increase. Body fat is most often measured by using special calipers to measure the skinfold thickness of the triceps and other parts of the body. *Skinfold thickness* is a measurement of the fleshy part of the body at a specified location. Because half of all body fat is under the skin, this method is quite accurate. Standards exist for comparing the measurements and using them to gauge not only percent body fat, but also overall nutritional status (protein and calorie nutrition). Other anthropometric measurements include mid-arm circumference, and mid-arm muscle circumference.

Biochemical Tests

Biochemical tests, or laboratory tests, can be very helpful in assessing a client's nutritional status. Some typical standards for interpreting these test values appear in Figure 8.8. The normal values for each of these tests are determined by the institution. Following are some of the laboratory tests with nutritional significance:

Serum albumin. More than half of all the protein in the blood is albumin. Serum albumin is a good indicator of nutritional status, particularly protein status, but it takes time to change. Therefore a client with a low serum albumin has been in poor nutritional status for some time. Serum albumin decreases in trauma, severe infection, or protein calorie malnutrition.

Serum transferrin. Like albumin, transferrin is a protein found in the blood. Transferrin carries iron to where red blood cells are made. Serum transferrin levels are considered a more sensitive indicator of protein deficiency than albumin because transferrin levels change more quickly in response to changes in nutritional status.

Serum prealbumin. This is a protein made by the liver, and is considered one of the most sensitive and reliable indicators of protein status. Unlike serum albumin, it is not affected by hydration. It is a good measure for effectiveness of nutrition support, because it will begin to change within approximately four days. Even though it is produced by the liver, prealbumin is not affected by most forms of liver disease.

Total lymphocyte count (TLC). Lymphocytes are white blood cells involved in fighting infection. In the case of protein deficiency, the total number of lymphocytes decreases. Certain drugs also decrease total lymphocyte count.

Hematocrit and hemoglobin. Hematocrit is the percent of red blood cells found in blood. Hemoglobin is the oxygen-carrying pigment of the red blood cells. A low hemoglobin level may indicate iron deficiency anemia.

Clinical Information

Some of the clinical information that can have a bearing on nutrition screening and assessment is available in the medical record. Certain diagnoses or

Figure 8.8

SELECTED LABORATORY TESTS WITH NUTRITIONAL SIGNIFICANCE

Serum Albumin (alb)
NORMAL RANGE*: 3.5-5.0 gm/dl (Centers for Medicaid Services uses 3.4 – 4.8 gm/dl for individuals over 60 years of age)
SIGNIFICANCE: Can measure protein status; 3.0 – 3.4 may indicate mild protein depletion; 2.1 – 2.9 may indicate moderate protein depletion. May appear high due to dehydration, which concentrates the blood. Takes about 2-3 weeks to change in response to protein status.

Serum Prealbumin (PAB)
NORMAL RANGE*: 16-35 mg/dl
SIGNIFICANCE: Can measure protein status; 11-15 mg/dl may indicate mild protein depletion; < 10 mg/dl suggests significant protein depletion. PAB takes only a few days to change in response to protein status. With adequate nutrition support of a malnourished client, this value should rise approx. 2 mg/dl each day.

Serum Transferrin
NORMAL RANGE*:180-380 gm/dl
SIGNIFICANCE: Can measure protein status; takes about 10 days to change in response to protein status; may be elevated with iron deficiency anemia

Total Lymphocyte Count (TLC)
NORMAL RANGE*: 3,000-5,000 cells/mm
SIGNIFICANCE: This is a count of lymphocyte cells in the immune system; can measure protein status; 1,500-1,800 may indicate mild protein depletion; 900-1,500 suggests moderate depletion. TLC may be high in infection.

Fasting Blood Sugar/Glucose (FBS or FBG)
NORMAL RANGE*: 80-120 mg/dl
SIGNIFICANCE: Elevated FBS suggests diabetes or poor control of blood sugar for a person with diabetes. Slight elevations may occur with age. Note that random blood sugar (e.g. after a meal) may be higher (up to about 140 mg/dl). BS of approx. 300 mg/dl is dangerously high, leading to severe confusion and possible coma. Very low BS (< 60 mg/dl) is hypoglycemia and requires immediate treatment.

Glycosylated Hemoglobin (HbA1c)
NORMAL RANGE*: < 5%
SIGNIFICANCE: This value indicates control of blood sugar over a recent period of several months. It is valuable in evaluating ongoing blood sugar control for a person with diabetes. A low figure indicates good control.

A high figure (e.g. > 7%) suggests blood sugar may have been consistently or frequently high.

Hemoglobin (Hgb or Hb)
NORMAL RANGE*: 12-15 g/dl (adult female); 14 - 17 g/dl (adult male)
SIGNIFICANCE: Low Hgb with low HCT together often indicate anemia due to inadequate iron, folate, vitamin B6, vitamin B12, or other nutrients in the body. It is also low following blood loss, e.g. from internal bleeding, trauma, or surgery, and during cancer. Slightly low levels may occur with aging.

Hematocrit (HCT)
NORMAL RANGE*: 36 - 46% (adult female); 41 - 53% (adult male)
SIGNIFICANCE: Measures number and size of red blood cells; low Hgb with low HCT together often indicate iron-deficiency anemia; may be high (or appear normal) in dehydration

Serum cholesterol (chol)
NORMAL RANGE*: < 200 mg/dl
SIGNIFICANCE: High levels represent risk of cardiovascular disease

High density lipoprotein (HDL) cholesterol
NORMAL RANGE*: 40 – 60 mg/dl +
SIGNIFICANCE: "Good" cholesterol; < 40 mg/dl represents risk of cardiovascular disease; high levels are desirable (see Chapter 6)

Low density lipoprotein (LDL) cholesterol
NORMAL RANGE*: < 100 mg/dl optimal; 100 – 129 mg/dl near optimal
SIGNIFICANCE: "Bad" cholesterol; elevated levels represent risk of cardiovascular disease (see Chapter 6)

Serum triglyceride (TG)
NORMAL RANGE*: < 150 mg/dl
SIGNIFICANCE: High levels may mildly increase risk for cardiovascular disease; very high levels may suggest a blood lipid disorder; can lead to fatty deposits in the body (e.g. in liver); can also suggest uncontrolled diabetes

SELECTED LABORATORY TESTS WITH NUTRITIONAL SIGNIFICANCE, *CONTINUED*

Serum potassium (K)
NORMAL RANGE*: 3.5 – 5.0 mEq/l
SIGNIFICANCE: Becomes elevated during renal failure and other conditions; may become low with medications (e.g. potassium-wasting diuretics) or diarrhea; elevated or very low levels can become life-threatening; important to monitor for a client placed on either a high or low potassium diet

Blood urea nitrogen (BUN)
NORMAL RANGE*: 8-20 mg/dl
SIGNIFICANCE: An important measure of renal function; high levels may indicate renal failure, dehydration, or other medical conditions

* Note that standards for normal ranges are set by institution and may vary slightly. Also note that many clinical factors, such as fluid retention, dehydration, medication regimens, diseases of major organs, and many others can affect laboratory value readings. Thus, it is important to review the entire clinical picture, and consult with other members of the healthcare team in interpreting laboratory values.

Sources: National Institutes of Health, Centers for Medicare & Medicaid Services (CMS), American Family Physician

conditions, for example, may indicate a need for nutritional evaluation. We've already reviewed the idea that pressure ulcers are one of these conditions. A client whose symptoms include ongoing diarrhea and/or fever would be another. A client on a tube feeding would be yet another example. Figure 8.9 lists medical and social factors that may affect nutritional status.

Yet another type of clinical information that is important in understanding the nutritional picture for any client is medications. The effects foods and drugs have on each other can determine whether medications do their jobs and whether the body gets the nutrients it needs. Medications can interfere with the way the body digests, absorbs, or uses a nutrient. A medication that causes taste changes or gastrointestinal discomfort may reduce a person's food intake over time. This may cause weight loss and/or loss of nutritional well-being. Conversely, dietary factors can affect how medicines function in the body. This interchange can be mild or life-threatening. It depends on the medication and many other factors. Figure 8.10 lists some commonly used drugs that may have nutrition-related effects.

Figure 8.9

NUTRITION-RELATED CLINICAL INFORMATION

MEDICAL FACTORS
Cancer

Diabetes

Heart and circulatory disease

High blood pressure

Kidney disease

Liver disease

Lung disease

Illness with increased metabolic needs:
burns, infection, trauma, protracted fever

Malabsorption syndromes

Surgery of gastrointestinal tract

Overweight

Underweight

Recent unplanned weight loss

Certain medications

Chemotherapy/radiation therapy

Pressure ulcers

Chewing/swallowing problems

Inadequate fluid intake

Declining cognition

SOCIAL FACTORS
Living and eating alone

Not enough money for food

Inadequate facilities for storing and preparing food

Problems shopping for food

Declining mobility

Diet History

A **diet history** is a unique assessment tool of the client's food intake patterns. A diet history has two features: 1) It describes actual food intake, and 2) It gives information about why the client makes certain food choices. It also includes a review of many factors that may have an impact on nutrition, such as lifestyle, social factors, medical conditions, and more.

A diet history usually begins with a series of questions. A dietitian or designated caregiver will ask things like:

- When do you usually eat?
- How often do you usually eat?
- Where do you usually eat?
- Do you eat by yourself, or with others?
- Who does the food shopping in your household?

DRUGS WITH POSSIBLE NUTRITION-RELATED EFFECTS

Drug	Possible Effects
ANALGESIC (PAIN-KILLER)	
Aspirin	Gastric pain or bleeding, nausea and vomiting
Acetaminophen	Gastrointestinal disturbance, liver toxicity
ANTIBIOTIC	
Amoxicillin	Diarrhea, nausea and vomiting
Ampicillin	Diarrhea, glossitis (inflammation of the tongue), stomatitis (mouth ulcers), nausea and vomiting
Cephalexin	Abdominal pain, diarrhea, nausea and vomiting
Erythromycin	Abdominal cramping, diarrhea, nausea and vomiting
Penicillin	Diarrhea, glossitis, stomatitis, nausea and vomiting
Tetracycline	Anorexia, diarrhea, dysphagia, glossitis, nausea and vomiting, decreases vitamin K synthesis
HIGH BLOOD PRESSURE	
Atenolol	Diarrhea, nausea
Propranolol	Abdominal cramping, constipation, diarrhea, nausea and vomiting, decreased carbohydrate tolerance
BRONCHODILATOR	
Theophylline	Anorexia, gastric irritation, nausea, vomiting
DIURETIC	
Chlorthalidone	Anorexia, constipation, cramping, diarrhea, gastric irritation, electrolyte imbalance
Furosemide	Abdominal cramping, anorexia, constipation, diarrhea, dry mouth, thirst, fluid and electrolyte imbalance, nausea and vomiting, decreased blood potassium, magnesium, sodium; increased urinary potassium, magnesium, sodium
Hydrochlorothiazide	Anorexia, constipation, diarrhea, gastrointestinal irritation and ulceration, nausea and vomiting
ESTROGEN REPLACEMENT THERAPY	
Estrogens	Abdominal cramping, bloating, edema, nausea and vomiting, carbohydrate intolerance
ULCER	
Cimetidine	Bitter taste, constipation, decreased absorption of calcium and iron
NON-STEROIDAL ANTIINFLAMMATORY	
Ibuprofen	Abdominal cramping, constipation, diarrhea, edema, flatulence, gastrointestinal bleeding and ulceration, heartburn, nausea and vomiting
Naproxen	Abdominal pain, constipation, diarrhea, gastrointestinal bleeding and ulceration, heartburn, nausea and vomiting, stomatitis
STEROIDAL ANTIINFLAMMATORY	
Prednisone	Abdominal distention, fluid and electrolyte imbalance, fluid and sodium retention, indigestion, nausea and vomiting, negative nitrogen balance, peptic ulcer, decreased carbohydrate tolerance, less vitamin D activity, increased appetite, increased weight

Source: US Public Health Service

▶ How is your appetite?

▶ Are you having any problems or concerns with eating?

▶ Are you having any problems in chewing?

▶ Are you having any problems in swallowing?

▶ Are you experiencing any digestive concerns, such as nausea, vomiting, or constipation?

▶ Have you experienced any weight changes within the past six months?

▶ Do you currently follow a special diet?

▶ Do you currently take any nutritional supplements?

▶ Are there any foods you avoid? If so, why?

Questions such as these and many others begin to build a picture of a person's overall dietary situation. A diet history may include one or more tools designed to develop a reasonably good snapshot of a client's eating habits. A dietitian may request a **food record**, which is a diary of food and beverages consumed. A common food record is kept for any number of days, such as one, two, three days, or longer. A meaningful food record must include all condiments and additions to foods—such as mayonnaise used on a sandwich, or margarine and jelly spread on toast. Also, measurements of foods consumed are important. If a client has to tell how many ounces of roast beef he consumed, for example, this can be challenging. Sometimes, it helps to go over measurements and reporting with a client before the record begins. Food models (pieces of plastic molded to look like real foods) are useful for explaining portion sizes. The food record is then reviewed with the client to be sure all foods are listed and all portion sizes and preparation methods are accurate. Figure 8.11 shows a sample food record form.

Another tool is a **food frequency questionnaire**. This is a checklist that identifies how often a client eats each of a variety of foods. This provides information about eating habits and preferences that may not show up on a brief food record. Figure 8.12 shows a sample food frequency questionnaire.

In addition to diet histories, the dietitian/dietary manager or nursing staff can record what the client eats and drinks for three days and then do a nutrient analysis to quantify intake of calories, protein, and/or other nutrients. This is called a **calorie count**, or *nutrient intake analysis*. Observing and/or recording actual intake is extremely important for understanding a client's nutritional needs. Industry research shows that about 75% of nursing home residents eat less than three-quarters of their food, which can have a tremendous impact on health.

Now, remember that water is a nutrient and that dehydration is a major risk among older Americans. Thus, monitoring fluid intake is important, too.

Figure 8.11

FOOD/BEVERAGE INTAKE RECORD

▶ Record all foods and beverages you consume. Include meals, snacks, juices, supplements, condiments, sugar, butter, and jelly.

▶ Describe the amount eaten (cc, oz, cup, etc.) and include careful measurements.

Your name: _____ Date: _____

Meal	Food or Beverage	Amount (oz, tsp, cups)	Where Eaten
Breakfast			
Lunch			
Supper			
Snack			
Snack			

Nursing staff and other team members may monitor fluid intake for certain patients. From a clinical perspective, they may also want to know more about how kidneys or other body organs are functioning. Thus, a typical review of fluid becomes an I/O record. An **I/O (in and out) record** is a document of all fluids consumed and all fluids excreted over a 24-hour time period.

In a healthcare setting, nursing, dietary, and other caregivers also review a resident's ability to eat and feed himself. **Meal observation** is a key assessment

Figure 8.12

SAMPLE FOOD FREQUENCY QUESTIONAIRE

FOOD GROUP	AVERAGE INTAKE:	NEVER	DAILY	WEEKLY	MONTHLY
Milk:	Whole				
	Skim				
	Low fat				
Cheese					
Cottage cheese					
Beef					
Pork					
Veal					
Chicken/turkey					
Fish					
Shellfish					
Lunch meats					
Peanut butter					
Eggs					
Fruit:	Citrus				
	Others				
Vegetables:	Deep green or leafy				
	Dark yellow				
	Potato				
	Dried peas or beans				
Cereals:	Hot				
	Cold				
Bread:	White				
	Whole grain				
Rice, pasta					
Margarine, oil					
Cakes, cookies, pie					
Candy					
Nuts					
Ice cream					
Frozen yogurt					
Jam or jelly					
Salt:	Cooking				
	Added				
Soups:	Cream				
	Broth base				
Alcohol:	Wine				
	Beer				
	Other				
Coffee					
Tea					
Soft drinks:	Regular				
	Sugar-free				

tool that helps to identify individuals who are having problems with appetite, chewing, swallowing, alertness, self-feeding, or many other factors that may influence nutritional well-being. Based on observations, members of the team may begin to form strategies for helping a client eat well and enjoy meals.

Finally, a nutrition assessment includes a broader background on lifestyle and social factors that may influence nutrition. Any of the factors described in Chapter 1—such as cultural influences, religious beliefs, attitudes, and more—may be relevant in a diet history. For example, a person's ability to shop for and prepare food at home is very important. Awareness of support systems and knowing who is responsible for meals sets groundwork for nutrition education that may be needed later in the nutrition care process. Developing a solid diet history usually involves gathering information directly from the medical record, from other caregivers in a healthcare institution, from the client, and sometimes from family or significant others, too. The ability to gather accurate information depends on interpersonal rapport and solid communication skills. Talking with others to gather information requires interviewing skills. Figure 8.13 lists tips for conducting effective interviews. Upon completion of a nutrition assessment, a caregiver lists all nutrition problems identified, and then recommends a plan for addressing each problem.

TIPS FOR CONDUCTING EFFECTIVE INTERVIEWS

- ▶ Plan questions in advance, and use a form to keep track.
- ▶ Introduce yourself by name and title.
- ▶ Be friendly and sincere.
- ▶ Establish rapport by taking a genuine interest in the client.
- ▶ Avoid yes-or-no questions. Instead, use open-ended questions, such as: "Tell me more about...."
- ▶ Remain neutral during the interview. Do not judge a client's dietary habits.
- ▶ Ask for more information or clarification when needed. This can be done by paraphrasing (summarizing and rephrasing what has been said).
- ▶ Allow the client time to give an answer. Silence can be helpful.
- ▶ Use nonverbal language to show the client you are listening. For example, maintain good eye contact, and lean slightly toward the client to demonstrate your attention.
- ▶ Avoid leading questions, which give the client the answer you expect. For example, do not ask, "You don't eat pizza often, do you?"
- ▶ Actively listen to the client and observe nonverbal responses.
- ▶ When closing the interview, express your appreciation to the client and review the next steps, if appropriate.

Figure 8.13

THE NUTRITION SCREENING INITIATIVE

Industry support for nutrition screening takes shape with an effort called the Nutrition Screening Initiative. The Nutrition Screening Initiative is a broad multi-disciplinary effort led by the American Academy of Family Physicians, the American Dietetic Association, the National Council on the Aging, Inc. and a coalition of over 25 national health, aging and medical organizations. Founded in 1989, the Initiative's goal is to accelerate the incorporation of nutrition screening and intervention into the nation's healthcare delivery system for older Americans. The Initiative views every point of healthcare for an elderly person as an opportunity to enhance cost-effective nutrition care. To this end, the Initiative maintains alliances with professionals working in nutrition, dentistry, pharmacology, mental health, managed care, home care, and community social services. The Initiative implements a multi-faceted strategy that includes research, professional education, consumer outreach and policy. The Nutrition Screening Initiative has developed a nutrition screening tool and related educational packet for older adults to help them identify some major nutrition risk factors. The checklist is called DETERMINE, which stands for Disease, Eating poorly, Tooth loss, Economic status, Referral to social support, Multiple medications, Involuntary weight loss, Need assistance to care for self, and Elderly—all potential risks. For more information about this effort, visit one of the Screening Initiative websites listed in Appendix A.

BEE AND NUTRIENT NEEDS

Yet another aspect of nutritional assessment is an estimation of nutrient needs. Some assessments involve comparing these estimations with actual intake, in order to evaluate whether a client is able to nourish himself adequately. Estimating nutrient needs also forms a foundation for planning individual menus and meals, as well as for planning tube feedings and parenteral nutrition regimens. Most often, the estimation of nutrient needs will be the responsibility of a registered dietitian. However, here is some background that helps to de-mystify these seemingly magic numbers.

BEE. Basal metabolism is a term that describes how much energy the body needs when it is completely at rest. **Basal energy expenditure (BEE)** is the energy (calories) needed to maintain functions such as breathing, maintaining brain function, and keeping the heart beating. It is usually expressed as calories per day. There are many formulas for calculating BEE, which differs between men and women and varies according to age. Figure 8.14 shows a sample set of formulas for adults. BEE calculations may also be automated through use of computer software.

BEE accounts for only about two-thirds of calories in an average person's daily needs. Above and beyond the total resting state, the body needs more calories for digesting food, for moving and exercising, for growing or healing, and more. When a fever is present, the body uses a tremendous amount of energy

Figure 8.14

FORMULAS FOR CALCULATING BEE

Men
HARRIS-BENEDICT EQUATION: BEE = 66 + (13.7 x weight in kg) + (5 x height in cm) – (6.8 x age in years)

ALTERNATE FORMULA: BEE = 1.0 x (wt. in kg) x 24

Women
HARRIS-BENEDICT EQUATION: BEE = 655 + (9.6 x weight in kg) + (1.8 x height in cm) – (4.7 x age in years)

ALTERNATE FORMULA: BEE = 0.9 x (wt. in kg) x 24

Notes: To convert pounds to kilograms, divide by 2.2 (1lb = 2.2kg). To convert inches to centimeters, multiply by 2.54 (1in = 2.54cm).

to produce the fever. A fever is heat, and heat is energy. A **caloric needs estimate** is an estimate that accounts for the total amount of calories needed, e.g. for one day. It is built on the BEE, but includes additional factors to account for other energy needs. As with BEE, there are many models and formulas for calculating this. Figure 8.15 identifies some guidelines. Note that these guidelines are for adults only and are quite general. Furthermore, an estimate is only an estimate. In practice, any nutritional plan must be monitored. Follow-up assessment always includes weight monitoring, and adjustments to an initial plan are common.

Other common clinical nutrition calculations include an estimation of protein needs (Figure 8.16) and an estimation of fluid needs (Figure 8.17). For additional nutrient needs estimates, the RNIs described in Chapter 3 provide guidance for healthy people. As you learned in Chapter 6, many medical conditions can alter the needs for calories, protein, fluids, and other nutrients. For fluids, it is particularly important to be aware of a physician's order. Fluid restrictions are common among healthcare clients.

Figure 8.15

CALORIC NEEDS ESTIMATE

ACTIVITY FACTORS (ADD THESE TO THE BEE)
0.2 x BEE for a patient who is in bed most of the time

0.3 x BEE for an individual who is ambulatory and/or moderately active

0.5 x BEE for an individual who is very active

INJURY FACTORS (ALSO ADD THESE TO THE BEE)
0.2 x BEE following surgery

0.35 x BEE following skeletal trauma (bone fractures)

0.1 – 0.4 X BEE following other trauma

0.1 x BEE for each degree (F) of fever

2.1 x BEE for severe burn

FOR PROTEIN CALORIE MALNUTRITION
Add an amount for weight gain/growth. This might be 500-1000 calories per day.

TO ACHIEVE WEIGHT LOSS (FOR AN OVERWEIGHT INDIVIDUAL)
Subtract 500-1,000 calories per day to promote a loss of 1-2 lbs/week.

Figure 8.16

ESTIMATING DAILY PROTEIN NEEDS

For a healthy adult: 0.8 grams x body weight in kg

For a malnourished client or patient with pressure ulcers: 1.2-1. 5 grams x body weight in kg

Following surgery: 1.0-2.0 grams x body weight in kg

Following trauma, severe burn, or multiple fractures: 2.0 grams x body weight in kg

Figure 8.17

ESTIMATING DAILY FLUID NEEDS

Adults: 30-35 cc x body weight in kg

▶ Nutrition screening is a systematic method for identifying individuals at risk for nutrition problems.

▶ Nutrition screening is applied to all clients entering an institution, according to regulatory standards and institutional policies and procedures.

▶ Nutrition screening relies on indicators to predict nutrition-related risks, and often uses a scoring system.

▶ Nutrition assessment is an in-depth evaluation of a person's nutritional well-being.

▶ Certain types of information may be used in nutrition screening and/or nutrition assessment. This information includes anthropometric measurements, biochemical (laboratory) tests, clinical information, and diet history.

▶ Nutritional status is a person's state of nutritional health.

▶ Ideal body weight (IBW) is an estimate of what would be a healthy weight for an individual.

▶ Actual weight may be compared with ideal body weight to give a figure called percent of IBW.

▶ Actual weight may be compared with a past weight to give a figure called percent weight change.

▶ A calorie count is a nutritional analysis of recorded food intake.

▶ An I/O record documents fluids consumed and excreted.

▶ Medications can interfere with the way the body digests, absorbs, or uses a nutrient. A medication that causes taste changes or gastrointestinal discomfort may reduce a person's food intake over time.

▶ Total estimated energy needs for a day include basal energy expenditure (BEE) plus factors to account for level of activity and/or injury. To promote weight gain or loss, we can add or subtract up to 1,000 calories per day from the calculated recommendation.

▶ Estimated fluid needs for adults are 30-35 cc x body weight in kg.

▶ What constitutes a safe and healthy fluid intake may change based on medical conditions.

Actual weight: what a person weighs at the time of measurement

Anthropometric measurements: measurements of the human body

Basal energy expenditure (BEE): daily calories needed when the body is at rest

Basal metabolism: a measure of how much energy the body needs when it is completely at rest

Body mass index (BMI): a standard for evaluating body weight; based on proportion of weight to height

Caloric needs estimate: an estimate of the total amount of calories needed for a given period of time

Calorie count: a record of what a person eats and drinks for a certain number of days, which can be followed by a nutrient analysis

Diet history: a description of a person's actual food intake, along with information as to why the person makes certain food choices

Food frequency questionnaire: a checklist that identifies how often a person eats each of a variety of foods

Food record: a diary of food consumed

Frame size: the thickness of bones, or underlying body build

Ideal body weight (IBW): an estimate of what would be a healthy weight for an individual

Indicators: pieces of information that might suggest a concern or risk

I/O (in and out) record: a document of all fluids consumed and all fluids excreted over a 24-hour time period

Lean body mass: the weight of all parts of the body that are not fat, e.g. muscle, bones, organs

Meal observation: an assessment tool that helps to identify individuals who are having problems with appetite, with chewing, swallowing, alertness, self-feeding, or many other factors that may influence nutritional well-being

Nutrition assessment: an in-depth evaluation of a person's nutritional well-being

Nutrition risk scoring system: a system that assigns each nutrition risk indicator a point value, and then totals the point values to identify the level of nutrition risk

Nutrition screening: a process that applies selected nutrition criteria to an entire group, in order to select members of that group who are candidates for further intervention

Nutritional status: a person's state of nutritional health

Percent of IBW: a description of how closely a person's actual weight resembles the ideal

Percent weight change: the proportion by which the body weight has changed over a certain period of time

1. The first step of the nutrition care process is:

   A. Calculating calorie needs
   B. Estimating fluid requirements
   C. Checking for food-drug interactions
   D. Conducting nutrition screening

2. Nutrition screening differs from nutrition assessment in that:

   A. Nutrition screening identifies individuals who need nutrition assessment.
   B. Nutrition screening uses anthropometric measurements, while nutrition assessment does not.
   C. Nutrition screening requires a food frequency questionnaire, while nutrition assessment does not.
   D. Nutrition screening is only appropriate for older Americans, while nutrition assessment covers all ages.

3. The goal of nutrition screening is to:

   A. Identify government standards for nutrition care
   B. Identify individuals who may be nutritionally at risk
   C. Identify the diet an individual has followed in the past
   D. Identify which member of the healthcare team should take over management of a patient

4. In a nursing home, nutrition screening should be performed on:

   A. Any individual who has lost more than 10% of body weight within the past six months
   B. Any individual who has lost more than 7.5% of body weight within the past 90 days
   C. Any individual who has lost more than 5% of body weight within the past month
   D. Every individual who is admitted to the nursing home

5. A BMI of 16 suggests:

   A. Obesity
   B. Underweight
   C. Iron deficiency anemia
   D. Dehydration

6. A patient weighs 150 lbs. His ideal body weight is 175 lbs. What is his *percent of IBW?*

   A. (150 ÷ 175) x 100 or 86%
   B. (175 ÷ 150) x 100 or 117%
   C. (150 x 175) or 26,250%
   D. (175 - 150) x 100 or 25%

7. A resident weighed 123 lbs a month ago, and now weights 118 lbs. Her ideal body weight is 120 lbs. What is her *percent weight change?*

   A. (123 lbs - 118 lbs) ÷ 123 x 100 or 4%
   B. (118 lbs - 123 lbs) x 100 or 500%
   C. (120 lbs - 118 lbs) or 2%
   D. (123 lbs - 120 lbs) or 3%

8. Which of the following is a good indicator of protein status?

   A. Blood glucose
   B. HDL level
   C. Prealbumin
   D. BEE

9. Which of the following is most likely to raise a person's daily energy needs?

   A. Being confined to bed for three days
   B. Having a fever of 103°F for three days
   C. Encountering minor bruises from a fall
   D. Having blood pressure checked

10. Which of the following is NOT a benefit of using computer software for nutrition screening and/or assessment?

    A. Software can automate the calculations involved.
    B. Software can eliminate the need to interview clients.
    C. In some institutions, software can automatically capture laboratory values or other indicators.
    D. Software can identify individuals at nutrition risk.

Calculating nutrient intake is a key component of nutritional evaluation and the monitoring of ongoing care.

After completing this chapter, you should be able to:

▶ Name the food components that contribute to calorie intake, and identify the contribution of each one.

▶ Calculate percent calories from carbohydrate, protein, and fat.

▶ Identify sources of nutrient information.

▶ Explain the uses of nutritional analysis software.

▶ Use a Nutrition Facts Label to identify nutrient intake.

▶ Use the Exchange Lists to calculate intake of carbohydrate, protein, fat, and calories.

▶ Use a carbohydrate counting system to express carbohydrate intake.

▶ Calculate fluid intake.

In Chapters 3 and 6, we learned that the percent of calories from carbohydrate, protein, and fat can make a difference in overall health. Recommendations for a healthy diet often use guidelines based on percentages of these nutrients. In addition, we've seen guidelines for percentages in diets to treat high blood cholesterol, diabetes, and other conditions. With so much focus on energy balance and caloric consumption, it's important for a dietary manager to be able to determine how many calories are in food. Sometimes, a summary of calories becomes important in evaluating a person's dietary habits. For a patient receiving medical care, the focus may be on consuming adequate calories to maintain nutritional status.

As you learned in Chapter 2, three macronutrients provide calories. These are:

Carbohydrate (CHO): 4 calories per gram

Fat: 9 calories per gram

Protein (PRO): 4 calories per gram

Also, alcohol provides calories at the rate of 7 calories per gram. Knowing this, we can calculate calories and percent calories in any food or diet, as long as we know the grams of carbohydrate, fat, and protein—and alcohol, if applicable. Figure 9.1 shows the formula for calculating total calories. Once we know total calories for any food, meal, or food record, it's easy to calculate the percent of calories contributed by each component. Percent of calories is simply a way to express the proportions, or how much each macronutrient (and alcohol, if applicable) is contributing to the total calories. This is also called caloric distribution. **Caloric distribution** describes what

Figure 9.1

CALCULATING TOTAL CALORIES

This formula works for a single food, a meal, or any food record.

STEP 1: FIND OUT HOW MANY GRAMS OF CARBOHYDRATE, FAT, PROTEIN, AND ALCOHOL ARE PRESENT.

_____ grams of carbohydrate

_____ grams of fat

_____ grams of protein

_____ grams of alcohol

STEP 2: MULTIPLY EACH BY ITS CALORIE CONTRIBUTION.

_____ grams of carbohydrate x 4 cal/gm = _____ cal from carbohydrate

_____ grams of fat   x 9 cal/gm = _____ cal from fat

_____ grams of protein   x 4 cal/gm = _____ cal from protein

_____ grams of alcohol   x 7 cal/gm = _____ cal from alcohol

STEP 3: ADD THE SUB-TOTALS YOU OBTAINED IN STEP 2.

_____ grams of carbohydrate x 4 cal/gm = _____ cal from carbohydrate +

_____ grams of fat   x 9 cal/gm = _____ cal from fat +

_____ grams of protein   x 4 cal/gm = _____ cal from protein +

_____ grams of alcohol   x 7 cal/gm = _____ cal from alcohol

TOTAL CALORIES   = _____

proportion of total calories comes from each macronutrient (and alcohol, if applicable). Figure 9.2 shows the math. Figure 9.3 shows a sample calculation of calories and percent calories.

To calculate caloric distribution for a meal, or a one-day menu, or a food record, you can use the same formulas shown in Figures 9.1 and 9.2. For the Figure 9.1 calculation, simply total grams of carbohydrate, fat, protein, and alcohol from all the foods in the diet for Step 1. Here are a few words of caution about interpreting the percent of calories information: We do not want to compare the caloric distribution of each individual food in a diet to the Dietary Guidelines for Americans or other standards. Let's say that we are aiming to achieve a caloric distribution of 50% of calories from carbohydrate, 20% of calories from protein, and 30% of calories from fat. Is it all right to eat the two graham crackers we examined in Figure 9.3? They do not meet this caloric distribution. The answer is: Yes. When applying caloric distribution guidelines, don't worry about individual foods. Simply review the total for the day.

Figure 9.2

CALCULATING PERCENT CALORIES OR CALORIC DISTRIBUTION

Take another look at Step 2 in Figure 9.1. Use the sub-totals you obtained in Column 1 of this calculation. Now, take a look at the total calories you obtained in Step 3 in Figure 9.1. Enter this figure (total calories) in Column 2 below.

COLUMN 1	COLUMN 2: TOTAL CALORIES	COLUMN 3: % CAL. FROM THIS COMPONENT
____ Cal from carbohydrate	____	Cal from carbohydrate ÷ Total calories = ____
____ Cal from fat	____	Cal from fat ÷ Total calories = ____
____ Cal from protein	____	Cal from protein ÷ Total calories = ____
____ Cal from alcohol	____	Cal from alcohol ÷ Total calories = ____

Now, round each figure to two decimal places. Next, remove the decimal point (or multiply by 100) to change each figure to a percentage.

To check your work, you can add the percentages together. Your total should come close to 100%. (Depending on rounding, you may obtain a total like 99% or 101%. This is OK.)

Figure 9.3

SAMPLE CALCULATION: CALORIES AND PERCENT CALORIES

We are determining calories for 2 full graham crackers. So far, we know that this serving contains 24 gm of carbohydrate, 3 gm of fat, and 2 gm of protein.

24 grams of carbohydrate x 4 Cal/gm = 96 Cal from carbohydrate +

3 grams of fat   x 9 Cal/gm = 27 Cal from fat +

2 grams of protein   x 4 Cal/gm = 8 Cal from protein =

Total calories   = 131 Cal

COLUMN 1	COLUMN 2: TOTAL CALORIES	COLUMN 3: PERCENT CALORIES FROM THIS COMPONENT
96 Cal from carbohydrate	131	96 ÷ 131 = 0.73 or 73%
27 Cal from fat	131	27 ÷ 131 = 0.21 or 21%
8 Cal from protein	131	8 ÷ 131 = 0.06 or 6%

To check the calculation, we can add the three percentages, and see if they total close to 100%:

73% + 21% + 6% = 100%

However, if you find daily totals are far off, it can be helpful to look at the caloric distribution of individual foods. For example, if the daily total is too high in fat, we might look at which individual food(s) provided the highest percentage of fat, and reduce portion sizes of these foods to bring the diet into balance.

SOURCES OF NUTRIENT INFORMATION

By now, you may be wondering where to obtain figures for these calculations. How do you determine grams of carbohydrate, fat, and protein in a food? A second question may be: What about all the other nutrients? As it turns out, there are many sources of nutrient information available to us. A convenient resource for many of the key nutrients is a Nutrition Facts Label from a food package, described below.

In addition, nutrient information is available from a book called *Bowes and Church's Food Values of Portions Commonly Used*, or the *USDA Nutrient Database for Standard Reference*, also called "Handbook 8," which contains over 6,600 foods. The USDA nutrient data is available in the form of free downloads from the Internet (see Appendix A). You can also do an online search of any food to retrieve its nutrient information. Or, you can display lists of foods containing a selected nutrient. The Web address for searching USDA data appears in Appendix A. Another option for obtaining nutrient information is to use the nutrient database provided in a nutrient analysis software program, as described later in this chapter.

To use any of these sources, it's helpful to know a little bit of background about nutrient data. Historically, almost all nutrient data came from laboratory research conducted by the USDA. Over the years, the USDA has vastly augmented its information, adding nutrients such as dietary fiber and trace minerals—and now, caffeine, lycopene, isoflavones (a food component in soybeans), trans-fatty acids, and many others. For the most part, nutrient data in other books and software programs comes from the USDA database. Following are six points to keep in mind with USDA data.

Much of the USDA data is available per 100 gram portion. For a small serving of meat, this might be realistic (just over 3 ounces). However, for some foods, it is not a "usual fit" with dietary habits. For instance, one cup of Cheerios cereal is only 30 grams. When using USDA data, be sure to check units of measure carefully and select a unit that applies to your need. Also, you may have to convert weights to volume measurements. If the data is not available in the format you need, you can use a conversion table from another source, such as *Food for Fifty*, a quantity food production cookbook.

Using USDA nutrient data requires careful attention to edible portion and/or product yield. Edible portion is the amount of a food you can actually eat after preparation is complete; product yield is the final volume of the cooked food. Consider that meat shrinks when it is cooked, and grain products like rice and pasta expand. If you want the nutrient values for a ground beef patty, you need to determine the final weight of the cooked patty, and match it to "cooked" ground beef in the database. Imagine you start with a 6-ounce patty, and it cooks down to 4 ounces. If you calculate nutrients based on USDA data for 6 ounces of cooked ground beef, you will over-report nutrients. You would want to match "4 ounces" and "cooked" to the nutrient database. Now consider macaroni. Nutrients for a cup of uncooked macaroni may be about three times higher than nutrients for a cup of cooked macaroni. You need to match macaroni to a weight or volume and then carefully select "dry" or "cooked".

Your calorie total and the USDA calorie total may not match. If you conduct your own calculation of total calories based on grams of carbohydrate, fat, and protein (as in Figure 9.1), your calorie total and the one you see in USDA data may not match perfectly. This is OK. USDA uses more highly refined techniques for determining calorie information.

USDA data is primarily built on individual foods. Each time you have a recipe or combination dish, the most accurate way to determine nutrients is to calculate them based on individual ingredients. This is a cumbersome process. However, USDA data does include some combination dishes. You may need to decide how closely a USDA item matches your own recipes or sources for foods.

Historically, USDA nutrient data was all for generic foods. Today, the USDA maintains quite a bit of information by brand name. This is useful, as many people eat not only brand-name foods—but also packaged and convenience foods that would be difficult to calculate any other way.

Some data simply is not available. Despite the massive research conducted by the USDA, the task of determining nutrient values for thousands of foods is no small feat! As a result, certain nutrient values may be absent. This can lead to *false zeroes*. A false zero is a report that a nutrient is absent in food, when in fact we just don't have the data.

Nutrient Analysis Software

Because calculating nutrients in a recipe, meal, or menu can be a great deal of work, many dietary professionals use software for the job. Nutrient analysis software is readily available within a range of budgets. Some programs are built into foodservice management software packages. This can be convenient because they draw on lists of foods and recipes that are already in the system. Be aware, though, that any software does initially require you to enter data, such as an inventory list, individual recipes, and menus. This can demand time.

If you are selecting a program for nutrient analysis, look carefully at the sources of nutrient data. Generally, nutrient databases are built on USDA data, which is freely available. Some packages use the USDA database in its entirety. Others use a small proportion of USDA data. So, look at the number of foods contained in a program's database. Also check whether you can add foods to the database yourself, using Nutrition Facts Labels.

In addition, some software developers invest immense effort into expanding the database by adding nutrient data available from food manufacturers, restaurants, and other sources. A database offering significantly more foods than USDA Handbook 8—such as 8,000 - 12,000 foods—has most likely undergone development to list more brand-name and convenience foods. In addition, some developers use sources beyond the USDA to eliminate false zeroes in the database through mathematical calculations and estimations. This eliminates the problem of under-reporting certain nutrients. Which nutrients and food components are included varies by software package.

Another consideration with software is portion sizes or units of measure. Some packages offer more choices for portion sizes and units of measure, as compared with the USDA database. This can improve accuracy and efficiency for a program user. If you are evaluating options, also take a look at how you find and enter foods. This should be a straightforward and convenient process. Finally, review the types of reports available. Most software will compare calculated totals with nutrient standards, such as the Food Guide Pyramid, RDAs, diabetic exchanges, and/or many others. Some reports are graphic and easy to read. Reports may be available for individual foods, recipes, menus, or averages for a series of days.

Let's look at how you might use the computer to get a nutrient analysis for one portion of a recipe. First, you may type the name of an ingredient (or part of the name), and the computer lists choices so that you can choose a match. Then you type in how much of that ingredient you want to be used in the analysis, such as one cup—or you select a measurement from a drop-down list. After entering all the ingredients, you can have the computer divide the results by the yield, such as 12 portions. Then the computer will tell you exactly how much of each nutrient (and the percent of the RDA) is contained in one portion. Most computer analysis programs can also give you a percentage breakdown of calories from protein, fats, carbohydrate, and alcohol. Of course, these figures can be printed on a printer and/or stored in the computer. A sample nutrient analysis for a recipe appears in Figure 9.4.

Nutrition Facts Labels

The Nutrition Labeling and Education Act of 1990 requires labeling for most foods, except meat and poultry. The FDA notes that Nutrition Facts Labels are designed to offer consumers the following:

- Nutrition information about almost every food in the grocery store
- Distinctive, easy-to-read formats that enable consumers to find the information they need to make healthful food choices
- Information about the amount of nutrients per serving
- Standardized serving sizes, which make nutritional comparisons of similar products easier

Figure 9.4

SAMPLE NUTRIENT ANALYSIS

Recipe: FRENCH TOAST (2 SL)
Serving size: 3.5 ounc

Recipe Number: 2002 FRENCH TOAST (2 SL)   Number of servings: 574

Calories	558.74 Kcal	20.7%	
Protein	11.67 gr	20.8%	
Fat	13.90 gr	15.4%	
Carbohydrate	98.53 gr	26.5%	
Calcium	179.71 mg	22.5%	
Iron	3.66 mg	36.6%	
Sodium	702.11 mg	26.0%	
Potassium	257.63 mg	5.6%	
Vitamin A	0.00 RE	0.0%	
Ascorbic Acid	0.17 mg	0.3%	
Folic Acid	47.67 mcg	11.9%	
Cholesterol	57.50 mg	19.2%	
Nutrient 13	0.00 mg	0.0%	
Nutrient 14	0.00 mg	0.0%	
Nutrient 15	0.00 mg	0.0%	

Do you want a bar chart for this data (1=Yes, 2=No, 99=End)? 1

Code No.	Item Name	Quantity Needed
47	MILK NON-FAT DRY	2 Pounds + 2.44 Ounces (weight)
179	WATER.COLD	2 Quarts + 1.74 Pints
96	EGGS FRESH EX LG	14 Pounds + 5.60 Ounces (weight)
68	SPICES NUTMEG	1.952 Ounces (weight)
48	SUGAR,CANE-GRAN DOMINO	5 Pounds + 11.84 Ounces (weight)
174	BK-FS BREAD, WHITE	140 Pounds + 10.08 Ounces (weight)
57	SYRUP PANCAKE MAPLE	8 Gallons + 2.44 Quarts
104	MARGARINE ONE LB SPEC PRNT	14 Pounds + 5.60 Ounces (weight)

DISSOLVE DRY MILK IN WATER
BEAT EGGS, ADD TO MILK
MIX SUGAR AND NUTMEG, ADD TO MIXTURE
DIP BREAD IN MIXTURE
FRY ON 375 F GRILL COVERED WITH MARGARINE
COOK TIL GOLDEN BROWN
SERVE WITH 2 OZ SYRUP

Nutritional Analysis

Name:	SAMPLE	Age:	23-50	
Date:	09-14-1984	Weight:	154 pounds	Activity Level: Light
Prescribed Diet:	RDA, Safe & Adequate	Height:	70 inches	Lactating: No
Recipe:	FRENCH TOAST (2 SL)	Sex:	Male	Pregnant: No

Nutritional Category	0	25	50	75	100	125
Calories	21%					
Protein	21%					
Fat	15%					
Carbohydrate	27%					
Calcium	22%					
Iron	37%					
Sodium	26%					
Potassium	6%					
Vitamin A	0%					
Ascorbic Acid	0%					
Folic Acid	12%					
Cholesterol	19%					
Nutrient 13	0%					
Nutrient 14	0%					
Nutrient 15	0%					

- Nutrient reference values, expressed as percent Daily Values, that help consumers see how a food fits into an overall daily diet
- Uniform definitions for terms that describe a food's nutrient content—such as "light," "low-fat," and "high-fiber"—to ensure that such terms mean the same for any product on which they appear
- Claims about the relationship between a nutrient or food and a disease or health-related condition, such as calcium and osteoporosis, or fat and cancer. These are helpful for people who are concerned about eating foods that may help keep them healthy.
- Declaration of total percentage of actual juice in juice drinks

A Nutrition Facts Label (Figure 9.5) must include information about: total calories, calories from fat, total fat, saturated fat, cholesterol, sodium, total carbohydrate, dietary fiber, sugars, protein, vitamin A, vitamin C, calcium, and iron. Optionally, a label may include: calories from saturated fat, polyunsaturated fat, monounsaturated fat, potassium, soluble fiber, insoluble fiber, sugar alcohols, other carbohydrate, percent of vitamin A present as beta-carotene, and other essential vitamins and minerals. If a label makes a claim regarding one of these optional items, then it must provide the nutrition facts for the item.

The label must express each nutrient as a percentage of the Daily Value. **Daily Values (DVs)** are reference intake levels devised specifically for nutrition facts labeling. In Chapter 3, you learned that government standards exist for recommended intake of most nutrients. These standards, however, are not the same for everyone. They vary based on age and sex. Iron needs, for example, are different for men versus women, and change at various ages. Thus, the dilemma becomes: How can a food manufacturer compare the amount of iron in a food to the amount that you, as a consumer, need? It would be much too complicated to develop a nutrition facts label that compares with the various RDAs for all age and sex groupings. So, the government has developed generalized figures for nutrients that can be applied to healthy people as a single group. These generalized references are Daily Values, and they are only for nutrition facts labeling. Think of them as a generic set of "one-size-fits-all" nutrient recommendations for consumers. When there is variation in actual RDAs, daily values for labeling tend to reflect the higher values within ranges.

There are two kinds of daily values: daily reference values and reference daily intakes. **Daily Reference**

Figure 9.5

SAMPLE NUTRITION FACTS LABEL

Nutrition Facts
Serving Size 1 cup (228g)
Servings Per Container 2

Amount Per Serving

Calories 250 Calories from Fat 110

	% Daily Value*
Total Fat 12g	18%
Saturated Fat 3g	15%
Cholesterol 30mg	10%
Sodium 470mg	20%
Total Carbohydrate 31g	10%
Dietary Fiber 0g	0%
Sugars 5g	
Protein 5g	

Vitamin A 4%	•	Vitamin C 2%
Calcium 20%	•	Iron 4%

* Percent Daily Values are based on a 2,000 calorie diet. Your daily values may be higher or lower depending on your calorie needs:

	Calories:	2,000	2,500
Total Fat	Less than	65g	80g
Sat Fat	Less than	20g	25g
Cholesterol	Less than	300mg	300mg
Sodium	Less than	2,400mg	2,400mg
Total Carbohydrate		300g	375g
Dietary Fiber		25g	30g

Calories per gram:
Fat 9 • Carbohydrate 4 • Protein 4

Values (DRVs) are the references used for fat, saturated fat, cholesterol, carbohydrate, protein, fiber, sodium, and potassium. **Reference Daily Intakes (RDIs)** are the references used for essential vitamins and minerals. Not all nutrients are addressed in a nutrition facts label. For nutrition facts labeling, the FDA has selected only some key nutrients that relate to common health concerns.

Why have two types of references? Remember that how much fat you should consume in a day depends on how many calories you consume. It's not really a "gram limit" alone. The recommendation for fat is expressed as a percentage of calories. If you eat 3,000 calories per day, you need to limit fat to 100 grams to stay within this limit. However, if you eat 1,500 calories per day, you should stop at about 50 grams of fat. It so happens that recommendations for all the nutrients that use DRVs correspond to calorie intake. The FDA sets DRVs based on consuming 10% of calories as protein, 30% of calories as fat, and 60% of calories as carbohydrate—*on a 2,000 calorie diet*. Seriously nutrition-oriented individuals who eat significantly more or less than 2,000 calories per day may need to convert these figures for personal reference, based on calorie intake. (Note that some nutrition facts labels provide DRVs for both 2,000 and 2,500 calorie diets.)

On the other hand, recommendations for the nutrients that use reference daily intakes tend to stay stable, even with lower or higher calorie intakes. You need the same amount of vitamin C or calcium, whether you eat 3,000 calories per day or 1,500 calories per day. This is the rationale for two sets of reference values.

As you can see, daily values used for nutrition facts labeling are less precise than RDAs. They are quite generalized. If you need to conduct detailed nutrient evaluation for an individual, your first choice of reference should be RDAs. However, nutrition facts labels do provide an excellent educational tool for consumers. They offer consistency and give consumers a way to compare nutritional values of foods. The label shows nutrient values based on a defined serving size. It also shows how many of this "serving" are in the package. This is very helpful for consumers, because not everyone would eat the same amount of a food at any given time. If you happen to eat a bowl of whole grain Total cereal, you will consume 3 grams of dietary fiber (based on a 2003 nutrition facts label for this product). However, that's only true if the bowl of cereal matches a defined serving size of ¾ cup. What if you eat 1 cup instead? You will receive proportionally more fiber: 4 grams.

Note that many labels also provide a set of nutrient information based on common serving or preparation practices. For cereal, you'll see values for the cereal alone, and for the cereal plus milk. For a bakery mix, you may see values for the mix alone (the contents of the package), and also for the mix prepared with added ingredients, according to preparation instructions on the package. Some labels vary based upon intended use. Infant formulas, for example, will not carry reference information about calories from fat, or cholesterol. The reason is to prevent parents from mistakenly believing that they should restrict infants' fat intake.

Finally, labeling standards govern the use of special terminology to describe foods. Figure 9.6 describes this terminology. Foods must meet specific criteria to make certain labeling claims. In addition, many terms have legal definitions when it comes to labeling statements. Just like the nutrition facts, these claims are based on per-serving information.

Now, let's consider the nutrition facts label as a source of nutrient information. Let's say you are planning a menu. You want to be sure it falls within certain dietary recommendations, and you want to be sure that the menu contains enough of key nutrients. You would like to include a frozen casserole—a convenience item. How can you identify the nutrients? If this product is not available in the USDA nutrient database (or in a nutrient analysis software system you use), you need to identify the nutrients from a label. Here are some pointers:

- First, compare the serving size. Determine whether it matches the serving size you will use. If not, use an adjustment factor. For example, imagine a product shows a serving size of ½ cup, but you plan to serve it as ¾ cup. You will need to adjust all the nutrients by a factor of 1.5. You will multiply each nutrient value by 1.5 to get the nutrients for your serving size.

- Next, use the label to obtain calories and any of the following: fat, saturated fat, cholesterol, sodium, carbohydrate, fiber, sugars, and protein. (These are nutrients that have DRVs).

- If you also want actual nutrient values—rather than just percent daily values—for other nutrients listed on the label, you will have to do some math. Iron, calcium, vitamin A, and vitamin C, for example, are expressed only as percentages of the daily values. To get an actual figure, such as 3 mg iron, you can convert based on the FDA's reference, which appears in Figure 9.7. Here is an example: A nutrition facts label for a frozen pasta dinner says that one serving provides 20% of the daily value for vitamin C. You check Figure 9.7 and find that the daily value for vitamin C is 60 mg. Working backwards, you can calculate that this dinner contains 20% of 60 mg of vitamin C. That's: 0.2 x 60 mg or about 12 mg of vitamin C. Are there alternatives? Yes. One is to contact your food supplier or the manufacturer and request more nutrient detail so you won't need to go through the work. Another, using nutrient analysis software, is to add the food to the database. Many programs have a feature that allows you to enter percent daily values from a food label. The software does the conversion.

Figure 9.6

FOOD LABEL DICTIONARY

Nutrient Content Claim . . . . . . .Definition

CALORIES
Calorie free .less than 5 calories
Low calorie .40 calories or less
Reduced or fewer calories . . . . .at least 25% fewer calories*
Light or lite . . . . .one-third fewer calories or 50% less fat*

SUGAR
Sugar free .less than 0.5 gram sugars
Reduced sugar or less sugar . . . . . . .at least 25% less sugars*
No added sugar . . . . .no sugars added during processing or packing, including ingredients that contain
                                             sugars, such as juice or dry fruit

FAT
Fat free . . . . .less than 0.5 gram fat
Low fat . . . . .3 grams or less of fat
Reduced or less fat . . . . .at least 25% less fat*
Light . . . . .one-third fewer calories or 50% less fat*

SATURATED FAT
Saturated fat free . . . . .less than 0.5 gram saturated fat and less than 0.5 grams of trans fat
Low saturated fat . . . . .1 gram or less saturated fat and no more than 15% of calories from saturated fat
Reduced or less saturated fat . . . . . .at least 25% less saturated fat*

CHOLESTEROL
Cholesterol free . . . . .less than 2 milligrams cholesterol and 2 grams or less of saturated fat
Low cholesterol . . . . .20 milligrams or less cholesterol and 2 grams or less of saturated fat
Reduced or less cholesterol . . . . . . .at least 25% less cholesterol* and 2 grams or less of saturated fat

SODIUM
Sodium free . . . . .less than 5 milligrams sodium
Very low sodium . . . . .35 milligrams or less sodium
Low sodium . . . . .140 milligrams or less sodium
Reduced or less sodium . . . . .at least 25% less sodium*
Light in sodium . . . . .50% less*

FIBER
High fiber .5 grams or more
Good source of fiber . . . . .2.5 to 4.9 grams
More or added fiber . . . . .at least 2.5 grams more*

OTHER CLAIMS
High, rich in, excellent source of . . . .20% or more of Daily Value*
Good source, contains, provides . . . .10% to 19% of Daily Value*
More, enriched, fortified, added . . . . .10% or more of Daily Value*
Lean** . . . . .less than 10 grams fat, 4.5 grams or less saturated fat, and 95 milligrams cholesterol
Extra lean** . . . . .less than 5 grams fat, 2 grams saturated fat, and 95 milligrams cholesterol

* As compared with a standard serving size of the traditional food

** On meat, poultry, seafood, and game meats

Source: FDA

Figure 9.7

FDA REFERENCE VALUES FOR NUTRITION FACTS LABELING

(Based on a 2000 Calorie Intake; for Adults and Children 4 or More Years of Age)

NUTRIENT	UNIT OF MEASURE	DAILY VALUES	NUTRIENT	UNIT OF MEASURE	DAILY VALUES
Total Fat	grams (g)	65	Niacin	milligrams (mg)	20
Saturated fatty acids	grams (g)	20	Vitamin B6	milligrams (mg)	2.0
Cholesterol	milligrams (mg)	300	Folate	micrograms (µg)	400
Sodium	milligrams (mg)	2400	Vitamin B12	micrograms (µg)	6.0
Potassium	milligrams (mg)	3500	Biotin	micrograms (µg)	300
Total carbohydrate	grams (g)	300	Pantothenic acid	milligrams (mg)	10
Fiber	grams (g)	25	Phosphorus	milligrams (mg)	1000
Protein	grams (g)	50	Iodine	micrograms (µg)	150
Vitamin A	International Unit (IU)	5000	Magnesium	milligrams (mg)	400
Vitamin C	milligrams (mg)	60	Zinc	milligrams (mg)	15
Calcium	milligrams (mg)	1000	Selenium	micrograms (µg)	70
Iron	milligrams (mg)	18	Copper	milligrams (mg)	2.0
Vitamin D	International Unit (IU)	400	Manganese	milligrams (mg)	2.0
Vitamin E	International Unit (IU)	30	Chromium	micrograms (µg)	120
Vitamin K	micrograms (µg)	80	Molybdenum	micrograms (µg)	75
Thiamin	milligrams (mg)	1.5	Chloride	milligrams (mg)	3400
Riboflavin	milligrams (mg)	1.7			

Source: FDA

CALCULATING NUTRIENTS BASED ON EXCHANGE LISTS

In some situations, a full-blown nutrient analysis is more than you really need. For example, if you are performing a calorie count for a nursing home resident, you may be interested in finding out how much protein and how many calories the resident consumes in a day. Or, if you are trying to evaluate whether a particular diet provides fewer than 30% of calories from fat, you may not need to pull out reference books or launch a software program. As you learned in Chapter 6, the exchange lists for meal planning group foods according to their content of carbohydrate, fat, protein, and calories. Any time you need a short-cut method of estimating these same four items, you can use the exchange lists. Here's how:

Step 1. Match the food(s) you wish to analyze to exchanges. Assign each food an exchange group, and identify how many exchanges it represents. For mixed dishes, you may be listing more than one exchange group. Do not count foods in the "Free foods" exchange list at all.

Step 2. Total the exchanges for each group.

Step 3. For each exchange group, multiply the total number of exchanges by the standard carbohydrate, fat, protein, and calorie figures for that exchange group.

The exchange lists appear in Appendix B. Figure 9.8 shows a worksheet for performing these steps, and Figure 9.9 shows an example of how you can apply it.

If you are obtaining a calorie count or calculating intake from a food record, your estimates will be only as good as the original records. Calorie counts in institutions can be challenging. To collect the best records possible:

- Inform everyone who may be involved in care that a calorie count is in progress. This includes the client, visitors, nurses, and other caregivers.

- Post a notice or make another visible reminder, as permitted by your policies and procedures.

- Keep printed menus or tray tickets from meal trays. Ask each person to record the *percent consumed* next to each menu item. Percents (rather than actual measurements) are useful. They do not require others to guesstimate portion sizes. However, you can refer to your actual menu and food production information to determine what the portion size is.

- If possible, review records frequently throughout the day. If a meal has not been recorded, check with the caregiver, or (if appropriate) with the client directly.

- Ask all caregivers to record any additional items the resident consumes, even if they are not printed on the menu. Example: A resident asks for a can of ginger ale. Or: A nurse offers a patient a cup of apple juice for taking medications. Or: A visitor brings in a cookie.

Obtaining a valid calorie count requires excellent communication, as well as vigilance and monitoring.

CARBOHYDRATE COUNTING

As explained in Chapter 6, carbohydrate counting may be used as a method of managing dietary concerns for an individual who has diabetes. This system revolves around one simple idea: Foods that contain carbohydrate become glucose in the body. Glucose is blood sugar. (Note that fiber does not become blood sugar because it is not digested.) In a diet for managing diabetes, the bottom line is often how much glucose enters the body—and how often.

Figure 9.8

WORKSHEET FOR CALCULATING MACRONUTRIENTS USING EXCHANGE LISTS

Step 1. Match the food(s) you wish to analyze to exchanges. Assign each food an exchange group, and identify how many exchanges it represents.

FOOD	SERVING SIZE	# OF EXCHANGES						
		STARCH	FRUIT	MILK*	OTHER CARB.	VEGETABLE	MEAT**	FAT

Step 2. Total the exchanges for each group:

TOTALS								

*To simplify calculations, this worksheet uses skim milk as the standard for milk. If you are listing 2% milk, please add 1 fat exchange. If you are listing whole milk, please add 2 fat exchanges.

**To simplify calculations, this worksheet assumes all meats are medium fat.

Step 3. For each exchange group, multiply the total number of exchanges by the standard carbohydrate, fat, protein, and calorie figures for that exchange group.

EXCHANGE GROUP	# OF EXCHANGES	CHO GM	YOUR TOTAL	PRO GM	YOUR TOTAL	FAT GM	YOUR TOTAL	CAL	YOUR TOTAL
Starch		x 15 =		x 3 =				x 80=	
Fruit		x 15 =						x 60=	
Milk		x 12 =		x 8 =				x 90=	
Other carb.		x 15 =						x 60=	
Vegetable		x 5 =		x 2 =				x 25=	
Meat				x 7 =		x 5 =		x 75=	
Fat						x 5 =		x 45=	
TOTALS									

Carbohydrate counting is based on a prescribed level of carbohydrate intake. For example, one client may be aiming for 220 gm carbohydrate per day; another may be aiming for 185. Generally, this carbohydrate intake needs to be distributed throughout the day to prevent major surges in blood glucose levels. How rigid this distribution needs to be is dictated by the diabetes itself and medication regimens. It varies tremendously among individuals. Carbohydrate

SAMPLE CALCULATION FOR A CALORIE COUNT

John is a resident in a nursing home. The healthcare team is not sure he is eating enough to maintain his nutritional health. You are conducting a calorie count. You have a food record of everything he has eaten over the course of a day, including breakfast, lunch, dinner, and snacks. Note that the exchange values for chicken noodle soup come from the combinations foods list. You enter each food into the worksheet, and calculate nutrients as shown below.

FOOD	SERVING SIZE=	# OF EXCHANGES STARCH	FRUIT	MILK*	OTHER CARB.	VEGETABLE	MEAT**	FAT
orange juice	½ cup		1					
toast	1 slice	1						
margarine	1 tsp							1
chicken noodle soup	1 cup				1			
applesauce	¾ cup		1.5					
meatloaf	1 oz						1	
TOTALS		1	2.5	0	1	0	1	1

EXCHANGE GROUP	# OF EXCHANGES	CHO GM	YOUR TOTAL	PRO GM	YOUR TOTAL	FAT GM	YOUR TOTAL	CAL	YOUR TOTAL
Starch	1	x 15 =	15	x 3 =	3			x 80=	80
Fruit	2.5	x 15 =	38					x 60=	150
Milk	0	x 12 =		x 8 =				x 90=	
Other carb.	1	x 15 =	15					x 60=	60
Vegetable	0	x 5 =		x 2 =				x 25=	
Meat	1			x 7 =	7	x 5 =	5	x 75=	75
Fat	1					x 5 =		x 45=	45
TOTALS			68 gm CHO		10 gm PRO		5 gm fat		410 calories

Conclusion: John's intake for this day was 68 gm carbohydrate, 10 gm protein, 5 gm fat, and a daily total of 410 calories.

counting is done in conjunction with blood glucose monitoring, and members of the healthcare team evaluate any necessary fine-tuning in carbohydrate totals and distribution.

To count carbohydrates, simply tally grams of carbohydrate in each food consumed. You need to count the carbohydrate in starches as well as sugars. Starchy foods include grain products, potatoes, dried beans, peas, and corn.

Foods with sugar include fruit, sweets, soft drinks, and milk. (Milk contains lactose, or milk sugar.) An easy way to track all of this is with exchange lists. You can use the same method shown in Figure 9.8 to count carbohydrate. Enter a food on the worksheet *only* if it contains carbohydrate. Omit foods that fall into the exchange lists for meats or fats. *Do count* foods that fall into these exchange groups: starch, fruit, milk, other carbohydrates, or vegetables. In the second chart shown in Figure 9.8, total the grams of carbohydrate. You do not need to calculate grams of protein or fat, or calories.

What if a food does not appear on the exchange lists? Nutrition facts labels can be useful. Check the product label for grams of carbohydrate. Count every 15 grams of carbohydrate shown as one exchange in the *Other Carbohydrates* group. Or, simply add the grams of carbohydrate from product labels to your tally.

CALCULATING FLUID INTAKE

Managing fluids is often a critical part of clinical care. It is important when there is a concern about dehydration—a common condition among those who are elderly, those who are eating poorly, and those who are undergoing various forms of medical stress. Certain conditions may require a diet order that includes an instruction to push fluids. Conversely, there are times when the body cannot rid itself of water adequately. For example, a person experiencing end stage renal failure is not able to excrete water. As water builds up in the bloodstream, it dilutes the rest of the blood's contents. It often raises blood pressure and disrupts the sensitive balance of electrolytes (chemicals) in the blood. Fluid restriction may be required to avoid potentially life-threatening conditions. Other conditions that may require fluid restriction include advanced liver failure, congestive heart failure, and certain hormonal disorders.

When a fluid restriction is needed, a physician specifies the restriction along with the rest of the diet order. Fluid restrictions are expressed in cubic centimeters, or cc. A cc may also be called a milliliter or ml. A number indicates how many cc's should be consumed per day. For example, a diet for an individual in renal failure may read:

60 gm protein, 2 gm Na, 2 gm K, 1000 cc.

This means the diet is limited to 60 grams of protein, 2 grams of sodium, 2 grams of potassium, and 1000 cc of fluid per day.

To honor an order such as this one, nursing and dietary staff must communicate and work together. Some of the fluid may be served with meals. Other fluid may take the form of a drink offered by the nurse, e.g. with medications. Thus, the first step in implementing a fluid-restricted diet order is to find out which part you should provide through dietary services. Your institution may have a universal standard—80% from dietary services and 20% from nursing services, for instance. That would be 800 cc from dietary services and 200 cc

Figure 9.10

FLUID CONVERSIONS

VOLUME	FLUID OZ	CC OR ML
1 cup	8 fluid oz	240 cc
¾ cup	6 fluid oz	180 cc
½ cup	4 fluid oz	120 cc
⅓ cup	2.7 fluid oz	80 cc
¼ cup	2 fluid oz	60 cc
2 T	1 fluid oz	30 cc

from nursing services. If there is no standard, you and a nurse may need to specify and agree upon a split. You will need to manage menus and trays meticulously to stay in compliance.

As you plan a day's worth of menus, how do you count fluid? First, you need a conversion factor. One cup or 8 fluid ounces = 240 cc. Figure 9.10 lists some related conversions. Next, you need to decide what menu items count as fluids. This is specified in the diet manual, and you should use the manual as a reference. Generally, however, anything that *looks* like a liquid at room temperature counts as fluid. Examples include: broth, juice, soft drinks, milk, shakes, coffee, tea, fruit ices, ice cream, sherbet, liquid nutritional supplements, gelatin, and popsicles. Pudding, custard, yogurt, hot cereal, and gravy do not count as fluid. Like calorie counting and carbohydrate counting, fluid counting is not 100% precise. We know, for example, that many fruits and vegetables contain water, but most systems do not count that as fluid.

If you are planning a fluid-restricted menu, consider menu needs. For example, most people want to have milk with cold cereal. Also, special portion sizes of fluid-containing items may be in order. The milk, for example, may be ½ cup instead of 1 cup. Fruits may come through as whole, fresh fruits or drained canned fruits rather than juice. As a practical matter, most dietary departments also provide a message on menus or tray tickets for fluid-restricted meals. One institution may use a red rubber stamp to mark "Fluid Restriction." Another may generate a special message through a software program that prints tray tickets. Usually, nursing staff also post an alert near a patient's bed.

Key Points

- The macronutrients in food provide calories as follows: carbohydrate – 4 cal/gm; protein – 4 cal/gm; fat – 9 cal/gm. Also, alcohol provides 7 cal/gm.

- We can calculate caloric distribution—or what proportion of calories are provided by each macronutrient. The number of calories provided by one macronutrient divided by the total number of calories gives percent of calories for that nutrient.

- Most information about the nutrients in foods comes from USDA nutrient data, and some may also be available from a food supplier or manufacturer.

- Software automates the calculations involved in nutrient analysis.

- When using nutrient data, it's important to match portion sizes, and to account for changes in the yield based on preparation methods.

- Nutrition Facts Labels provide simplified nutrition information for consumers, and make it easy to compare foods.

- Nutrient standards used on nutrition facts labels are called Daily Values.

- There are two types of Daily Values (DVs): Daily Reference Values (DRVs) for fat, saturated fat, cholesterol, carbohydrate, protein, fiber, sodium, and potassium; and Reference Daily Intakes (RDIs) for essential vitamins and minerals.

- Food label claims such as "light" or "reduced" are governed by regulations, and have uniform definitions for all food labels.

- Exchange lists provide a shortcut for estimating the carbohydrate, protein, fat, and calories in any meal, menu, or food record.

- Exchange lists can also be used to plan and track carbohydrate for a carbohydrate counting diet.

- Fluid restricted diets should be implemented based on a physician's order and standards in an institution's diet manual. One cup equals 240 cc or 240 ml.

Key Terms

Caloric distribution: the proportion of total calories that comes from each macronutrient consumed

Daily Reference Values (DRVs): references used for fat, saturated fat, cholesterol, carbohydrate, protein, fiber, sodium, and potassium in a Nutrition Facts Label

Daily Values (DVs): reference intake levels devised specifically for nutrition facts labeling

Reference Daily Intakes (RDIs): the references used for essential vitamins and minerals in nutrient facts labeling

1. A particular 7-oz steak contains 50 gm of protein. How many calories is that protein worth?

    A. 50 cal
    B. 100 cal
    C. 200 cal
    D. 360 cal

2. That same steak contains 40 gm of fat. How many calories is that fat worth?

    A. 50 cal
    B. 100 cal
    C. 200 cal
    D. 360 cal

3. Jim eats 1000 calories in a day. Of these, 500 calories come from fat. What is the percent of fat in his diet for that day?

    A. 10%
    B. 20%
    C. 40%
    D. 50%

4. Which of the following is true about using USDA nutrient data?

    A. You can find the information online free of charge.
    B. You should always select 100 gm portion sizes.
    C. You should re-check all calorie values with a calculator.
    D. You cannot use this data in software.

5. You are performing a calorie count for a resident of a nursing home, and notice nothing has been recorded for the lunch meal. You should:

    A. Count it as though the resident consumed all foods.
    B. Check with a nurse and ask how many ounces of meat the resident consumed.
    C. Check with a nurse and ask what percentage of each food the resident consumed.
    D. Call the physician and ask what the resident was supposed to consume.

6. You are analyzing a food record with exchange lists. How should you count one cup of tuna noodle casserole? (Tip: Use the exchange lists in Appendix B.)

    A. 2 carbohydrate exchanges plus 2 meat exchanges
    B. 3 carbohydrate exchanges
    C. 1 carbohydrate exchange plus 1 meat exchange
    D. 2 fat exchanges

7. In the same example, how would you count one half cup of tuna noodle casserole?

   A. 2 carbohydrate exchanges plus 2 meat exchanges
   B. 3 carbohydrate exchanges
   C. 1 carbohydrate exchange plus 1 meat exchange
   D. 2 fat exchanges

8. You are analyzing a food record with exchange lists. How should you count 1 carton (8 oz) of 2% milk?

   A. 1 milk exchange
   B. 1 milk exchange plus 1 fat exchange
   C. 1 milk exchange plus 2 fat exchanges
   D. 2 milk exchanges

9. You are counting carbohydrates. How should you count 1 cup of skim milk, 1 banana, and 5 vanilla wafers?

   A. 10 + 12 + 15 = 37 gm
   B. 15 + 15 + 15 = 45 gm
   C. 12 + 15 + 15 = 42 gm
   D. 0 + 15 + 15 = 30 gm

10. You are counting fluid at a lunch meal. How will you count 6 oz. cranberry juice?

   A. 120 cc
   B. 140 cc
   C. 180 cc
   D. 240 cc

A dietary manager needs to interpret nutritional data in order to support the entire process of nutrition assessment and planning.

After completing this chapter, you should be able to:

- Explain the role of a dietary manager in interpreting nutritional data.
- Classify the types of information that are relevant to nutrition care.
- Name sources for relevant information.
- Explain the rationale for reviewing medications.
- Compare nutrient intake to nutrient standards.
- Describe how nutritional data relates to dietary management.

One of the responsibilities of a dietary manager in a healthcare institution is to support nutrition care. Food and meal services are one component of this support. Clinical nutrition care is another. Meals and the clinical activities that support each client's individual needs go hand-in-hand to ensure that clients are well nourished and in the best possible state of health. *Clinical nutrition* tasks that may appear on a dietary manager's job description include: nutrition screening, obtaining a diet history, reviewing medical records for information relevant to nutrition, calculating nutrient intake, planning individualized menus according to diet orders, documenting nutrition care, counseling clients about basic dietary restrictions, and communicating with the client and the healthcare team. Dietary managers work with dietitians (and sometimes related personnel) to provide this care. In many longterm care institutions, a dietary manager attends to nutrition-related needs on a daily basis, while a part-time or con-sulting dietitian provides intermittent assessment and planning. Often, the dietary manager will be the first to identify a nutrition-related concern, and may bring it to the attention of others. Providing clinical nutrition care requires an understanding of what information to look for—and a sense of what it means.

NUTRITION-RELATED INFORMATION

By now, you probably already have a list of ideas in your mind. You know from Chapter 8 that nutrition-related information may take the form of anthropo-metric measurements, biochemical tests, clinical information, and diet histories. Sources for this information include the medical record (discussed in Chapter 11), direct observations and interviews, nutrition care documents, and communications with the healthcare team (described in Chapter 12). Let's examine the process of gathering information from these sources.

Medical record. The medical record contains the formal documentation of all aspects of care for each individual patient or resident. Members of the health-care team record their activities here. This includes the dietary manager. In

Figure 10.1

NUTRITION-RELATED INFORMATION IN THE MEDICAL RECORD

Diet order

Diagnosis

Medical history

Social history

Laboratory tests

Height and weights

Laboratory values

List of medications

Care plan

Progress notes

Nursing intake notes

Nursing notes

Minimum Data Set (MDS form described in Chapter 11)

addition, the record contains all orders written by the physician. Diet order is one of these. The medical record is the first document a dietary manager will review in performing nutrition screening. Pertinent data here includes a report of laboratory tests performed, as well as history forms completed by the physician, the nurse, and other team members. Be alert to overlaps in these records with some of the pertinent questions for a diet history. For example, a nurse may note the patient's concerns with eating, and previous diet patterns. Height and weight are usually in the medical history and/or the nursing intake notes. How the record is organized is somewhat unique to each institution. However, your job is to become familiar with it, and use it as a resource for information on an ongoing basis. Figure 10.1 summarizes information to check in the medical record.

Direct observation and interviews. In a healthcare institution, personal visits and direct observation are crucial to an understanding of a client's nutrition-related problems and progress. As much as possible, it's a good idea to visit at meal times. Figure 10.2 summarizes what to look for. Meal time is an excellent time to chat with a client about food-related concerns, too, because the focus is already on food. A client may not enjoy certain food choices, and you can discuss alternatives. A client may not understand why bacon is not being offered on his low sodium diet, and you can explain this. In addition, it's important to observe food intake. If a client does not consume 25% or more of food for two out of three days, or does not consume all/almost all of fluids for two out of three days, there is cause for concern. When a visual observation of intake suggests a problem, the next step is often a calorie count, and review with the healthcare team.

Nutrition care documents. In most institutions, the dietary department maintains its own detailed documents for managing day-to-day nutritional care. The system varies, but may include a nutrition care plan or kardex card. Here, the dietitian, dietary manager, and other dietary personnel note information that

Figure 10.2

KEY MEAL TIME OBSERVATIONS

Is the client eating the meal? How much?

Is the client avoiding certain foods? Which ones?

Is the client enjoying certain foods? Which ones?

Is the client drinking fluids? How much?

Is the client able to initiate eating, or does he need a cue?

Is the client able to position himself for a meal, or does he need assistance?

Is the client able to open/handle food packages?

Is the client able to use utensils provided?

Is the client able to feed himself safely?

Is the client experiencing any problems with chewing, drinking, or swallowing?

Is there any coughing, drooling, or choking occurring?

Is there any unusual behavior, e.g. loss of attention, disorientation, wandering?

Does the client appear to be uncomfortable in any way?

Does the client have any questions or concerns regarding the diet?

Is the client consuming any other food (not provided by the institution)?

will help with planning and meal management. A diet history may be recorded here. A dietary manager or dietitian may copy pertinent facts from the medical record to this plan. A weight record is important. Each weight should be recorded with a date for ongoing monitoring. If you are monitoring certain laboratory values, you may also record these here. Meal planning details that appear in a nutrition care document include: the physician's diet order, a list of food likes and dislikes, a meal plan (if the client is following an exchange system diet or other meal pattern), and any special requests or needs. Dietary staff use this information when planning individual menus for each meal. In some longterm care facilities, food preferences are recorded on a tray card, which accompanies a tray along a conveyor during tray assembly. In other institutions, nutrition care documents are maintained in a dietary computer system. The menu itself is also a critical nutrition care document. Whether by computer or by hands-on intervention, dietary staff review menu offerings for clients and assure that each meal served meets the diet order and client preferences.

Communications with the healthcare team. Healthcare involves the cooperative efforts of many professionals. Each contributes expertise to address a broad range of needs for clients. Each team member has direct contact with the client, as well as with family and others. Each has observations to share. Nutrition-related information is always a piece of a bigger picture. Direct communication with team members helps a dietary manager become aware of nutrition-related issues, gain perspective and implement nutrition care effectively.

FOOD-DRUG INTERACTIONS

A dietary manager needs to devote specific attention to the topic of food-drug interactions. As explained in Chapter 8, the effects foods and drugs have on each other can determine whether medications do their jobs, and whether the body receives the nutrients it needs. The extent of interaction between foods and drugs depends on the drug dosage and on the individual's age, size, and specific medical condition. In general, though, the presence of food in the stomach and intestines can influence a drug's effectiveness by slowing down or speeding up the time it takes the medicine to go through the gastrointestinal tract to the site in the body where it is needed.

Food also contains natural and added chemicals that can react with certain drugs in ways that make the drugs virtually useless. Alternately, components in foods can enhance the action of certain drugs, sometimes triggering a medical crisis or, in rare instances, even death.

A major way food affects drugs is by impeding absorption of the drug into the bloodstream. A classic interaction is the one between tetracycline compounds and dairy products. The calcium in milk, cheese, and yogurt impairs absorption of tetracycline. The solution is to avoid dairy products close to the time of taking tetracycline. Another example is a drug called Fosamax. It must be taken without food, especially coffee and orange juice. Otherwise, it may not be used by the body. In general, it is unwise to take drugs with soft drinks or acid fruit or vegetable juices. These beverages can result in excess acidity that may cause some drugs to dissolve quickly in the stomach instead of in the intestines, where they can be more readily absorbed into the bloodstream.

Excessive consumption of foods high in vitamin K, such as liver and leafy green vegetables, may hinder the effectiveness of anticoagulants. Vitamin K, which promotes clotting of the blood, works in direct opposition to these drugs, which are intended to prevent blood clotting.

Some of the potassium-sparing diuretics (drugs that remove excess water from the body) can interact with large quantities of potassium in the diet. As potassium builds up in the bloodstream, heartbeat can become irregular. Even though high-potassium foods are ordinarily a great idea, a patient taking one of these medications must moderate potassium intake by avoiding excess orange juice, bananas, potatoes, tomatoes, and other high-potassium foods. However, other types of diuretic drugs remove potassium from the body. These are called potassium-wasting diuretics. Clients taking these drugs need to boost potassium intake to help maintain safe blood potassium levels.

Figure 10.3

FOODS TO AVOID ON A LOW TYRAMINE DIET

Sharp or aged cheese

Other aged foods such as pickled herring, fermented sausages, salami, and pepperoni

Yogurt and sour cream

Beer

Chianti wine, sherry, other wines in large quantities

Chicken and beef livers

Canned figs, bananas, avocados

Soy sauce

Active yeast preparations

Broad beans such as fava beans

Note: MAO inhibitors may also react adversely with cola beverages, coffee, chocolate, and raisins.

Perhaps the most hazardous food-drug interaction is the one between monoamine oxidase (MAO) inhibitors, drugs prescribed for depression and high blood pressure, and tyramine in foods. Figure 10.3 lists foods that are high in tyramine. The reaction can raise blood pressure to dangerous levels, sometimes causing severe headaches, brain hemorrhage, and, in extreme cases, death. To prevent a possible reaction, anyone taking MAO inhibitor drugs should avoid high tyramine foods.

Alcohol, which is a drug itself, does not mix well with a wide variety of medications, such as antibiotics; anticoagulants; hypoglycemic drugs, including insulin; antihistamines; high blood pressure drugs; MAO inhibitors; and sedatives. Alcohol combined with antihistamines, tranquilizers, or antidepressants causes excessive drowsiness that can be especially hazardous to someone driving a car, operating machinery, or performing some other task that requires mental alertness. Alcohol can also dissolve coatings on time-released medications. The result is that a medication surges into the bloodstream too quickly.

Just as some foods can affect the way drugs behave in the body, some drugs can affect the way the body uses food. Drugs may act in various ways to impair proper nutrition by hastening excretion of certain nutrients, by hindering absorption of nutrients, or by interfering with the body's ability to convert nutrients into usable forms. Nutrient depletion of the body occurs gradually, but for those taking drugs over long periods of time, these interactions can lead to deficiencies of certain vitamins and minerals, especially in children, the elderly, those with poor diets, and the chronically ill.

Some drugs inhibit nutrient absorption by their effect on the walls of the intestines. Among these are colchicines, drugs prescribed for gout, and mineral oil, an ingredient used in some over-the-counter laxatives. Mineral oil can interfere with absorption of vitamin D, vitamin K, and carotene.

A number of drugs affect specific vitamins and minerals. The antihypertensive drug hydralazine and the antituberculosis drug INH can deplete the body's supply of vitamin B6. They can do this by inhibiting production of the enzyme necessary to convert the vitamin into a form the body can use, or by combining with the vitamin to form a compound that is excreted. Similarly, anticonvulsant drugs that are used to control epilepsy can lead to deficiencies of vitamin D and folic acid because they increase the turnover rate of these vitamins in the body.

Quite a few drugs—such as the antibiotic neomycin and oral hypoglycemic agents—can impair absorption of vitamin B12. But because most Americans have good stores of B12 in their livers, it takes prolonged ingestion of these drugs to cause a deficiency. Anticonvulsant medications, such as dilantin, reduce the body's supplies of vitamin D and folacin. To prevent deficiency, clients may need to drink more milk, eat folacin-rich foods, and/or take vitamin supplements. Drugs readily available without prescription can also lead to nutrition problems. For example, chronic use of antacids can cause phosphate depletion, a condition that in its milder form produces muscle weakness and in more severe form leads to a vitamin D deficiency. Aspirin can cause vitamin C loss. Modifying the diet to include more foods rich in the vitamins and minerals that may be depleted by certain drugs generally is preferable to taking vitamin or mineral supplements. In fact, supplements of some vitamins can counter the effectiveness of certain drugs.

COMPARING NUTRIENT INTAKE TO STANDARDS

Often, a dietary manager needs to use the results of nutrient calculations to support an assessment of nutritional needs. In Chapter 3, you became familiar with standards for evaluating a diet. In Chapter 9, you learned how to calculate nutrients in a diet. Let's explore how these ideas come together.

Let's say you have calculated the results of a one-day food record for a client. You need to make some comments about whether the intake would meet her nutritional needs. The first step is to select nutrients you need to report. Using the same nutrients ordinarily displayed on a nutrition facts label is usually a good approach. For each nutrient, identify the RDA for your client's age and sex. Then, calculate total intake as a percentage of the RDA. To calculate percentage, divide the actual intake of a nutrient by the recommended intake of the nutrient. Remove the decimal point. Here is an example. Mary consumes 11 mg of iron in one day. Her RDA is 18 mg of iron. Percentage of RDA is 11 ÷ 18 = 0.61 or 61%. For calories, you can estimate energy needs (as in Chapter 8), and then compare.

Is it necessary to have 100% of the RDAs for each nutrient? Not always. Consider Mary again, with the low iron intake for one day. Here are conclusions we *cannot* draw:

> Mary is deficient in iron.
>
> Mary never eats enough iron.

What can we conclude? Here is a conclusion we can draw:

> Mary's intake of iron for one day was marginal.

What's next? Other information that would help in evaluating Mary's iron situation includes:

- ◗ **Laboratory data.** Serum hemoglobin and hematocrit will help to determine whether Mary actually has iron-deficiency anemia.
- ◗ **Physician's diagnosis.** Does the physician say Mary has iron deficiency anemia?
- ◗ **Diet history.** More than a single day, we would like to know whether Mary frequently consumes less iron than the RDA. We may want to check food intakes for other days, or even calculate an average intake over many days.
- ◗ **Food frequency.** We can examine how often Mary eats iron-rich foods.

In many situations, a comparison with the Food Guide Pyramid is a convenient and meaningful tool for evaluation, too. You can tally the number of servings a client has consumed from each food group, and compare these with recommended servings.

NUTRITIONAL DATA AND DIETARY MANAGEMENT

By now, it's clear that a dietary manager needs to consider many factors at once to provide effective dietary care. Let's consider another example. Connie has Type 2 diabetes, as well as hypertension. What kinds of information do we need to review to understand her nutritional care? Here are some pieces of data that will be especially important:

- ◗ **Blood sugar levels.** By noting blood sugar levels first thing in the morning (fasting blood sugar), and following meals, we can find out whether Connie's diabetes is under control on a daily basis.
- ◗ **Blood pressure readings.** Usually part of the nurse's notes, blood pressure readings help us understand whether Connie's blood pressure is under control.
- ◗ **Meal time observation.** We need to know how well Connie is tolerating and following her therapeutic diet.

▶ **Weight, percent body weight, weight changes.** If Connie happens to be overweight, weight reduction is likely to improve management of both the diabetes and the hypertension.

If blood sugar or blood pressure consistently run too high, team members may confer to decide on adjustments. Solutions may involve changes in medication and/or diet. It's important to recognize that these are closely intertwined. In addition, decisions are based on an understanding of the unique person receiving care. A physician makes a final decision, based on input from team members. What can you offer as a dietary manager? You can note how well Connie understands and complies with her diet, and give your judgment as to how effective a dietary change might be, based on the information you've collected. For example, if you find that she is not tolerating her diet well, you may not recommend further restrictions. A physician may then decide to accomplish more with medications.

Let's imagine Connie is a resident in a longterm care facility. Since admission six months ago, she has paid careful attention to her diet and has lost 17 lbs. Now, you notice that her blood sugar levels and blood pressure levels are making a gradual decline. In the past few days, she has had two episodes of hypoglycemia (very low blood sugar), and the nurse has given her juice to bring her blood sugar back up to safe levels. This could be a signal that Connie's weight loss has improved her health, and it may be time for an adjustment to her care plan. Can you as a dietary manager be absolutely certain? Can you make changes on your own? The answer to both questions is: No. The reasoning is that the nutrition-related data you are reviewing is not quite the whole clinical picture. It's always possible that there are other medical factors at play. The physician is responsible for an actual diagnosis and medical assessment. What is your role as a dietary manager in this situation? Because you have the background and expertise to focus on the nutrition-related information, you are the prime candidate to point out Connie's weight changes, to highlight a possible relationship between her weight and clinical changes, and alert other team members. Your information may signal a need for further evaluation and possible adjustments to the overall treatment plan.

Let's consider another situation. Ricky is a resident of a longterm care facility, and has been bedridden for more than a year. He developed two pressure ulcers (stage I) several months ago. At the time, you noted that he was underweight and his serum transferrin level was below normal. You and the dietitian agreed that Ricky was experiencing some protein calorie malnutrition. He has been following a high protein, high calorie diet. What information is most pertinent to understanding his nutritional needs today? Here are some ideas:

▶ **Weight.** You need to monitor his weight to see whether it is going up or down or remaining stable.

- **Serum transferrin** (or other blood indicator of protein status preferred in your institution). You want to determine whether his protein status is improving in response to the diet.

- **Pressure ulcers.** You want to know whether the pressure ulcers have improved, remained stable, or advanced to another stage. You want to know whether any new ulcers have developed.

- **Diet tolerance/intake.** To balance the above information with the overall nutrition care, you need to know whether Ricky is eating his food and tolerating it comfortably.

- **Calorie count.** If your observations raise concern, you may perform a calorie count to quantify the situation. You can compare his intake of calories and protein with estimated needs.

All of this information feeds into the ongoing monitoring of Ricky's nutritional status. It becomes critical in planning and adjusting his clinical care to assure that his nutritional status is raised and maintained at optimal levels. We already know that nutritional status is a major factor in the development and healing of pressure ulcers.

Here is one more scenario. Marilyn is a resident of a nursing home. She entered in excellent nutritional status, and was also in the early stage of Alzheimer's disease. She was also following a diet to manage high blood cholesterol levels. Since her admission, she has experienced an advancement of Alzheimer's and has lost more than 6% of her body weight within the past month. As you monitor her ongoing nutritional care, you may be concerned with:

- **Weight.** You want to know how Marilyn's actual weight compares with her ideal body weight. You need to monitor weight and percent weight change as indicators of overall nutritional status.

- **Serum transferrin** (or other blood indicator of protein status preferred in your institution). You want to evaluate protein status and find out whether she is maintaining or losing lean body mass.

- **Clinical information.** You need to know what stage her Alzheimer's disease is in, and whether any new symptoms have arisen.

- **Diet tolerance/intake.** Mealtime observation is essential to find out how Marilyn is eating and drinking—and whether the Alzheimer's disease is affecting her food intake. She may be inattentive to meals, or may be exhibiting behaviors that interfere with nutritional intake. You also may wish to evaluate whether dietary restrictions for high blood cholesterol are affecting her nutrient intake.

- **Calorie count.** If your observations raise concern, you may perform a calorie count to quantify the situation. You can compare her intake of calories and protein with estimated needs.

Notice that Marilyn's blood cholesterol levels are not high on the priority list now. This is a matter of clinical judgment. Because of her rapid weight loss, her nutritional status has advanced to the forefront as a nutritional concern. Her protein calorie status takes priority. With a decline or threatened decline in nutritional status, it's much more important to protect her overall and immediate health. Most likely, one of your suggestions for Marilyn will be to liberalize her diet. You may need more flexibility in offering high-fat foods to provide a diet that is dense in calories.

Each institution may have its own policies, regulatory concerns, and standards that influence a dietary manager's actions in providing nutrition care. Some standards of practice or standards of quality management actually dictate what information will be reviewed in monitoring clinical conditions. Regulations addressing financial reimbursement to the institution may require specific monitoring and documentation. Concerns for residents' rights will affect how strong a role a resident plays in making decisions about his or her own care. An institutional policy and/or regulatory requirements may identify the role of the dietary manager slightly differently in various locales.

Key Points

- The dietary manager focuses on nutrition care, examining and interpreting a variety of information that reflects nutritional well-being, as well as the effectiveness of dietary care.

- Sources of nutrition-related information include the medical record, direct observations and interviews, nutrition care documents, and communications with the healthcare team.

- A dietary manager needs to devote specific attention to the topic of food-drug interactions.

- The dietary manager works closely with other members of the healthcare team.

- The physician makes diagnoses, and orders treatments such as diet order and medications.

- The dietary manager can provide ongoing feedback and insight about nutrition-related issues for clients.

- The dietary manager may take the initiative to recommend a diet change or liberalization of the diet.

1. Which of the following is a good source for a patient's current and past weights?

   A. The medical record
   B. The laboratory report
   C. The physician's orders
   D. A table of ideal body weights

2. You are visiting a resident at breakfast and discover she likes to have hot cocoa rather than coffee. You will record this information where?

   A. In the physician's diet orders
   B. In a list of food preferences in your nutrition care document
   C. In the nurse's notes of the medical record
   D. On a post-it note kept on your desk

3. You are planning tomorrow's menus for a resident who follows an exchange system diet. Where will you find the meal plan that shows how many exchanges to serve at each meal?

   A. In your nutrition care document
   B. In the nurse's notes of the medical record
   C. In the physician's diet orders
   D. In a nutrition textbook

4. Upon reviewing a calorie count for a resident, you calculate that he is consuming 45% of the RDA for protein. What is the most logical conclusion?

   A. His body has a protein deficiency.
   B. He is not consuming enough protein.
   C. He is probably in prime nutritional condition, as most Americans eat too much meat.
   D. He is uncooperative.

5. The same resident described in Question 4 is undergoing cancer treatment. Your meal observations show that he is eating scrambled eggs but avoiding hot meat entrees. What would you suggest to improve protein intake?

   A. Offer more non-meat sources of protein such as cheese, eggs, and bean dishes; try cold entrees.
   B. Offer more fruits at breakfast to replace the eggs, because eggs are high in cholesterol.
   C. Avoid between-meal snacks so that he will eat more meat at meal times.
   D. Take no action; poor dietary habits are just his choice.

6. Upon interviewing a patient, you find that she avoids milk because it gives her cramps and gas. You notice that one of her diagnoses is osteoporosis. What could you suggest to help with her dietary calcium intake?

   A. Eat more bananas and oranges.
   B. Drink milk anyway because the calcium is important.
   C. Try low-lactose dairy products.
   D. Eat more red meats.

7. A patient is taking an MAO inhibitor drug. Which of the following foods is NOT acceptable on his diet?

   A. Lettuce
   B. Hot oatmeal
   C. Applesauce
   D. Sharp cheddar cheese omelet

8. A patient is taking a potassium-wasting diuretic. Which foods would be best to include in her diet to replace potassium?

   A. Bananas and oranges
   B. Iceberg lettuce
   C. English muffins
   D. Soft drinks

9. A resident is taking an anticoagulant drug to prevent blood clots. Which nutrient should he avoid?

   A. Potassium
   B. Vitamin K
   C. Fat
   D. Magnesium

10. A client has been following an exchange system diet to manage diabetes, and is also eating poorly. What information would be most valuable in helping you decide whether to recommend liberalizing her diet order?

    A. Blood sugar levels and weight records
    B. Blood cholesterol levels
    C. Blood hemoglobin and hematocrit
    D. Blood pressure readings and medication list

Documentation of nutritional data is a critical tool for medical management as well as regulatory compliance.

After completing this chapter, you should be able to:

- Describe reasons for documenting nutrition-related care.
- Explain the uses of common documents, including a kardex, a medical record, and an MDS form.
- List types of information to document.
- Explain the organizational system of a problem-oriented medical record.
- Outline the flow of information involved in communicating and documenting a diet order and other meal-related information.
- Translate commonly used abbreviations into medical terms.
- Explain the use of the Resident Assessment Instrument (RAI), and its components: Minimum Data Set (MDS) and Resident Assessment Protocols (RAPs).
- Describe the impact of HIPAA regulations on medical documentation.

In a healthcare environment, it is not enough to provide excellent care. It is also crucial to document all medical care, including nutrition-related care. Why? Documentation serves a number of purposes. Among them:

- Documentation provides a reference that you and other caregivers can use on an ongoing basis as you provide care. It helps you focus details about how you are implementing a plan of care. It also helps you compare information from one time to another, to track changes in nutritional status.
- Documentation becomes a communication tool with other members of the healthcare team. This is important because you need to work together to accomplish high-quality care for any individual.
- Documentation is required by government agencies, and is mandatory for healthcare institutions.
- Documentation lays groundwork for a healthcare institution to receive reimbursement for the services it provides (e.g. from insurance companies and Medicare).
- Documentation is a legal record.
- Documentation is part of quality standards for healthcare institutions.
- Documentation is also a resource for monitoring quality of services.

As you can see, documentation has a multi-faceted rationale. The need to document care applies not only to dietary managers, but also to all members of the healthcare team. In fact, most care documents are shared by members of the team. It is also apparent that when you write down what you do, you are not writing just for yourself. Much of what you document will be read and used by others. Thus, you need to follow certain guidelines that are universally used and understood in the healthcare professions. Furthermore, documentation is guided by policies and procedures in your own place of employment. While the principles are universal, details about how, where, and what to document vary. Wherever you work, it is an excellent idea to become familiar with all policies and procedures about documentation and to follow them closely.

What types of documents does a dietary manager use and maintain? Among the most common are: a medical record, a dietary reference card, and an MDS form (used in longterm care).

MEDICAL RECORD

A **medical record** is a formal, legal account of a patient's health and disease. It contains findings, test results, diagnoses, and treatment plans. A medical record may also be called a *medical chart* or a *chart*. Although each institution has its own procedures and guidelines for recording in the medical record, many use the **problem-oriented medical record (POMR)**. The POMR is a system of collecting data and planning client care that focuses on the client's problems. It was devised by Dr. Lawrence Weed. He first published the system in 1969, and it was received enthusiastically within the medical community. Besides improvement in the standardization and organization of the patient record, the main purpose of the problem-oriented medical record is to give a clear view of the care provider's line of reasoning. Much of the information in a POMR is organized according to problems. It is immediately clear to which problem any findings and treatment plan pertain. The POMR includes:

- Collection of data
- A problem list
- Plans for addressing each problem
- Evaluations of care plans

Initially, an information source is developed about the client, including such data as:

- Client's diagnosis
- Past medical history
- Client background
- Physical examination
- Results of laboratory tests and other diagnostic tests

From this data, caregivers generate a problem list. A *problem* is any condition (health, socioeconomic, personal) the client has that the healthcare team will need to treat. The problem list is continually updated. Physicians and professionals from various disciplines (nursing, nutrition, physical therapy, etc.) write progress notes in the chart. A progress note summarizes a client's progress related to a specific problem. A **progress note** is a notation in the medical record by a health professional. For example, imagine a client has a problem identified as: poor nutritional status (protein and calories). A progress note will review this problem, evaluate effectiveness of the plan for improving nutritional status, and state how the condition has changed. Progress notes are written at key intervals during the course of a patient's stay in a healthcare institution.

Using the POMR method, notes in the client's chart are usually structured according to the SOAP format. **SOAP** is an acronym for information types. It stands for: Subjective, Objective, Assessment, and Plan:

- **S- Subjective** information is what the client, client's family, or significant others tell you about how the client/family feels, what the client wants, and the client's perception of his/her condition and problems.
- **O- Objective** information includes results of laboratory tests, height, weight, and any other measureable information that has direct bearing on the client's medical status and treatment.
- **A- Assessment** describes professional judgments based on the subjective and objective information.
- **P- Plan** is the caregiver's recommended actions, which usually fall into one of three categories: obtain more information, treat, and/or educate.

Figure 11.1 provides examples of nutrition-related components for SOAP notes. Figure 11.2 lists rules for keeping good nutrition-related records, and Figure 11.3 shows a sample SOAP note. It is always important to sign your entries in the medical record, and include your credentials. Also, keep in mind that if you do not document something, it has—for legal and regulatory purposes—not occurred. So, think carefully about what you need to write down. Do not overlook anything important or relevant.

You should also document to show what information you have reviewed and looked for. For example, the sample note in Figure 11.3 indicates that you have tried to find out the usual weight for a client and were not able to do so. It also shows that you have reviewed a list of the client's medications to see if any might be affecting the patient's nutritional status. These notations are important to demonstrate that you did not simply forget or overlook important aspects of nutrition care. As a shortcut, healthcare professionals use many abbreviations for medical and clinical terms in medical records. Figure 11.4 lists some common abbreviations. In any institution, accepted standards for abbreviations may vary slightly.

Figure 11.1

NUTRITION-RELATED COMPONENTS OF SOAP NOTES

SUBJECTIVE INFORMATION
- Eating habits and patterns
- Food preferences
- Appetite
- Reaction/adherence to diet
- Problems chewing or swallowing
- Food allergies
- Usual weight
- Changes in eating habits
- Changes in weight
- Previous diets and instructions
- Habits—activity, sleep, bowel
- Use of vitamin/mineral supplements
- Use of medications

Examples:

Client reports feeling nauseated and wants less food.

Client reports feeling better and is requesting more food.

Client reports difficulty swallowing due to sore mouth. Has requested liquids or soft foods only.

ASSESSMENT
- Evaluation of weight as it compares to standards and usual past weight
- Evaluation of appropriateness of prescribed diet
- Evaluation of nutrient and drug interactions
- Evaluation of laboratory values
- Evaluation of diet history
- Evaluation of eating/feeding ability
- Evaluation of client's compliance with diet
- Evaluation of any other problems that are nutritionally related

Examples:

Client is able to make menu selections consistent with 4 gram sodium diet.

Diet history shows client's daily intake of sodium is over 10 grams due to frequent consumption of high sodium foods.

Client's low albumin indicates significant malnutrition.

OBJECTIVE INFORMATION
- Height
- Actual weight
- Ideal body weight
- Percent weight change
- Diet order
- Pertinent laboratory values
- Nutritional needs: calories and protein
- Calorie count or food intake information
- Medications (as they pertain to nutrition)
- Observed feeding or eating ability
- Diet history taken
- Diet instruction given

Examples:

Client is blind.

Diet order is 1,800 cal ADA.

Client given diet instruction on fat-controlled diet.

PLAN
- Weight goal
- Initiate/recommend supplemental feedings
- Initiate/recommend vitamin/mineral supplements
- Initiate/recommend diet instruction prior to discharge
- Initiate/recommend calorie counts (intake records)
- Request more laboratory tests
- Request daily weights
- Referral to other health team members

Examples:

Will provide liquid, complete nutritional supplement between meals.

Will design 1,800 calorie diabetic diet with client.

Start calorie count tomorrow AM.

Figure 11.2

RULES FOR KEEPING GOOD CLIENT RECORDS

▶ Use the color ink your institution requires. (Usually, this is black.)

▶ Include direct quotes from clients (marked with quotation marks) as appropriate in the *Subjective* portion of a SOAP note.

▶ Aside from documenting subjective information obtained from a client, place only facts in the medical record. Do not speculate.

▶ Complete all blocks and spaces on forms.

▶ Use facility-approved abbreviations; do not invent your own.

▶ Date all entries accurately.

▶ Refer to days of the week as dates.

▶ Write legibly and spell words correctly.

▶ Do not erase anything. If you need to make a correction, just cross through it and write "error" above it.

▶ Document missed appointments or any other acts of poor compliance.

▶ Do not be uncomplimentary in remarks about the client or client's family.

▶ Do not record anything in the record that does not pertain to the client.

▶ Do not use the medical record to criticize others.

▶ Be complete and accurate.

▶ Be as brief as possible. Remember that others have to read your notes, and everyone is busy. Complete sentences are not necessary.

▶ Do not make (or appear to make) a diagnosis of a medical condition, as this is the physician's role.

▶ Always sign your entries with your name and your credentials.

▶ Document all relevant information. If you don't document something, it is presumed it did not occur.

Adapted from a presentation by James G. Zimmerly at 1984 American Dietetic Association Annual Meeting, Washington, DC.

Finally, remembering that the medical record is also a legal document, do not criticize others or appear to be assuming a role you are not qualified for in a progress note. For example, you would not want to write:

> *Patient did not receive her lunch tray because nurse forgot to pass it.*

or

> *I think this patient has diabetes – please check.*

Another charting format is DAP, which stands for: Data, Assessment, and Plan. It is similar to SOAP without the "subjective" component. DAP components are:

> **D- Data** includes diet, supplements, tube feedings, and compliance based on diet history; weight, height, usual weight, percent IBW and weight trends if pertinent; protein, calorie, and fluid needs

Figure 11.3

SAMPLE SOAP NOTE

S: Client states, "I can't eat like I used to. Nothing tastes good." Also states she does not know her weight, but clothes feel baggy.

O: 84 y.o. female
Height: 5'5"
IBW: 130 lbs.
Weight: 119 lbs.; 92% IBW
Usual weight: not available
Serum albumin: 2.8
Diet order: General
Meds with possible effects on taste: none

A: Recent weight loss likely. Low serum alb. consistent with malnutrition. Currently below IBW. May be losing some sense of taste.

P: Work with client to follow food preferences; provide more highly seasoned menu selections and hot foods. Monitor eating patterns at meal time. Follow up in three days.

---

compared to actual intakes; tube feeding breakdown for calories, protein, fat, and fluids.

> **A- Assessment** includes an assessment of the risk level with background reasons, a listing of nutrition problems, and food-drug interactions.
>
> **P- Plan** lists goals and approaches.

In this format, follow-up notes include problems, assessment, and plan (PAP). Problems are listed as identified on the care plan. In the assessment section, discuss progress in achievement of care plan goals. Add any supportive data which specifically relate to the problem. Also include changes in risk level and any new problems. The plan section includes information on changes in goals or approaches and recommendations for the physician.

DAR is another charting format, which stands for:

> **D-** Data
>
> **A-** Action
>
> **R-** Response

No matter which charting format a facility uses, the total content of the chart notes should be very similar. In longterm care facilities, care plans are written up separately. The care plan form is used by all disciplines, such as nursing and physical therapy. Writing in the progress notes and in the care plan is often the responsibility of the dietitian. State regulations vary as to who is responsible for writing progress notes and care plans. In some states, the dietary manager may

COMMON ABBREVIATIONS FOR MEDICAL RECORDS

ABC	Ambulatory/Bed/Chair	**FBS**	Fasting Blood Sugar	**prn**	As necessary
A/C	Alert/Confused	**fl**	Fluid	**PT**	Physical Therapy
ac	Before food or meals	**g/c**	Geriatric chair	**pt**	Patient
ADL	Activities of Daily Living	**gd**	Good	**qAM**	Every morning
ADR	Adverse Drug Reaction	**GI**	Gastrointestinal	**qd***	Every day
ad lib	As desired	**gm**	Gram	**qh**	Every hour
AHD or ASHD		**GTT**	Glucose Tolerance Test	**qid**	Four times a day
	Arteriosclerotic Heart Disease	**hb/Hg/Hgb**		**resp**	Respiration
alb	Albumin		Hemoglobin	**ROM**	Range of Motion
bid	Two times daily	**Hct**	Hematocrit	**Rx**	Treatment
BM	Bowel Movement	**hs***	Bedtime	$\overline{s}$	without
BP	Blood Pressure	**IV**	Intravenous	**sob**	Shortness of breath
BUN	Blood Urea Nitrogen	**K**	Potassium	**stat**	Immediately
$\overline{c}$	with	**liq**	Liquid	**supp**	Suppository
CBC	Complete Blood Count	**mg**	Milligram	**tab**	Tablet
cc*	Cubic centimeter	**ml**	Milliliter	**tid**	Three times a day
CHF	Congestive Heart Failure	**Na**	Sodium	**URI**	Upper Respiratory Infection
co, c/o	Complains of	**noc**	At night	**UTI**	Urinary Tract Infection
CRF	Chronic Renal Failure	**NPO**	Nothing by Mouth	**via**	By way of
CV	Cardiovascular	**OOB**	Out of Bed	**WBC**	White Blood Count
Dx	Diagnosis	**OT**	Occupational Therapy	**WNL**	Within Normal Limits
ECG, EKG		**OTC**	Over the Counter Medication	**wt**	Weight
	Electrocardiogram	**PH**	Past History		
eg	For example	**po**	By mouth		

Avoid these if subject to JCAHO standards, per new guidance Jan. 2004.

update care plans and chart in the medical record. State regulations also vary as to how often the progress notes and care plans must be updated. It may be 30 days, 60 days, or another interval of time.

MEAL-RELATED DOCUMENTS

In a healthcare institution, a designated dietary team member reviews the diet order. A diet order is the diet prescribed by the physician for an individual client. This is usually a written order in the medical record. Often, it is the responsibility of a nurse or someone on the nursing staff to notify the dietary department of a diet order. Although diet orders most often are transmitted via an internal document called a diet sheet, sometimes they are transmitted by phone, in what is called a verbal order. Verbal orders from the nursing units should be discouraged, because they do not provide solid documentation. Both nursing and dietary units need to develop and jointly approve a policy and procedure for communicating and documenting diet order transmission. If

Figure 11.5

SAMPLE DIETARY KARDEX CARD

Diet Order			Nourishments	
Physician	J.S. Werner, M.D.		AM	
Diagnosis	Cardiac and Cerebral		PM	
	Arteriosclerosis		HS	
Allergies				

DATE	INT	DIET ORDERED
11/10/03	RM	Mecanical Soft, NAS

	Carbohydrates	Dairy	Fruit	Meat	Vegetable
Likes					
Dislikes					

Beverage   Room

B _____   Dining Room

L _____   Usual Servings

D _____   Small ☐

                  Medium ☐

                  Large ☐

Room No.	Name	Current Diet Order
306	H.K. Smith	Mechanical Soft, no added salt

policies and procedures where you work permit verbal orders, the names of the persons transmitting and receiving the diet order and the time it is received should be written down. Such orders should be verified in writing before the next meal, to confirm accuracy.

In almost all healthcare institutions, diet orders are written by the physician. As explained in Chapter 6, a physician should order only diets listed in the facility's approved diet manual. In a typical healthcare institution, the diet manual is reviewed and/or updated on a regular basis and approved by the registered dietitian and the medical director of the facility.

Now that the diet order has been sent to dietary services, it must be recorded in dietary department records. Within a dietary department, nutrition caregivers usually maintain an internal record of the meal-related information. This may be maintained as a card in a kardex system (a small, portable file system), or it may be maintained on a computer system. Typically, a kardex card lists food preferences, allergies or intolerances, and meal planning patterns used in meal

Figure 11.6

SAMPLE TRAY CARDS

Name: _____

Room: _____

Diet: _____

Comments:

Likes	Dislikes

Border is color-coded to indicate required diets. (For example, regular diet may be on blue, soft diet on red, etc.)

Name _____

Room No. _____

1,500 Calorie Diabetic or
Restricted Calorie Diet

BREAKFAST EXCHANGES
Fruit	1
Bread/Cereal	2
Egg	1
Fat	1
Milk, whole	1
Coffee or tea	

DINNER EXCHANGES
Meat	2 ounces
Potato	1
Bread	1 slice
Vegetable	1
Fat	1
Fruit	1
Milk, whole	½
Coffee or tea	

SUPPER EXCHANGES
Meat	2
Potato/Sub.	1
Vegetable	1
Bread	1 slice
Fat	1
Fruit	1
Coffee or tea	

BEDTIME EXCHANGE
Milk, whole	½
Bread	1 slice

service. It also lists the diet order, as copied from the physician's order in the medical record. It may also contain other information about the plan of care and relevant clinical data used in monitoring nutritional status. A sample appears in Figure 11.5.

Alternately, some longterm care operations maintain tray cards or meal cards indicating preferences and diet-related guidelines for individual residents' meals, as shown in Figure 11.6. Tray cards and menus may be color-coded to indicate a specific diet. The color-coding helps foodservice workers assemble trays quickly, as they can glance ahead at the color and anticipate which foods are needed. Documents such as these exist primarily as a convenience for carrying out meal service. Maintaining a kardex card or tray card does not substitute for formal, legal documentation as required of the entire healthcare team.

FEDERAL REGULATIONS CONCERNING NUTRITION AND DOCUMENTATION IN NURSING FACILITIES

Nursing facilities participating in the Medicare and Medicaid programs must follow federal regulations developed by the Centers for Medicare & Medicaid Services (CMS). Regulations address quality of care. CMS requires certain documentation in a standardized format. Both institutional licensure and reimbursement for services depend on proper documentation. Individual states enforce the regulations, and sometimes adapt them. States also enforce regulations controlling licensure for the institutions. Thus, in any state where you work, you need to become familiar with the standards.

A centerpiece of the CMS regulations is the **Resident Assessment Instrument (RAI)**. This is a specialized form of medical documentation required of every healthcare institution that is receiving funding from Medicare and/or Medicaid. The RAI helps healthcare team members assess and plan high-quality care. Its documentation process is a tool to help clinicians, and the documentation is required above and beyond the medical record that is already being maintained. The RAI includes these two components: the Minimum Data Set (MDS) and Resident Assessment Protocols (RAPs). Each is discussed below.

Minimum Data Set (MDS)

The MDS is a standardized reporting form used by members of the healthcare team to do an assessment of each resident. Members of the healthcare team work together to complete the form, which may be maintained on paper or in a computerized system. Regulations require an institution to transmit MDS forms to CMS on a regular basis. By current regulations, this transmission is an electronic (not paper) process.

The **Minimum Data Set (MDS)** form outlines a minimum amount of data (information) that caregivers must collect and use. It is designed for use by a number of healthcare professionals, as an interdisciplinary care tool. The MDS includes a face sheet and a full assessment form that is used upon admission and once a year or more often if there is a significant change in the resident's condition. A shortened version of the MDS, called the MDS Quarterly Assessment Form, is filled out every three months. The MDS form collects basic information such as:

- Disease diagnoses
- Health conditions
- Physical and mental functional status

- Sensory and physical impairments
- Nutritional status and requirements
- Special treatments or procedures
- Mental and psychosocial status
- Discharge potential
- Dental condition
- Activities potential
- Drug therapy

The dietitian/dietary manager fills out Section K, "Oral/Nutritional Status," on the MDS 2.0, and may become involved in helping with nutrition-related components in other sections of the MDS form as well. A sample page from the MDS form appears in Figure 11.7.

Some basic rules for filling out the MDS are as follows:

- When the box is blank, you must fill in a number or letter, according to the code given.
- When there is a letter in the box, check if the condition applies.
- Once an MDS has been completed, you can't change the information written on it. Changes should be written in the clinical record.
- According to the facility's policy, the person(s) completing the MDS must sign with their title, date, and section they completed (Section K) on the face sheet.

Section K asks for information on the following:

1. Oral problems
2. Height and weight
3. Weight change
4. Nutritional problems
5. Nutritional approaches
6. Parenteral or enteral intake

The intent of this section is to prevent malnutrition and dehydration, and to ensure the appropriate use of feeding tubes. The CMS Guidelines for Section K appear in detail in Figure 11.8.

Figure 11.7

Sample Page from the MDS 2.0 Form

Resident _____

Numeric Identifier _____

2.	PAIN SYMPTOMS	(Code the **highest level of pain** present in the **last 7 days**)		
		a. FREQUENCY with which resident complains or shows evidence of pain 0. No pain (*skip to J4*) 1. Pain less than daily 2. Pain daily	**b. INTENSITY** of pain 1. Mild pain 2. Moderate pain 3. Times when pain is horrible or excruciating	

3.	PAIN SITE	(*If pain present*, **check all sites** that apply in **last 7 days**)				
		Back pain	a.	Incisional pain	f.	
		Bone pain	b.	Joint pain (other than hip)	g.	
		Chest pain while doing usual activities	c.	Soft tissue pain (e.g., lesion, muscle)	h.	
		Headache	d.	Stomach pain	i.	
		Hip pain	e.	Other	j.	

4.	ACCIDENTS	(**Check all that apply**)				
		Fell in **past 30 days**	a.	Hip fracture in **last 180 days**	c.	
		Fell in **past 31-180 days**	b.	Other fracture in **last 180 days**	d.	
				NONE OF ABOVE	e.	

5.	STABILITY OF CONDITIONS	Conditions/diseases make resident's cognitive, ADL, mood or behavior patterns unstable—(fluctuating, precarious, or deteriorating)	a.
		Resident experiencing an acute episode or a flare-up of a recurrent or chronic problem	b.
		End-stage disease, 6 or fewer months to live	c.
		NONE OF ABOVE	d.

SECTION K. ORAL/NUTRITIONAL STATUS

1.	ORAL PROBLEMS	Chewing problem	a.
		Swallowing problem	b.
		Mouth pain	c.
		NONE OF ABOVE	d.

2.	HEIGHT AND WEIGHT	Record (**a.**) height in inches and (**b.**) weight in pounds. Base weight on most recent measure in **last 30 days**; measure weight consistently in accord with standard facility practice—e.g., in a.m. after voiding, before meal, with shoes off, and in nightclothes
		a. HT (in.) [ ] [ ] **b.** WT (lb.) [ ] [ ] [ ]

3.	WEIGHT CHANGE	**a. Weight loss**—5 % or more in **last 30 days**; or 10 % or more in **last 180 days** 0. No 1. Yes
		b. Weight gain—5 % or more in **last 30 days**; or 10 % or more in **last 180 days** 0. No 1. Yes

4.	NUTRI-TIONAL PROBLEMS	Complains about the taste of many foods	a.	Leaves 25% or more of food uneaten at most meals	c.
		Regular or repetitive complaints of hunger	b.	*NONE OF ABOVE*	d.

5.	NUTRI-TIONAL APPROACH-ES	(**Check all that apply in last 7 days**)			
		Parenteral/IV	a.	Dietary supplement between meals	f.
		Feeding tube	b.	Plate guard, stabilized built-up utensil, etc.	g.
		Mechanically altered diet	c.	On a planned weight change program	h.
		Syringe (oral feeding)	d.	*NONE OF ABOVE*	i.
		Therapeutic diet	e.		

6.	PARENTERAL OR ENTERAL INTAKE	(*Skip to Section L if neither 5a nor 5b is checked*)
		a. Code the proportion of **total calories** the resident received through parenteral or tube feedings in the **last 7 days** 0. None 3. 51% to 75% 1. 1% to 25% 4. 76% to 100% 2. 26% to 50%
		b. Code the average **fluid intake** per day by IV or tube in **last 7 days** 0. None 3. 1001 to 1500 cc/day 1. 1 to 500 cc/day 4. 1501 to 2000 cc/day 2. 501 to 1000 cc/day 5. 2001 or more cc/day

SECTION L. ORAL/DENTAL STATUS

1.	ORAL STATUS AND DISEASE PREVENTION	Debris (soft, easily movable substances) present in mouth prior to going to bed at night	a.
		Has dentures or removable bridge	b.
		Some/all natural teeth lost—does not have or does not use dentures (or partial plates)	c.
		Broken, loose, or carious teeth	d.
		Inflamed gums (gingiva); swollen or bleeding gums; oral abscesses; ulcers or rashes	e.
		Daily cleaning of teeth/dentures or daily mouth care—by resident or staff	f.
		NONE OF ABOVE	g.

SECTION M. SKIN CONDITION

1.	ULCERS (Due to any cause)	(*Record the number of ulcers at each ulcer stage—regardless of cause. If none present at a stage, record "0" (zero). Code all that apply during **last 7 days**. Code 9 = 9 or more.*) [**Requires full body exam.**]	Number at Stage
		a. Stage 1. A persistent area of skin redness (without a break in the skin) that does not disappear when pressure is relieved.	
		b. Stage 2. A partial thickness loss of skin layers that presents clinically as an abrasion, blister, or shallow crater.	
		c. Stage 3. A full thickness of skin is lost, exposing the subcutaneous tissues - presents as a deep crater with or without undermining adjacent tissue.	
		d. Stage 4. A full thickness of skin and subcutaneous tissue is lost, exposing muscle or bone.	

2.	TYPE OF ULCER	(*For each type of ulcer, **code for the highest stage in the last 7 days** using scale in item M1—i.e., 0=none; stages 1, 2, 3, 4*)	
		a. Pressure ulcer—any lesion caused by pressure resulting in damage of underlying tissue	
		b. Stasis ulcer—open lesion caused by poor circulation in the lower extremities	

3.	HISTORY OF RESOLVED ULCERS	Resident had an ulcer that was resolved or cured **in LAST 90 DAYS** 0. No 1.Yes	

4.	OTHER SKIN PROBLEMS OR LESIONS PRESENT	(**Check all that apply** during **last 7 days**)	
		Abrasions, bruises	a.
		Burns (second or third degree)	b.
		Open lesions other than ulcers, rashes, cuts (e.g., cancer lesions)	c.
		Rashes—e.g., intertrigo, eczema, drug rash, heat rash, herpes zoster	d.
		Skin desensitized to pain or pressure	e.
		Skin tears or cuts (other than surgery)	f.
		Surgical wounds	g.
		NONE OF ABOVE	h.

5.	SKIN TREAT-MENTS	(**Check all that apply** during **last 7 days**)	
		Pressure relieving device(s) for chair	a.
		Pressure relieving device(s) for bed	b.
		Turning/repositioning program	c.
		Nutrition or hydration intervention to manage skin problems	d.
		Ulcer care	e.
		Surgical wound care	f.
		Application of dressings (with or without topical medications) other than to feet	g.
		Application of ointments/medications (other than to feet)	h.
		Other preventative or protective skin care (other than to feet)	i.
		NONE OF ABOVE	j.

6.	FOOT PROBLEMS AND CARE	(**Check all that apply** during **last 7 days**)	
		Resident has one or more foot problems—e.g., corns, callouses, bunions, hammer toes, overlapping toes, pain, structural problems	a.
		Infection of the foot—e.g., cellulitis, purulent drainage	b.
		Open lesions on the foot	c.
		Nails/calluses trimmed during **last 90 days**	d.
		Received preventative or protective foot care (e.g., used special shoes, inserts, pads, toe separators)	e.
		Application of dressings (with or without topical medications)	f.
		NONE OF ABOVE	g.

SECTION N. ACTIVITY PURSUIT PATTERNS

1.	TIME AWAKE	(**Check appropriate time periods over last 7 days**) Resident awake all or most of time (i.e., naps no more than one hour per time period) in the:			
		Morning	a.	Evening	c.
		Afternoon	b.	*NONE OF ABOVE*	d.

(If resident is comatose, skip to Section O)

2.	AVERAGE TIME INVOLVED IN ACTIVITIES	(**When awake and not receiving treatments or ADL care**) 0. Most—more than 2/3 of time 2. Little—less than 1/3 of time 1. Some—from 1/3 to 2/3 of time 3. None

3.	PREFERRED ACTIVITY SETTINGS	(**Check all settings** in which activities are **preferred**)			
		Own room	a.		
		Day/activity room	b.	Outside facility	d.
		Inside NH/off unit	c.	*NONE OF ABOVE*	e.

4.	GENERAL ACTIVITY PREFER-ENCES (adapted to resident's current abilities)	(**Check all PREFERENCES** whether or not activity is currently available to resident)			
		Cards/other games	a.	Trips/shopping	g.
		Crafts/arts	b.	Walking/wheeling outdoors	h.
		Exercise/sports	c.	Watching TV	i.
		Music	d.	Gardening or plants	j.
		Reading/writing	e.	Talking or conversing	k.
		Spiritual/religious activities	f.	Helping others	l.
				NONE OF ABOVE	m.

MDS 2.0 September, 2000

Figure 11.8

CMS Guidelines for Completing the MDS – Section K

SECTION K. ORAL/NUTRITIONAL STATUS

Residents in nursing facilities challenge the staff with many conditions that could affect their ability to consume food and fluids to maintain adequate nutrition and hydration. Early problem recognition can help to ensure appropriate and timely nutritional intervention. Prevention is the goal, and early detection and modification of interventions is the key. Section K, oral and Nutritional Status, should assist the nursing facility staff in recognizing nutritional deficits that will need to be addressed in a resident's care plan. Nurse assessors will need to collaborate with the dietitian and dietary staff to ensure that some items in this section have been assessed and calculated accurately.

Keep in mind that Section 1.13 states that the RAI must be conducted or coordinated with the appropriate participation of health professionals…facilities have flexibility in determining who should participate in the assessment process, as long as it is accurately conducted. A facility may assign responsibility for completing the RAI to a number of qualified staff members. In most cases, participants in the assessment process are licensed health professionals. It is the facility's responsibility to ensure that all participants in the assessment process have the requisite knowledge to complete an accurate and comprehensive assessment.

K1. ORAL PROBLEMS (7-DAY LOOK BACK)
Intent:
To record any oral problems present in the last seven days.

Definition:
a. Chewing Problem—Inability to chew food easily and without pain or difficulties, regardless of cause (e.g., resident uses ill-fitting dentures, or has a neurologically impaired chewing mechanism, or has temporomandibular joint [TMJ] pain, or a painful tooth). Code chewing problem even when interventions have been successfully introduced.

b. Swallowing Problem—Dysphagia. Clinical manifestations include frequent choking and coughing when eating or drinking, holding food in mouth for prolonged periods of time, or excessive drooling. Code swallowing problem even when interventions have been successfully introduced.

c. Mouth Pain—Any pain or discomfort associated with any part of the mouth, regardless of cause. Clinical manifestations include favoring one side of the mouth while eating, refusing to eat, refusing food or fluids of certain temperatures (hot or cold).

d. NONE OF ABOVE (Not Used on the MPAF)

Process:
Ask the resident about difficulties in these areas. Observe the resident during meals. Review the medical record for staff observations about the residents; e.g., "pockets food," etc. Inspect the mouth for abnormalities that could contribute to chewing or swallowing problems or mouth pain.

Coding:
Check all that apply. If none apply, check NONE OF ABOVE.

K2. HEIGHT AND WEIGHT (30-DAY LOOK BACK)
Intent:
To record a current height and weight in order to monitor nutrition and hydration status over time; also, to provide a mechanism for monitoring stability of weight over time. For example, a resident who has had edema can have an intended and expected weight loss as a result of taking a diuretic. Or weight loss could be the result of poor intake, or adequate intake accompanied by recent participation in a fitness program.

A. HEIGHT
Process:
New Admissions—Measure height in inches.

Current Resident—Check the clinical records. If the last height recorded was more than one year ago, measure the resident's height again.

Coding:
Round height upward to the nearest whole inch. Measure height consistently over time in accord with standard facility practice (shoes off, etc.)

FIGURE 11.8 CONT'D...MDS GUIDELINES—SECTION K

B. WEIGHT

Process:

Check the clinical records. If the last recorded weight was taken more than one month ago or previous weight is not available, weigh the resident again. If the resident has experienced a decline in intake at meals, snacks, or fluid intake, weigh the resident again. If the resident's weight was taken more than once during the preceding month, record the most recent weight.

Coding:

Round weight upward to the nearest whole pound. Measure weight consistently over time in accord with standard facility practice (after voiding, before meal, etc.). There may be circumstances when a resident cannot be weighed, for example: extreme pain, immobility, or risk of pathological fractures. If, as a matter of professional judgment, a resident cannot be weighed, use the standard no-information code (-). Document rationale on resident's record.

K3. WEIGHT CHANGE (30 AND 180-DAY LOOK BACKS)

Intent:

To record variations in the resident's weight over time.

A. WEIGHT LOSS

Definition:

Weight Loss in Percentages (e.g., 5% or more in last 30 days, or 10% or more in last 180 days).

Process:

New Admission—Ask the resident or family about weight changes over the last 30 and 180 days. Consult physician, review transfer documentation and compare with admission weight. Calculate weight loss in percentages during the specified time periods.

Current Resident—Review the clinical records and compare current weight with weights of 30 and 180 days ago. Calculate weight loss in percentages during the specified time periods.

Coding:

Code "0" for No or "1" for Yes. If there is no weight to compare to, enter the unknown code (-).

B. WEIGHT GAIN

Definition:

Weight Gain in Percentages (i.e., 5% or more in last 30 days, or 10% or more in up to the last 180 days).

Process:

New Admission—Ask the resident or family about weight changes over the last 30 and 180 days. Consult physician, review transfer documentation and compare with admission weight. Calculate weight gain during the specified time periods.

Current Resident—Review the clinical records and compare current weight with weights of 30 and 180 days ago. Calculate weight gain during the specified time periods.

Coding:

Code "0" for No or "1" for Yes. If there is no weight to compare to, enter a dash (-)

Clarifications:

The first step in calculating percent weight gain or loss is to obtain the actual weights for the 30-day and 180-day time periods from the resident's clinical record. Calculate percentage for weight loss and weight gain based on the resident's actual weight. Do not round the actual weight. The calculation is as follows:

> 1. Start with the resident's weight from 30 days ago and multiply it by the proportion (0.05). If the resident has gained or lost more than 5%, code a "1" for Yes.

> 2. Start with the resident's weight from 180 days ago and multiply it by the proportion (0.10). If the resident has gained or lost more than 10%, code a "1" for Yes.

Residents experiencing a 7½% weight change (gain or loss) 90 days ago must be evaluated to determine how much of the 7½% weight change occurred over the last 30 days.

Figure 11.8 cont'd...MDS Guidelines—Section K

There are no specific regulations that address the desirable weight and time frames for weight gain or weight loss. However, there is some general information in the interpretive guidelines and in the Nutritional RAP that may provide guidance in this area. The amount of weight gain or loss is reflective of individual differences. Guidelines related to acceptable parameters of weight gain and loss are addressed in the OBRA regulations at 42 CFR 483.25, nutrition (F325 and F 326) and 483.20(b)2(xi), resident assessment nutritional status and requirements (F 272), which corresponds to the MDS 2.0 Section K, Oral/Nutritional status.

The parameters for weight loss identified in the guidelines referenced above are:

> 1 month 5% significant >5% severe
> 3 months 7.5% significant >7.5% severe
> 6 months 10% significant >10% severe

The measurement of weight is a guide in determining nutritional status. Therefore, the evaluation of the significance of weight gain or loss over a specific time frame is a crucial part of the assessment process.

However, if the resident is losing/gaining a significant amount of weight, the facility should not wait for the 30 or 180-day timeframe to address the problem. Weight changes of 5% in one month, 7.5% in three months, or 10% in six months should prompt a thorough assessment of the resident's nutritional status. For example, a 10% loss/gain within 4 months should also be coded here, and carefully evaluated. An adequate assessment should result in a comprehensive care plan for each resident that includes measurable objectives and timetables to meet a resident's needs and expressed desires.

K4. NUTRITIONAL PROBLEMS (7-DAY LOOK BACK)

Intent:
To identify specific problems, conditions, and risk factors for functional decline present in the last seven days that affect or could affect the resident's health or functional status. Such problems can often be reversed and the resident can improve.

Definition:
a. Complains About the Taste of Many Foods—The sense of taste can change as a result of health conditions or medications. Also, complaints can be culturally based—e.g., someone used to eating spicy foods may find nursing facility meals bland.

b. Regular or Repetitive Complaints of Hunger—On most days (at least 2 out of 3), resident asks for more food or repetitively complains of feeling hungry (even after eating a meal).

c. Leaves 25% or More of Food Uneaten at Most Meals—Eats less than 75 percent of food (even when substitutes are offered) at least 2 out of 3 meals a day. This assumes the resident is receiving the proper amount of food to meet their daily requirements and not excessive amounts above and beyond what they could be expected to consume.

d. NONE OF ABOVE

Process:
Consult resident's records (including current nursing care plan), dietary/fluid intake flow sheets, and dietary progress notes/assessments. Consult with direct-care staff, dietary staff and the consulting dietitian. Ask the resident if he or she experienced any of these symptoms in the last seven days. Sometimes a resident will not complain to staff members because he or she attributes symptoms to "old age." Therefore, it is important to ask the resident directly. Observe the resident while eating. If he or she leaves food or picks at it, ask, "Why are you not eating? Would you eat if something else was offered?" Observe if resident winces or makes faces while eating. NOTE: Facilities are required to offer substitutions when residents do not eat or like the food being served. Observe whether or not residents have refused offers for substitute meals.

Coding:
Check all conditions that apply. If no conditions apply, check NONE OF ABOVE.

Figure 11.8 cont'd...MDS Guidelines—Section K

K5. NUTRITIONAL APPROACHES (7-DAY LOOK BACK)

Definition:

a. Parenteral/IV—Intravenous (IV) fluids or hyperalimentation, including total parenteral nutrition, given continuously or intermittently. This category also includes administration of fluids via IV lines with fluids running at KVO (Keep Vein Open), or via heparin locks. Do not code IV "push" medications here. Do include the IV fluids in IV piggybacks. IV medications dissolved in a diluent, as well as IV push medications are captured as IV medications in P1ac. Do not include IV fluids that were administered as a routine part of an operative procedure or recovery room stay.

b. Feeding Tube—Presence of any type of tube that can deliver food/nutritional substances/fluids/medications directly into the gastrointestinal system. Examples include, but are not limited to, nasogastric tubes, gastrostomy tubes, jejunostomy tubes, percutaneous endoscopic gastrostomy (PEG) tube

c. Mechanically Altered Diet—A diet specifically prepared to alter the consistency of food in order to facilitate oral intake. Examples include soft solids, pureed foods, ground meat, and thickened liquids. A mechanically altered diet should not automatically be considered a therapeutic diet. Determine whether or not the therapeutic diet should be coded based on the definition in Item K5e below.

d. Syringe (Oral Feeding)—Use of syringe to deliver liquid or pureed nourishment directly into the mouth. All efforts should be made to utilize other feeding methods (e.g., rubber tipped spoon) as this can result in lowered resident dignity.

e. Therapeutic Diet—A diet ordered to manage problematic health conditions. Examples include calorie-specific, low-salt, low-fat lactose, no added sugar, and supplements during meals.

f. Dietary Supplement Between Meals—Any type of dietary supplement provided between scheduled meals (e.g., high protein/calorie shake, or 3 p.m. snack for resident who receives q.a.m. dose of NPH insulin). Do not include snacks that everyone receives as part of the unit's daily routine.

g. Plate Guard, Stabilized Built-Up Utensils, Etc.—Any type of specialized, altered, or adaptive equipment to facilitate the resident's involvement in self-performance of eating.

h. On Planned Weight Change Program—Resident is receiving a program of which the documented purpose and goal are to facilitate weight gain or loss (e.g., double portions; high calorie supplements; reduced calories; 10 grams fat).

i. NONE OF ABOVE (Not Used on the MPAF)

Coding:

Check all that apply. If none apply, check NONE OF ABOVE.

Clarification:

If the resident receives fluids by hypodermoclysis and subcutaneous ports in hydration therapy, code these nutritional approaches in this item. The term parenteral therapy means "introduction of a substance (especially nutritive material) into the body by means other than the intestinal tract (e.g., subcutaneous, intravenous)." If the resident receives fluids via these modalities, also code Items K6a and b, which refer to the caloric and fluid intake the resident received in the last 7 days. Additives such as electrolytes and insulin which are added to the resident's TPN or IV fluids should be counted as medications and documented in Section O1, Number of Medications AND P1ac, IV Medications.

K6. PARENTERAL OR ENTERAL INTAKE (7-DAY LOOK BACK)

Skip to Section L on the MDS if neither Item K5a nor K5b is checked.

Intent:

To record the proportion of calories received and the average fluid intake, through parenteral or tube feeding in the last seven days.

A. PROPORTION OF TOTAL CALORIES

Definition:

Proportion of Total Calories Received—The proportion of all calories ingested during the last seven days that the resident actually received (not ordered) by enteral or tube feedings. Determined by calorie count.

FIGURE 11.8 CONT'D...MDS GUIDELINES—SECTION K

Process:

Review Intake record. If the resident took no food or fluids by mouth, or took just sips of fluid, stop here and code "4" (76%-100%). If the resident had more substantial oral intake than this, consult with the dietitian who can derive a calorie count received from parenteral or tube feedings.

Coding:

Code for the best response:

    0. None
    1. 1% to 25%
    2. 26% to 50%
    3. 51% to 75%
    4. 76% to 100%

EXAMPLE OF CALCULATION FOR PROPORTION OF TOTAL CALORIES FROM IV OR TUBE FEEDING

Mr. H has had a feeding tube since his surgery. He is currently more alert, and feeling much better. He is very motivated to have the tube removed. He has been taking soft solids by mouth, but only in small to medium amounts. For the past week he has been receiving tube feedings for nutritional supplementation. As his oral intake improves, the amount received by tube will decrease. The dietitian has totaled his calories per day as follows:

Step #1:		Oral		Tube
	Sun.	500	+	2000
	Mon.	250	+	2250
	Tues.	250	+	2250
	Wed.	350	+	2250
	Thurs.	500	+	2000
	Fri.	800	+	800
	Sat.	800	+	1800
	TOTAL	3450	+	14350

Step #2: Total calories = 3450 + 14350 = 17800

Step #3: Calculate percentage of total calories by tube feeding. $14350/17800 = .806 \times 100 = 80.6\%$

Step #4: Code "4" for 76% to 100%

B. AVERAGE FLUID INTAKE

Definition:

Average fluid intake per day by IV or tube feeding in last seven days refers to the actual amount of fluid the resident received by these modes (not the amount ordered).

Process:

Review the Intake and Output record from the last seven days. Add up the total amount of fluid received each day by IV and/or tube feedings only. Also include the water used to flush as well as the "free water" in the tube feeding (based upon the percent of water in the specific enteral formula). The amount of heparinized saline solution used to flush a heparin lock is not included in the average fluid intake calculation, while the amount of fluid in an IV piggyback solution is included in the calculation. Divide the week's total fluid intake by 7. This will give you the average of fluid intake per day.

Coding:

Code for the average number of cc's of fluid the resident received per day by IV or tube feeding. Record what was actually received by the resident, not what was ordered.

    Codes: 0. None
              1. 1 to 500 cc/day
              2. 501 to 1000 cc/day
              3. 1001 to 1500 cc/day
              4. 1501 to 2000 cc/day
              5. 2001 or more cc/day

FIGURE 11.8 CONT'D...MDS GUIDELINES—SECTION K

EXAMPLE OF CALCULATION FOR AVERAGE DAILY FLUID INTAKE

Ms. A has swallowing difficulties secondary to Huntington's disease. She is able to take oral fluids by mouth with supervision, but not enough to maintain hydration. She received the following daily fluid totals by supplemental tube feedings (including water, prepared nutritional supplements, juices) during the last 7 days.

Step #1:

Sun.	1250 cc
Mon.	775 cc
Tues.	925 cc
Wed.	1200 cc
Thurs.	1200 cc
Fri.	1200 cc
Sat.	1000 cc
TOTAL	7550 CC

Step #2:   7550 divided by 7 = 1078.6 cc

Step #3:   Code "3" for 1001 to 1500 cc/day

Clarifications:

The basic TPN solution itself (that is, the protein/carbohydrate mixture or a fat emulsion) is not counted as a medication. The use of TPN is coded in Item K6a. When medications such as electrolytes, vitamins, or insulin have been added to the TPN solution, they are considered medications and should be coded in O1.

The amount of heparinized saline solution used to flush a heparin lock is not included in the average fluid intake calculation. The amount of fluid in an IV piggyback solution is included in the calculation.

Source: CMS's RAI Version 2.0 Manual (August 2003), Chapter 3: Item-By-Item Guide to the MDS

Resident Assessment Protocols (RAPs)

RAPs are the second part of the Resident Assessment Instrument (RAI). A resident is assessed at a greater level for problems (or potential problems) identified through the MDS. These problems are called *triggers*. A list of the 18 defined triggers appears in Figure 11.9. A **Resident Assessment Protocol (RAP)** is a set of guidelines for assessment of specific problems identified through these triggers. There are established guidelines for each RAP. These guidelines help members of the team examine possible causes and effects of clinical conditions. The team documents a complete assessment in the medical record. RAPs must be completed within 14 days.

As an example, if the MDS identifies dehydration, a Resident Assessment Protocol (RAP) addressing this is the next step. Each trigger is coded to one or more items in the MDS. Figure 11.10 lists items covered on the MDS form that identify the Nutritional Status RAP. A dietary manager may become involved in assessment for a number of different triggers. Nutritional status is an obvious one, but nutritional factors and dietary care may also play key roles in the assessment and care plans of many of the other triggers as well.

After the initial assessment, additional assessments must be completed as follows:

> Quarterly Assessment—Every three months, the MDS Quarterly Assessment Form must be completed. This form is not as long or in-depth as the full assessment form.

> Annual Reassessment—Every 12 months, the Resident Assessment Instrument must be re-done.

> Significant Change in Status Reassessment—If a significant change in a resident's status takes place, the Resident Assessment Instrument must be re-done.

A significant change is defined as a major change in the resident's status that is not self-limiting, has an impact on more than one area of the resident's health status, and requires interdisciplinary review or revision of the care plan. Examples include unplanned weight loss of 5% or more in 30 days or 10% in 180 days; emergence of a pressure ulcer at stage II or higher (where no ulcers were previously present at Stage II or higher); a need for extensive assistance or total dependence in eating; or a condition in which the resident is judged to be unstable.

TRIGGERS FOR RAPS

Delirium	Falls
Cognitive loss/dementia	Nutritional status
Visual function	Feeding tubes
Activities of Daily Living (ADL) function/rehabilitation	Dehydration/fluid maintenance
Urinary Incontinence and indwelling catheter	Dental care
Psychosocial well-being	Pressure ulcers
Mood state	Psychotropic drug use
Behavior symptoms	Physical restraints
Activities	

Figure 11.9

EXAMPLE: MDS FORM ITEMS THAT FLAG THE NUTRITIONAL STATUS RAP

K3a weight loss	K5c syringe feeding
K4a taste alterations	K5e therapeutic diet
K4c leaves 25% or more of food	M2a pressure ulcer
K5a parenteral feeding	

Figure 11.10

Like the nutrition screening and nutrition assessment processes described in Chapter 8, the MDS form and RAPs work together. The MDS, although very detailed, is functioning as a screening tool for clinical problems. When a particular problem is identified, a RAP guides the healthcare team through in-depth assessment. Together, these tools (the *Resident Assessment Instrument*) help caregivers develop an effective, individualized care plan for each resident. They help members of the team make good decisions.

Documentation should support your decision-making regarding whether to proceed with a care plan for a triggered RAP and if so, the type(s) of care plan interventions that are appropriate for a particular resident. Documentation may appear anywhere in the clinical record (e.g. progress notes, consults, flow-sheets, etc.), as dictated by the charting policies and procedures of your own facility.

For each triggered RAP, indicate whether a new care plan, care plan revision, or continuation of current care plan is necessary to address the problem(s) identified in your assessments. The Care Planning Decision column must be completed within seven days of completing the Resident Assessment Instrument (MDS and RAPs).

To summarize, when a RAP is triggered, the dietitian/dietary manager must participate in an additional assessment using the RAP Guidelines. Some institutions use computer-based systems that automatically identify triggers based on the MDS data. Some facilities also use RAP modules. RAP modules list questions contained in the RAP, to which "yes" or "no" answers are usually used, to document that the guidelines have been reviewed. RAP modules can speed up the process, but answering the questions is not enough. The dietitian/dietary manager must still document the nature of the condition, risk factors, factors to consider in care planning, referrals, and the reasons to proceed or not proceed with care planning.

Excerpts from the RAP Keys for Nutritional Status, Feeding Tubes, and Dehydration/Fluid Maintenance appear in Figures 11.11, 11.12, and 11.13, respectively. Each of these outlines an assessment process for a RAP. It tells healthcare team members what information to look for, and suggests questions to ask in the process of investigating this condition.

In addition to these three RAPs that are directly related to dietary services, there are several other RAPs that may require dietary services interventions.

- Cognitive Loss or Dementia. Cognitive loss may put residents at risk for eating problems.
- ADL Function Rehabilitation Potential. A resident may have difficulties feeding himself or herself.

- ◗ Mood State. A mood state problem may cause loss of appetite and weight.

- ◗ Activities. Offering nutrition supplements can be part of an activity program.

- ◗ Dental Care. A resident's teeth/dentures affect his or her ability to eat.

- ◗ Pressure Ulcer. Pressure ulcers have nutritional implications.

- ◗ Psychotropic Drugs. Drugs can decrease appetite or change a resident's ability to taste and smell foods.

Assessments On Return Stay/Readmission

If a facility has discharged a resident without the expectation that the resident would return, then the returning resident is considered a new admission (return stay) and would require an initial admission RAI comprehensive assessment within 14 days of admission. This typically occurs when a resident bed has not been held while they are out of the facility.

If a resident returns to a facility following a temporary absence for hospitalization or therapeutic leave, it is considered a readmission. Facilities are not required to assess a resident who is readmitted, unless a significant change in the resident's condition has occurred. In these situations, follow the procedures for significant change assessments.

RAI Versions and References

The December 2002 Revised Long Term Care Resident Assessment Instrument (RAI) User's Manual for the Minimum Data Set (MDS) Version 2.0 was last revised in August 2003 (at the time of publication of this book). CMS states that it is in process of developing new RAPs, as well as revising the MDS form. As of the time of this publication, a draft of the proposed MDS version 3.0 was released in April, 2003 and is under continuing revision. CMS indicates version 3.0 may become the standard in 2004. MDS 3.0, in its initial draft, includes a new component for evaluating quality of life, as reported by the resident. The new section includes the resident's answers to questions such as: *Can you find a place to be alone when you wish? Do you like the food here? Do you enjoy mealtimes here? Do you feel safe and secure?* In Section K, the draft incorporates new guidelines for assessing swallowing ability. It streamlines data for parenteral and enteral intake. In addition, the Section L draft includes information about oral status and disease prevention, as recommended by the American Dietetic Association. The draft also reorganizes several items, changes diseases and diagnoses (including nutritional deficiency), and incorporates revisions for easier coding.

Check the CMS Web site regularly for updates at: http://cms.hhs.gov/medicaid/mds20 or http://cms.hhs.gov/quality/mds30. Or, check with administrators in your own place of employment to be sure you are using the most current forms, standards, and guidelines.

Figure 11.11

RESIDENT ASSESSMENT PROTOCOL: NUTRITIONAL STATUS

I. PROBLEM

Malnutrition is not a response to normal aging; it can arise from many causes. Its presence may signal the worsening of a life-threatening illness, and it should always be seen as a dramatic indicator of the resident's risk of sudden decline. Severe malnutrition is, however, relatively rare, and this RAP focuses on signs and symptoms that suggest that the resident may be at risk of becoming malnourished. For many who are triggered, there will be no obvious, outward signs of malnutrition. Prevention is the goal, and early detection is the key.

Early problem recognition and care planning can help to ensure appropriate and timely nutritional intervention. For many residents, simple adjustments in feeding patterns may be sufficient. For others, compensation or correction for food intake problems may be required.

Within a nutrition program, food intake is best accomplished via oral feedings. Tube (enteral) feeding is normally limited to residents who have a demonstrated inability to orally consume sufficient food to prevent major malnutrition or weight loss. Parenteral feeding is normally limited to life-saving situations where both oral and enteral feeding is contraindicated or inadequate to meet nutrient needs. Oral feeding is clearly preferred. Depending on the nature of the problem, residents can be encouraged to use finger foods; to take small bites; to use the tongue to move food in the mouth from side to side; to chew and swallow each bite; to avoid food that causes mouth pain, etc. Therapeutic programs can also be designed to review for the need for adaptive utensils to compensate for problems in sucking, closing lips, or grasping utensils; to help the confused resident maintain a fixed feeding routine, etc.

II. TRIGGERS

Malnutrition problem suggested if one or more of following observed. (The item in brackets corresponds to a notation on the MDS Form.)

> Weight Loss [K3a = 1]
> Taste Alterations [K4a = checked]
> Leaves 25% or More Food Uneaten at Most Meals [K4c = checked]
> Parenteral/IV Feeding(a) [K5a = checked]

Mechanically Altered Diet [K5c = checked]
Syringe (Oral Feeding) [K5d = checked]
Therapeutic Diet [K5e = checked]
Pressure Ulcer(b) [M2a = 2, 3, or 4]

(a) Note: These items also trigger on the Dehydration/Fluid Maintenance RAP.

(b) Note: These items also trigger on the Pressure Ulcer RAP.

III. GUIDELINES
RESIDENT FACTORS THAT MAY IMPEDE ABILITY TO CONSUME FOOD
Reduced Ability to Feed Self
Reduced ability to feed self can be due to arthritis, contractures, partial or total loss of voluntary arm movement, hemiplegia or quadriplegia, vision problems, inability to perform activities of daily living without significant assistance, and coma.

Chewing Problems
Residents with oral abscesses, ill-fitting dentures, teeth that are broken, loose, carious or missing, or those on mechanically altered diets frequently cannot eat enough food to meet their calorie and other nutrient needs. Significant weight loss can, in turn, result in poorly fitting dentures and infections that can lead to more weight loss.

Losses from Diarrhea or an Ostomy

Swallowing Problems
Swallowing problems arise in several contexts: the long-term result of chemotherapy, radiation therapy, or surgery for malignancy (including head and neck cancer); fear of swallowing because of COPD/emphysema/asthma; stroke; hemiplegia or quadriplegia; Alzheimer's disease or other dementia; and ALS.

Possible Medical Causes
Numerous conditions and diseases can result in increased nutrient requirements (calories, protein, vitamins, minerals, water, and fiber) for residents. Among these are cancer and cancer therapies, Parkinson's disease with tremors, septicemia, pneumonia, gastrointestinal influenza, fever, vomiting, diarrhea and other forms of malabsorption including excessive nutrient loss from ostomy, burns, pressure ulcers, COPD/

FIGURE 11.11 CONT'D...RAP: NUTRITIONAL STATUS

emphysema/asthma, Alzheimer's disease with concomitant pacing or wandering, and hyperthyroidism.

Malignancy and Nutritional Consequences of Chemotherapy, Radiation Therapy/Surgery—For the resident undergoing therapy aimed at remission or cure, aggressive nutritional support is necessary to achieve the goal; for the resident with incurable malignancy who is undergoing palliative therapy or is not responding to curative therapy, aggressive nutritional support is often medically inappropriate.

> Have the wishes of the resident and family concerning aggressive nutritional support been ascertained?

Anemia (nutritional deficiency, not malnutrition) —A hematocrit of less than 41% is predictive of increased morbidity and mortality for residents.

> Are shortness of breath, weakness, paleness of mucous membranes and nailbeds, and/or clubbing of nails present?

Chronic COPD—Increases calorie needs and can be complicated by an elevated fear of choking when eating or drinking.

Shortness of Breath (frequently seen with congestive heart failure, hypertension, edema, and COPD/emphysema/asthma)—This is another condition that can cause a fear of eating and drinking, with a consequent reduction in food intake.

Constipation/Intestinal Obstruction/Pain—Can inhibit appetite.

Drug-Induced Anorexia—Often causes decreased or altered ability to taste and smell foods.

Delirium

PROBLEMS TO BE REVIEWED FOR POSSIBLE RELA- TIONSHIP TO NUTRITIONAL STATUS PROBLEM (CAUSAL LINK)
Mental Problems
Mental retardation, Alzheimer's or other dementia, depression, paranoid fears that food is poisoned, and mental retardation

can all lead to anorexia, resulting in significant amounts of uneaten food and subsequent weight loss.

Behavior Patterns and Problems
Residents who are fearful, who pace or wander, withdraw from activities, cannot communicate, or refuse to communicate, often refuse to eat or will eat only a limited variety and amount of foods. Left untreated, behavior problems that result in refusal to eat can cause significant weight loss and subsequent malnutrition.

> Does resident use food to gain staff attention?
> Is resident unable to understand the importance of eating?

Inability to Communicate
For most residents, enjoying food and mealtimes crucially affects quality of life. Inability to make food and mealtime preferences known can result in a resident eating poorly, losing weight, and being unhappy. Malnutrition due to poor communication usually indicates substandard care. Early correction of communication problems, where possible, can prevent malnutrition.

> • Does the area in which meals are served lend itself to socialization among residents? Is it a place where social communication can easily take place?
> • Has there been a failure to provide adequate staff and/or adequate time in feeding or assisting residents to eat?
> • Has there been a failure to recognize the need and supply adaptive feeding equipment for residents who can be helped to self-feed with such assistance?
> • Is the resident capable of telling staff that he/she has a problem with the food being served e.g., finds it to be unappetizing or unattractively presented?

Amputation
Weight loss may be due to an amputation.

Source: CMS's RAI Version 2.0 Manual, Appendix C, current as of August, 2003

RESIDENT ASSESSMENT PROTOCOL: FEEDING TUBES

I. PROBLEM

The efficacy of tube feedings is difficult to assess. When the complications and problems are known to be high and the benefits difficult to determine, the efficacy of tube feedings as a long-term treatment for individuals requires careful evaluation.

Where residents have difficulty eating and staff have limited time to assist them, insertion of feeding tubes for the convenience of nursing staff is an unacceptable rationale for use. The only rationale for such feedings is demonstrated medical need to prevent malnutrition or dehydration. Even here, all possible alternatives should be explored prior to using such an approach for long-term feeding, and restoration to normal feeding should remain the goal throughout the treatment program.

Use of nasogastric and nasointestinal tubes can result in many complications including, but not limited to: agitation, self-extubation (removal of the tube by the patient), infections, aspiration, unintended misplacement of the tube in the trachea or lungs, inadvertent dislodgment, and pain.

This RAP focuses on reviewing the status of the resident using tubes. The Nutritional Status and Dehydration/Fluid Maintenance RAPs focus on resident needs that may warrant the use of tubes. To help clarify the latter issue, the following guidelines indicate the type of review process required to ensure that tubes are used in only the exceptional and acceptable situation. As a general rule, residents unable to swallow or eat food and unlikely to eat within a few days due to physical problems in chewing or swallowing (e.g., stroke or Parkinson's disease) or mental problems (e.g., Alzheimer's depression) should be assessed regarding the need for a nasogastric or nasointestinal tube or an alternative feeding method. In addition, if normal caloric intake is substantially impaired with endotracheal tubes or a tracheostomy, a nasogastric or nasointestinal tube may be necessary. Finally, tubes may be used to prevent meal-induced hypoxemia (insufficient oxygen to blood), which occurs with patients with COPD or other pulmonary problems that interfere with eating (e.g., use of oxygen, broncholdilators, tracheostomy, endotracheal tube with ventilator support).

1. Assess causes of poor nutritional status that may be identified and corrected as a first step in determining whether or not a nasogastric tube is necessary (see Nutritional Status RAP).

(a) Eating, swallowing and chewing disorders can negatively affect nutritional status (low weight in relation to height, weight loss, serum albumin level, and dietary problems) and the initial task is to determine the potential causes and period of time such problems are expected to persist. Recent lab work should also be reviewed to determine if there are electrolyte imbalances, fluid volume imbalances, BUN, creatinine, low serum albumin, and low serum protein levels before treatment decisions are made. Laboratory measurement of sodium and potassium tell whether or not an electrolyte imbalance exists. Residents taking diuretics may have potassium losses requiring potassium supplements. If these types of imbalances cannot be corrected with oral nutrition and fluids or intravenous feedings, then a nasogastric or nasointestinal tube may be considered.

(b) Determine whether fluid intake and hydration problems are short term or long term.

(c) Review for gastrointestinal distention, gastrointestinal hemorrhage, increased gastric acidity, potential for stress ulcers, and abdominal pain.

(d) Identify pulmonary problems (e.g., COPD and use of endotracheal tubes, tracheostomy, and other devices) that interfere with eating or dehydration.

(e) Review for mental status problems that interfere with eating such as depression, agitation, delirium, dementia, and mood disorders.

(f) Review for other problems such as cardiovascular disease or stroke.

2. Determine the need for such a tube. Examine alternatives.

Alternatives to nasogastric and nasointestinal tubes should always be considered. Intravenous feedings should be used for short-term therapy as a treatment of choice or at least a first option. Jejunostomy may have some advantages for long-term

FIGURE 11.12 CONT'D...RAP: FEEDING TUBES

therapy, although may increase the risk for infection. A gastrostomy is better tolerated by agitated patients and those requiring prolonged therapy (more than 2 weeks). Gastrostomy with bolus feedings is preferable to nasogastric or nasointestinal tubes for long-term therapy for comfort reasons and to prevent the dislodgement and complications associated with nasal tubes. It is also less disfiguring as it can be completely hidden under clothing when not in use.

3. Assure informed consent and right to refuse treatment. Informed consent is essential before inserting a nasogastric or nasointestinal tube. Potential advantages, disadvantages, and potential complications need to be discussed. Resident preferences are normally given the greatest weight in decisions regarding tube feeding. State laws and judicial decisions must also be taken into account. If the resident is not competent to make the decision, a durable power of attorney or living will may determine who has the legal power to act on the resident's behalf. Where the resident is not competent or no power of attorney is in effect, the physician may have the responsibility for making a decision regarding the use of tube feeding. In any case, when illness is terminal and/or irreversible, technical means of providing fluids and nutrition can represent extraordinary rather than ordinary means of prolonging life.

4. Monitor for complications and correct/change procedures and feedings when necessary. Periodic changing of the nasogastric and intestinal tubes is necessary, although the appropriate interval for changing tubes is not clear. Assessment and determination of continued need should be completed before the tube is reinserted. Specific written orders by the physician are required.

5. Determine if the assessment for the resident's needs (calories, protein, and fluid) is met by the physician's enteral order (formula and flush). Determine if the actual formal and flush delivered is the same as ordered. Determine if there is a safe and sanitary handling of the feeding tube.

Individuals at risk of pulmonary aspiration (such as those with altered pharyngeal reflexes or unconsciousness) should be given a nasointestinal tube rather than a nasogastric tube, or other medical alternative. Those at risk for displacement of a nasogastric tube, such as those with coughing, vomiting, or endotracheally intubated, should also be given a nasointestinal tube rather than a nasogastric tube or other medical alternative.

II. TRIGGER
Consider efficacy and need for feeding tubes if (The item in brackets corresponds to a notation on the MDS Form.):

Feeding Tube Present* [K5b = checked]

* Note: This item also triggers on the Dehydration RAP.

III. GUIDELINES
COMPLICATIONS OF TUBE FEEDING
To reiterate, serious potential negative consequences include agitation, depression, mood disorders, self-extubation (removal of the tube by the patient), infections, aspirations, misplacement of tube in trachea or lung, pain, and tube dysfunction. Abnormal lab values can be expected and should be reviewed.

Infection in the Trachea or Lungs
Gastric organisms grow as a result of alkalizing (raising) the gastric pH. Gastric colonization results in transmission of gastric organisms to the trachea and the development of nosocomial pneumonia. In one study, colonization in 89% of patients within 4 days in ventilated patients with enteral nutrition was found with nosocomial respiratory infection in 62% of the patients studied. Symptoms of respiratory infections to be monitored include coughing, shortness of breath, fever, chest pain, respiratory arrest, delirium, confusion, and seizures.

Aspiration of Gastric Organisms into the Trachea and the Lungs
The incidence is difficult to determine, but most studies suggest it is relatively high.

Inadvertent Respiratory Placement of the Tube
This is the most common side effect of tube placement. In one study, 15% of small-bore nasogastric tubes and 27-50% of nasointestinal tubes were found to be out of their intended position upon radiographic examination without any other evidence of displacement.

Figure 11.12 cont'd...RAP: Feeding Tubes

Respiratory placement can occur in any patient, but is most likely in those who are neurologically depressed, heavily sedated, unable to gag, or endotracheally intubated. Detecting such placement is difficult; the following comments address this issue:

Radiologic detection is the most definitive means to detect tube displacement. Under this procedure, pneumothorax and inadvertent placement in the respiratory tract can be avoided by first placing the feeding tube in the esophagus with the tip above the xiphoid process and then securing the tube and confirming placement with a chest x-ray. Then the tube may be advanced into the stomach and another x-ray taken to confirm the position. The stylet can then be removed and tube feeding begun.

Unfortunately, nursing facilities are highly unlikely to have appropriate radiological technology and it is normally unreasonable to expect them to make arrangements to have patients transported to available radiology.

pH testing of gastric aspirates to determine whether a tube is in the gastric, intestine, or the respiratory area is a promising method for testing feeding tube placement. However, parameters for various secretions from the three areas have not yet been clinically defined.

Aspiration of visually recognizable gastrointestinal secretions, although a frequently used method of determining placement of tubes, is of questionable value as the visual characteristics of secretions can be similar to those from the respiratory tract.

Auscultatory method: although "shooshing" or gurgling sounds can indicate placement in the stomach, the same sounds can occur when feeding tubes are inadvertently placed in the pharynx, esophagus and respiratory tract. Although small-bore tubes make the auscultatory method more difficult to use, large-bore nasogastric tubes may also be placed inadvertently in the respiratory tract producing false gurgling.

Inadvertent Dislodgement of the Tubes
Nonweighted tubes appear to be more likely to be displaced than weighted tubes (with an attached bolus of mercury or tungsten at the tip).

Other Complications Include:
Pain, epistaxis, pneumothorax, hydrothorax, nasal alar necrosis, nasopharyngitis, esophagitis, eustachitis, esophageal strictures, airway obstruction, pharyngeal and esophageal perforations. Symptoms of respiratory infections are to be reviewed.

Complications of Gastric Tract Infections and Gastric Problems
Symptoms include abdominal pain, abdominal distention, stress ulcers, and gastric hemorrhage. There is also a need to monitor for complications including diarrhea, nausea, abdominal distention, and asphyxia. Such complications signal the need for a change in the type of formula or diagnostic work for other pathology.

Complications for the Cardiovascular Systems
Symptoms of cardiac distress or arrest to be monitored include chest pain, loss of heartbeat, loss of consciousness, and loss of breathing.

Periodic Tests to Assure Positive Nitrogen Balance During Enteral Feeding
Where positive balance is not achieved, a formula with high nitrogen density is needed. The absorptive capacity is impaired in many elderly patients so that serum fat and protein should be monitored. Effective nutrients should result in positive nitrogen balance, maintenance or increases in body weight, triceps skinfold and midarm muscle circumference maintenance, total iron binding capacity maintenance, and serum urea nitrogen level maintenance. Caloric intake and resident weight should be monitored on a regular basis.

Source: CMS's RAI Version 2.0 Manual, Appendix C, current as of August, 2003

RESIDENT ASSESSMENT PROTOCOL: DEHYDRATION/FLUID MAINTENANCE

I. PROBLEM

Water is necessary for the distribution of nutrients to cells, elimination of waste, regulation of body temperature, and countless other complex processes. On average, one can live only four days without water. Dehydration is a condition in which water or fluid loss (output) far exceeds fluid intake. The body becomes less able to maintain adequate blood pressure, deliver sufficient oxygen and nutrients to the cells, and rid itself of wastes. Many distressing symptoms can originate from these conditions, including:

>**Dizziness on Sitting/Standing** (blood pressure insufficient to supply oxygen and glucose to brain);
>**Confusion or Change in Mental Status** (decreased oxygen and glucose to brain);
>**Decreased Urine Output** (kidneys conserve water);
>**Decreased Skin Turgor,** dry mucous membranes (symptoms of dryness);
>**Constipation** (water insufficient to rid body of wastes); and
>**Fever** (water insufficient to maintain normal temperature).

Other possible consequences of dehydration include: decreased functional ability, predisposition to falls (because of orthostatic hypotension), fecal impaction, predisposition to infection, fluid and electrolyte disturbances, and ultimately death.

Nursing facility residents are particularly vulnerable to dehydration. It is often difficult or impossible to access fluids independently; the perception of thirst can be muted; the aged kidney can have a decreased ability to concentrate urine; and acute and chronic illness can alter fluid and electrolyte balance.

Unfortunately, many symptoms of this condition do not appear until significant fluid has been lost. Early signs and symptoms tend to be unreliable and nonspecific; staff will often disagree about the clinical indicators of dehydration for specific cases; and the identification of the most crucial symptoms of the condition are most difficult to identify among the aged. Early identification of dehydration is thus problematic, and the goal of this RAP is to identify any and all possible high-risk cases, permitting the introduction of programs to prevent the condition from occurring.

When dehydration is in fact observed, treatment objectives focus on restoring normal fluid volume, preferably orally. If the resident cannot drink a minimum recommended 1500 cc's of fluid every 24 hours, water and electrolyte deficits can be made up in a timely fashion via other routes to prevent dehydration. Fluids can be administered intravenously, subcutaneously, or by tube until resident is adequately hydrated and can take and retain sufficient fluids orally.

II. TRIGGERS

Dehydration suggested if one or more of following present (The item in brackets corresponds to a notation on the MDS Form.):

>Dehydration [J1c = checked]
>Insufficient Fluid/Did Not Consume All Liquids Provided [J1d = checked]
>UTI [I2j = checked]
>Dehydration Diagnosis [I3 = 276.5]
>Weight Fluctuation of 3+ Pounds [J1a = checked]
>Fever [J1h = checked]
>Internal Bleeding [J1j = checked]
>Parenteral/IV(a) [K5a = checked]
>Feeding Tube(b) [K5b = checked]
>Taking Diuretic [O4e = 1-7]

(a) Note: This item also triggers on the Nutritional Status RAP.

(b) Note: This item also triggers on the Feeding Tube RAP.

III. GUIDELINES
RESIDENTS FACTORS THAT MAY IMPEDE ABILITY TO MAINTAIN FLUID BALANCE
Moderate/Severely Impaired Decision-Making Ability

>Has there been a recent unexplainable change in mental status?
>Does resident seem unusually agitated or disoriented?
>Is resident delirious?
>Is resident comatose?

FIGURE 11.13 CONT'D...RAP: DEHYDRATION

Does dementia, aphasia or other condition seriously limit resident's understanding of others, or how well others can understand the resident?

Comprehension/ Communication Problems

Body Control Problems

Does resident require extensive assistance to transfer?
Does resident freely move on the unit?
Has there been recent ADL decline?

Hand Dexterity Problem

Can resident grasp cup?

Bowel Problems

Does the resident have constipation or a fecal impaction that may be interfering with fluid intake?

Swallowing Problems

Does resident have mouth sore(s) ulcer(s)?
Does resident refuse food, meals, meds?
Can resident drink from a cup or suck through a straw?

Use of Parenteral/IV

Are feeding tubes in use?

RESIDENT DEHYDRATION RISK FACTORS

Dehydration risk factors can be categorized in terms of whether they **decrease fluid intake** or **increase fluid loss**. The higher the number of factors present, the greater the risk of dehydration. Ongoing fluid loss through the lungs and skin occurs at a normal rate of approximately 500 cc/day and increases with rapid respiratory rate and sweating. Therefore, decreased fluid intake for any reason can lead to dehydration.

Purposeful Restriction of Fluid Intake

Has there been a decrease in thirst perception?
Is resident unaware of the need to intake sufficient fluids?
Has resident or staff restricted intake to avoid urinary incontinence?
Are fluids restricted because of diagnostic procedure or other health reason?
Does sad mood, grief, or depression cause resident to refuse foods/liquids?

Presence of Infection, Fever, Vomiting/Diarrhea/ Nausea, Excessive Sweating (e.g., a Heat Wave)

Frequent Use of Laxatives, Enemas, Diuretics

Excessive Urine Output (Polyuria)

Excessive urine output (polyuria) may be due to:

Drugs (e.g., lithium, phenytoin), alcohol abuse
Disease (e.g., diabetes mellitus, diabetes insipidus)
Other conditions (e.g., hypoaldosteronism, hyper-parathyroidism)

Other Test Results

Relevant test results to be considered:

Does systolic/diastolic blood pressure drop 20 points on sitting/standing?
On inspection, do oral mucous membranes appear dry?
Does urine appear more concentrated and/or decreased in volume?

Source: CMS's RAI Version 2.0 Manual, Appendix C, current as of August, 2003

HIPAA

In April, 2003, a new security regulation called HIPPA took effect. HIPAA stands for **Health Insurance Portability and Accountability Act**, a federal law intended to protect the privacy of healthcare clients, while also standardizing exchange of healthcare information. If you work in a healthcare institution, the manner in which you handle medical records and related documents will be guided, in part, by HIPAA.

HIPAA dictates that patient information and health-related data will be kept secure. "Secure" as defined in the law refers to two key ideas:

- Patient privacy and the right to keep personal and medical information confidential
- Safeguarding information, such as computer files, from physical and technical hazards

Thus, if you maintain a computer system that holds clients' nutrition care records, you need to be sure that access is limited and protected and be sure the system itself is safely maintained. Here are some examples of how you might accomplish these tasks:

- Control access to computers by requiring a login with user names and passwords. Do not keep a written record of these (or keep one in a highly secured location).
- Control availability of user names and passwords, and delete access if, for example, someone leaves employment.
- If client information is held on laptops, personal digital assistants, or other portable computers, make sure these computers are secured and locked to prevent unauthorized use.
- Maintain routine back-ups of computer data. Use virus and worm protection, as well as other safeguards, to prevent data destruction.

On a more general level, you and every employee of a healthcare institution must adhere to an established policy addressing privacy. You will need to refrain from discussing client information in public areas, where others could overhear it. If you destroy client records, you may need to shred them. If you carry a kardex, you may need to keep it under your direct supervision at all times, and secure it when it is not in use. You will also need to handle all documents in such a way that individual records, care plans, MDS forms, etc. cannot be seen by others (except authorized members of the healthcare team). For example, you cannot lay a printout with patient names and diagnoses on a chair while you are chatting with a patient and a family member.

Another fundamental HIPAA concept is called *chain of trust*. Healthcare institutions and related organizations have to exchange data in order to accomplish many tasks, such as insurance reimbursement. An organization must establish a chain of trust with others, meaning that it transmits data only to other organizations who have committed to following HIPAA regulations.

To develop a plan for complying with HIPAA, you can first examine where security of information is vulnerable. Then, you develop procedures for protecting information at each of these points. HIPAA compliance strategies and policies are still fairly new in the industry, and are evolving rapidly. If you work in a healthcare institution, you will want to become familiar with HIPAA-related policies and procedures and follow them carefully. You may be called upon to help develop policies and procedures related to records in the dietary department. Any time there is a change in the way you handle health information, you will need to re-evaluate and possibly revise the HIPAA policies and procedures.

Key Points

- Documentation of nutrition-related care serves many purposes. It can be a reference and communication tool, a legal document, a mandatory component of regulatory compliance, a resource for reimbursement to an institution, and a resource for monitoring quality of services.

- A medical record is a formal, legal account of a patient's health and disease. It contains findings, test results, diagnoses, and treatment plans.

- A common format for collecting and recording information in a medical record is the problem-oriented medical record (POMR), which organizes information according to a list of problems.

- Using the POMR method, notes in the client's chart are usually structured according to the SOAP format. SOAP is an acronym for: Subjective, Objective, Assessment, Plan.

- Alternate charting formats include DAP, which stands for: Data, Assessment, and Plan; and DAR, which stands for: Data, Action, and Response.

- In almost all healthcare institutions, diet orders are written by the physician. A diet order is communicated to the dietary department and is usually maintained in dietary records. Examples of dietary records include a kardex card or a tray card.

- Nursing facilities participating in the Medicare and Medicaid programs must follow federal regulations developed by the Centers for Medicare & Medicaid Services (CMS), which include documentation requirements.

- The CMS requires use of a Resident Assessment Instrument (RAI). The RAI is composed of two parts: the Minimum Data Set (MDS) and Resident Assessment Protocols (RAPs).

- A dietitian/dietary manager fills out Section K, "Oral/Nutritional Status," and may also assist with other sections of the MDS form.

▶ Based on defined criteria, certain coding on the MDS form flags the need for comprehensive assessment for certain triggers. The RAPs guide this process.

▶ HIPAA regulations dictate that patient information and health-related data will be kept secure. This affects confidentiality practices, how a dietary manger handles any medical documentation, and how computer systems that contain patient information are managed.

Health Insurance Portability and Accountability Act (HIPAA): Federal law that dictates patient information and health-related data will be kept secure. This addresses privacy of information, confidentiality, and the idea that computerized information must be kept safe from harm or damage.

Medical record: A formal, legal account of a patient's health and disease. It contains findings, test results, diagnoses, and treatment plans.

Minimum Data Set (MDS): A form that outlines a minimum amount of data (information) that caregivers must collect and use. It is designed by CMS for use by a number of healthcare professionals, as an interdisciplinary care tool.

Problem-oriented medical record (POMR): a common format for collecting and recording information in a medical record; organizes information according to a list of problems

Progress note: A notation in the medical record by a health professional. In a problem-oriented medical record, it summarizes a client's progress related to a specific problem.

Resident Assessment Instrument (RAI): A specialized form of medical documentation required of every healthcare institution that is receiving funding from Medicare and/or Medicaid. The RAI is composed of two parts: the Minimum Data Set (MDS) and Resident Assessment Protocols (RAPs).

Resident Assessment Protocols (RAPs): a set of guidelines for assessment of specific problems identified through problems (or potential problems) identified in the MDS

SOAP: an acronym for Subjective, Objective, Assessment, Plan; a method of organizing information for a progress note in a medical record

1. Which of the following is NOT a reason to document medical and nutrition-related care?

   A. Documentation helps you focus the care plan and provides details about how you are implementing a plan of care.
   B. Documentation is a communication tool among members of the healthcare team.
   C. Reimbursement for services is based on the number of pages of a medical record; the government reimburses a set dollar amount for every page.
   D. Documentation is a legal record of care provided.

2. Which of the following is NOT true about a problem-oriented medical record?

   A. The original concept was invented by Socrates in ancient Greece.
   B. It organizes information according to a list of problems.
   C. It involves collection of data.
   D. It includes evaluations of care plans.

3. Which of the following information should you include in the "S" component of a SOAP note?

   A. Serum transferrin
   B. Ideal body weight
   C. Diagnosis
   D. A client's observation about his appetite

4. Which of the following information should you include in the "O" component of a SOAP note?

   A. Serum transferrin
   B. Your plan of treatment
   C. Evaluation of nutrient and drug interactions
   D. The client's observation about his condition

5. If you make a mistake when you are writing in the medical record, you should:

   A. Cross through it and write "error" above it
   B. Erase it
   C. Use white-out on it
   D. Make a correction on an MDS form

6. Where should you record the current diet order in a SOAP note?

   A. Under "S"
   B. Under "O"
   C. Under "A"
   D. Under "P"

7. A kardex card or tray card is a good place to record:

   A. The RAPs for a resident of a skilled nursing facility
   B. Food preferences
   C. Insurance coding information
   D. Section K of the MDS form

8. HIPAA dictates that patient information will be kept:

   A. On a laptop
   B. Confidential and secure
   C. Paper-clipped to the MDS
   D. In a public area

9. Certain items marked on an MDS form may trigger a deeper evaluation, called a(n):

   A. Resident Assessment Protocol (RAP)
   B. MDS 3.0
   C. Resident Assessment Instrument (RAI)
   D. Problem-oriented medical record

10. Which of the following indicates a need to perform a new assessment?

   A. Weight loss of 1% or more within 180 days
   B. Weight loss of 5% of more within 30 days
   C. Weight loss of 5% or more in 180 days
   D. Disappearance of a pressure ulcer

In high-quality care, there is ongoing communication among members of the healthcare team. This assures that the team effectively evaluates the needs of each client and develops cohesive, workable plans for care.

After completing this chapter, you should be able to:

- List members of the healthcare team, and identify their roles.
- Describe how members of the team gather information.
- Explain how team members communicate with each other.
- Describe a dietary manager's role in a care conference.

Providing medical care is a complex task. It requires many different types of expertise. This expertise is contributed by professionals in many healthcare disciplines. The **healthcare team** is the group of professionals, each with unique training and expertise, who contribute to the overall care of a client. Thus, a dietary manager who works in a healthcare institution works closely with others. Let's take a look at some typical roles and a partial list of responsibilities, particularly as they relate to nutrition care. Additional responsibilities of a dietary manager appear in Figure 12.1.

Administrator (in a Nursing Home)

- Ensures that a nutritional screening/assessment system exists
- Ensures adequacy of staffing to implement and maintain the system
- Supports all staff members in performing their duties

Dietitian

- Assumes primary responsibility for nutrition screening and assessment and resident nutrition care planning
- Selects and sets up a nutrition screening/assessment system (in cooperation with the nursing service and facility administration); trains facility staff as needed
- Monitors the screening system
- Performs in-depth nutritional assessments
- Develops nutrition care plan
- Records assessment findings, recommendations, and follow-up plans in medical record and resident care plan
- Alerts other team members to any part of the nutritional care plan needing their cooperation
- Defines the role of a dietary manager and provides training

- Provides nutrition counseling
- Monitors the accuracy of diet service
- Participates in quality management

Director of Dietary Services/Dietary Manager

- Interviews clients for diet history
- Conducts routine nutrition screening/assessment
- Calculates nutrient intake
- Implements diet plans
- Documents nutrition information on clients' medical records
- Counsels clients on basic diet restrictions; specifies standards and procedures for food preparation to comply with diet restrictions
- Evaluates effectiveness of nutrition care plans
- Assists in nutrition care process according to established policies and procedures

Nurse

- Assesses client needs; develops, implements, and monitors care plan
- Delivers direct nursing care
- Ensures that resident consumes food: organizes the resident feeding responsibilities, distributes the workload, determines need for adaptive eating devices with input from occupational therapist
- Assists with mealtimes and feeding
- Records accurate and meaningful information about client's food and fluid intake
- Provides education to clients

Occupational Therapist

- Evaluates needs related to fine motor skills
- Often recommends assistive eating devices and other techniques to help patients feed themselves
- Provides therapy to develop fine motor skills

Physician

- Evaluates medical conditions and develops diagnoses
- Plans, oversees, and monitors treatment
- Bears major responsibility for the nutritional status of the resident (in conformance to acceptable standards of practice)
- Writes diet orders and/or approves protocol for standard orders

▶ Orders other treatments which affect nutritional status

▶ Utilizes information provided by other members of the healthcare team

Social Worker

▶ Evaluates social and support needs

▶ Assists patients and families with decision-making

▶ Helps clients and families plan care upon discharge from a healthcare institution

▶ Assists with applying for other healthcare services, such as home-delivered meals or home care

▶ Identifies resources

▶ Provides counseling

Speech Pathologist

▶ Evaluates the chewing and swallowing function of residents

▶ Recommends appropriate therapy for dysphagia

▶ Provides evaluation and therapy for speech-related needs

ADDITIONAL TASKS OF A DIETARY MANAGER

▶ Supervises production and distribution of food

▶ Ensures that food is palatable and attractive, diets are served accurately, and substitutions are appropriate

▶ Manages a sanitary foodservice environment

▶ Purchases, receives, and stores food following established quality standards

▶ Interviews, hires, and trains employees

▶ Develops work schedules/assignments

▶ Conducts employee performance appraisals and recommends wage adjustments

▶ Supervises, disciplines, and terminates employees

▶ Supervises business operations of the dietary department

▶ Develops budget and operates within budget parameters

▶ Plans and conducts meetings/inservice programs

Source: DMA

Figure 12.1

Policies and procedures must be developed and followed for optimal nutrition care. Whether dealing with clients in a hospital, longterm care facility, or other healthcare setting, the nutrition care process uses the same methods and principles. However, depending on your institution's policies and procedures and state regulations, the dietary manager's exact role in the nutrition care process will vary.

Note that in client care, the client and family members or significant others also play crucial roles. The client, for example, has a great deal of information and insight to offer in developing an understanding of his condition and needs. The client also has the right to contribute to care planning, and to play a well-informed role in deciding upon care. Ultimately, the client must participate in care for it to be effective.

GATHERING AND SHARING INFORMATION

As each member of the team contributes specialized training, knowledge, and experience to the care of clients, all members participate in such basic tasks as:

- Assessing client needs
- Developing a plan of care
- Evaluating a plan of care
- Providing education to clients

While the details of a nutrition care plan may differ from the details of a nursing care plan or a speech therapy care plan, the overall objectives are in unison. For example, team members may work together to improve a client's nutritional status as follows:

- A physician orders a diet.
- A dietary manager conducts a diet history to find out how the client usually eats and to determine food preferences and intolerances.
- A speech therapist recommends an appropriate diet for dysphagia and specifies techniques to manage a swallowing disorder.
- An occupational therapist helps a client develop the strength and skills to feed himself effectively.
- A nurse provides hands-on set-up and assistance at mealtime, and encourages a client to eat—or feeds a client.
- Both a nurse and a dietary manager may help to monitor diet tolerance and food intake.
- A dietary manager develops a menu and manages food production to ensure that the client receives appropriate foods, and that they are appetizing and wholesome.

All team members participate in monitoring how well the plan of care works. A nurse is involved in obtaining routine weights for the client. A dietary manager and/or dietitian are involved in monitoring indicators of nutritional status, such as weight and laboratory values. A dietary manger may also implement a calorie count to evaluate actual intake. A nurse may make observations and suggestions about the mealtime experience, and may relate food preferences or suggestions to the dietary team. These are just some examples of how team roles coordinate to achieve an overall goal of improving nutritional status.

To attain the best outcomes, team members have to share information. As each views the client's needs from a unique perspective, each has observations and ideas to offer. Thus, sharing information and communicating effectively are critical to clinical care. How do team members share information? As you learned in Chapter 11, one means is through the medical record itself. A good starting point is the list of problems (if a problem-oriented medical record system is used). Each team member documents assessments, plans, and progress in the record. Each time any team member works with a client, the first step is to open the medical record and review the documentation provided by other members of the team.

To gather information in a medical record, you must first become acquainted with how records are organized in your institution. Some institutions maintain records electronically, on a computer system. Most small healthcare institutions use paper-based systems. A typical medical record includes the following components:

- An admission sheet listing patient information, admission date, reason for admission, and names and contact details for family members
- A section for physicians' orders, including diet, medications, tests, and treatments
- A page listing problems
- A section for test results
- A section for progress notes from all disciplines

Some medical record systems use a unique section for nursing flow charts, vital signs checklists, and nursing notes, which are recorded on a daily basis. Weights may be periodically recorded on a flow chart, or on a special form developed just for weights. If you work in an institution that does MDS recording, find out where these and related forms are maintained as well. By learning how records are organized, you can become proficient at finding the information you need.

A second way team members share information is simply by talking with each other. Solid working relationships built on mutual respect are essential. In the course of a work day, a dietary manager interacts with many members of the team. This provides an opportunity to ask questions and relate observations. Informal communication can play a strong role in client care. However, these interactions must be managed professionally. Team members need to exert care to protect client confidentiality at all times. They need to avoid discussing client needs in public areas. A third way team members share information is through care conferences, discussed below.

Care Conferences

A **care conference** is a meeting of healthcare team members, with the objective of planning and evaluating care for specific clients. In longterm care facilities, client care conferences are held at least quarterly (or more often for high risk clients) to discuss the progress of the client. The meeting is planned in advance and each department receives a list of the clients to be reviewed at the care conference. The number of clients reviewed may vary, depending on the facility and the length of the meeting. All departments responsible for the care of the client are represented at the meetings. These usually include the nursing unit, dietary services, activities, social service departments, and others. The client and/or family may be present at the client care conference as well.

The organization of the meetings varies. In an initial client care conference, team members review the social history of the client. This may include a synopsis of a client's life situation, the names of family members and others who are important in a client's life, and related information. Each department reviews findings from its assessment. Team members identify problems, discuss them, and determine how various factors interplay in the client's care. As a group, the team lists problems. Then, the team develops goals and approaches or strategies for solving problems.

In follow-up, the client's progress is reviewed periodically to determine if the plan is appropriate. At these meetings, the problems and goals established at the previous conference are reviewed and evaluated. If a problem has been resolved, a notation is made in the plan to indicate this. The problems not resolved may be listed again with a new approach suggested. New problems or needs of the client are also addressed. For each new problem, a goal is set and an approach is planned. The department that will be working with the client to accomplish the goal is identified.

To prepare for client care meetings, the dietitian/dietary manager should review the client's nutritional status and have knowledge of the client's eating abilities, meal completion, fluid intake, and any areas of concern. It is important to bring related documentation for reference—such as nutritional status information, diet history details, calorie count results, and any other information that may be needed. In a care conference, a dietary manager should be prepared to relate specific facts and observations that will contribute to the evaluation and planning of client care.

During the meeting, each member of the team listens to others to understand the comprehensive clinical picture. Each member contributes ideas to help meet a client's needs. During the planning component, a dietary manager (or dietitian) recommends ways to address nutrition-related problems. Following a meeting, a dietary manager and each member of the team supports the plan as developed in the meeting. Diligence and follow-through are critical to success.

- Providing medical care is a complex task. It requires many different types of expertise. This expertise is contributed by professionals in many healthcare disciplines.

- A dietary manager who works in a healthcare institution works closely with others.

- The precise role of a dietary manager in a healthcare institution may vary, based on local regulations and institutional policies and procedures.

- All healthcare team members participate in assessing clients and planning care.

- Team members share information through the medical record, personal interaction, and care conferences.

- A dietary manager should prepare for a care conference by gathering all nutrition-related information, and should be prepared to share facts and answer questions.

- During a care conference, each team member needs to listen carefully to others, and participate in developing a plan for care.

- A care plan lists problems, goals, and approaches or strategies.

- After a care conference, each team member needs to follow through and support the plan developed.

Care conference: a meeting of healthcare team members, with the objective of planning and evaluating care for specific clients

Healthcare team: the group of professionals, each with unique training and expertise, who contribute to the overall care of a client

1. Which of the following healthcare team members plays a role in nutritional care?
   A. Dietary manager
   B. Nurse
   C. Speech pathologist
   D. All of the above

2. The member of the healthcare team who orders a diet is the:
   A. Dietary manager
   B. Dietitian
   C. Physician
   D. Nurse

3. The member of the healthcare team who evaluates swallowing disorders is the:
   A. Dietary manager
   B. Social worker
   C. Occupational therapist
   D. Speech pathologist

4. The member of the healthcare team who helps with discharge planning is the:
   A. Dietary manager
   B. Social worker
   C. Occupational therapist
   D. Speech pathologist

5. The member of the healthcare team who evaluates needs related to fine motor skills is the:
   A. Speech pathologist
   B. Social worker
   C. Administrator
   D. Occupational therapist

6. What is a client's role in the healthcare team?
   A. To take orders from everyone else
   B. To stay in bed as much as possible
   C. To help provide information and make informed decisions
   D. To make all members of the team cooperate with each other

7. Which of the following is the best way to obtain a client's current weight?
   A. Ask the client
   B. Check the designated section of the medical record
   C. Ask the speech therapist
   D. Eyeball it and make an estimate

8. The chief objective of a care conference is to:
    A. Plan and evaluate care for specific clients
    B. Introduce members of the healthcare team to each other
    C. Provide a break from working directly with clients
    D. Develop reports for CMS

9. If you are participating in a conference about a client with pressure ulcers, which of the following would be most useful to bring?
    A. A copy of the client's home telephone number
    B. A diet manual
    C. A copy of your own job description
    D. A kardex card identifying recent lab values and weights

10. You would like to check in with a nurse to find out how a client tolerated meals today. Which of the following would be a good place to talk about this?
    A. In a secluded section of the nurses' break area
    B. In an elevator
    C. In the cafeteria
    D. In the lobby as you are walking out of the building together

Regulations and standards governing the healthcare industry require that planning, documentation, and ongoing clinical care follow prescribed models. A dietary manager plays a role in compliance to provide optimal care.

After completing this chapter, you should be able to:

▶ Explain the purpose of a care plan, and describe how it is used.

▶ Describe the concept of a comprehensive care plan.

▶ List the steps involved in developing a nutrition care plan.

Clinical care revolves around a care plan. Every good outcome hinges on some advance planning. Imagine a simple everyday task, such as going to the grocery store. If you make a plan for what you will do there, you can be more effective. Let's say you want to buy food to prepare dinner this evening. If you go unprepared, you won't know what you need. When you get home, you might not be able to complete dinner preparation. Meanwhile, grocery aisles may tempt you with things you don't need. You may spend money on impulse items, yet not accomplish your original objective of being able to cook this evening.

If planning what you will do is useful for a mundane task like grocery shopping, imagine how critical it can be to providing medical care, where the stakes are high and the outcomes affect the quality of clients' lives profoundly. This is why a cornerstone of medical care is a care plan. A **care plan** is a written plan for medical care. It identifies objectives for helping a client reach the best possible physical, mental, social, and/or spiritual well-being. It describes steps members of the healthcare team will take to accomplish this.

A care plan essentially charts the course for actions that members of the healthcare team will take to support and improve an individual's well-being. All members of the team use it as a focal point and driving force in their routine of care for clients. The care plan assures that team members' actions contribute toward established clinical needs and objectives that are entirely customized to each client. A care plan actually makes the work that each team member performs more effective. We will examine the idea of a comprehensive care plan, and then examine the steps involved in developing a plan of care that specifically addresses nutrition.

COMPREHENSIVE CARE PLANS

In today's healthcare environment, emphasis on teamwork is high. Healthcare standards call for:

- Interdisciplinary contributions to the care planning process
- Coordination among members of the team, to assure they all work towards common objectives
- Ongoing communication among members of the team

As team members develop a care plan together, this becomes essentially a master plan that drives some of the details carried out by individual professionals. A care plan developed by members of a coordinated healthcare team and that addresses the multi-faceted needs of a client is called a **comprehensive care plan**.

The effectiveness of this interdisciplinary process is well recognized in the industry, and is a stipulation of every quality standard today.

The Joint Commission on Accreditation of Healthcare Institutions, a non-government organization that provides accreditation for healthcare institutions, also emphasizes interdisciplinary coordination in developing care plans and providing care to patients.

Let's take a closer look at comprehensive care plans, as explained in CMS regulations. These regulations set guidelines as follows:

The facility must develop a comprehensive care plan for each resident that includes measurable objectives and timetables to meet a resident's medical, nursing, and mental and psychosocial needs, which are identified in the comprehensive assessment. The plan of care must deal with both the relationship of services ordered to be provided (or withheld), and the facility's responsibility for fulfilling other requirements in these regulations.

According to CMS, a comprehensive care plan must be:

- Developed within seven days after the completion of the comprehensive assessment
- Be prepared by an interdisciplinary team that includes the attending physician, a registered nurse with responsibility for the resident, and other appropriate staff disciplines as determined by the resident's needs, and to the extent practicable, the participation of the resident, the resident's family, or the resident's legal representative
- Reviewed periodically and revised by a team of qualified persons after each assessment

CMS regulations further stipulate that an interdisciplinary team, in conjunction with the resident, resident's family, surrogate, or representative, as appropriate, should develop quantifiable objectives for the highest level of functioning the resident may be expected to attain, based on the comprehensive assessment. The interdisciplinary team should show evidence in the RAP summary of the clinical record that they considered the development of care planning interventions for all RAPs triggered by the MDS. (Remember, RAP is a resident assessment protocol, explained in Chapter 11, and MDS is the minimum data set.) The care plan must reflect intermediate steps for each outcome objective if identification of those steps will enhance the resident's ability to meet his/her objectives. Facility staff will use these objectives to follow resident progress. Facilities may, for some residents, need to prioritize needed care. This should be noted in the clinical record or on the plan of care.

The requirements reflect the facility's responsibility to provide necessary care and services to attain or maintain the highest practicable physical, mental, and psychosocial well-being, in accordance with the comprehensive assessment and plan of care. However, in some cases, a resident may refuse certain services or treatments that professional staff believe may be indicated. Desires of the resident should be documented in the comprehensive assessment and reflected in the plan of care.

Following are some questions to consider when care planning:

- Does the care plan address the needs, strengths, and preferences identified in the resident assessment, including the RAPs?
- Is the care plan oriented toward preventing a decline in functioning?
- How does the care plan try to manage risk factors?
- Does the care plan build on the resident's strengths?
- Does the care plan reflect standards of current dietetic practice?
- Do treatment objectives have measurable goals?
- Does the care plan contain the resident's wishes for treatment and opinions about goals?
- If the resident refuses treatment, does the care plan explain alternatives to address the problem?
- Is the care plan evaluated and revised as the resident's status changes?

To summarize, the comprehensive care plan is completed seven days after completion of the RAI. Developing a comprehensive care plan is the responsibility of the interdisciplinary team. Although the physician must participate as part of the interdisciplinary team, he or she may arrange with the facility for alternative methods, other than attending care planning conferences, such as one-on-one discussions and conference calls.

Although the MDS and supplemental assessments give much information about the resident's problems, they won't always identify or trigger them all. One purpose of the care plan conference is to help identify additional problems or needs. The dietitian and/or dietary manager needs to identify a resident's nutrition-related problems, set measurable goals with time limits, and determine appropriate interventions.

In longterm care, the care plan, which is part of the client's medical record, is updated at least quarterly and as the resident's condition changes. The date of the quarterly review is entered on the care plan. When a problem is no longer a problem, this needs to be noted on the care plan by highlighting it (with a yellow highlighter pen) and writing, "Resolved" with the date of resolution next to it.

STEPS IN DEVELOPING A NUTRITION CARE PLAN

As you will remember from Chapter 8, the nutrition care process involves screening patients for nutrition risk, assessing each patient identified by the screening process as being at risk, and then developing a nutrition care plan for each patient.

All care planning relates to a list of specified problems. These problems are pinpointed by various members of the healthcare team as they complete their respective assessments. As described above, members of the team tackle this list together. Aspects of the care plan are tightly interwoven among disciplines, and many plans require the efforts of multiple disciplines to succeed. Completing the detail of a plan is often up to the individual professionals involved. Once a plan is developed, the specifics of how it will be implemented follow. Afterwards, it is important to evaluate the effectiveness of care, as described in Chapter 14. Here are some basic steps for the nutrition care planning process.

Step 1. Identify nutrition problems.

Examples of nutrition problems include pressure sores, significant weight loss, complications related to tube feedings, or inability to chew food. The following guidelines can help you develop a meaningful statement of the problem:

- Be as specific as possible.
- State the problem as it relates to the client.
- Identify possible reasons for the problem.
- Identify any strengths the client has that will help in overcoming the problem.

For example, a problem statement may say, "Current weight is 80% of ideal body weight."

Step 2. Determine calorie, protein and fluid needs.

Developing care plans requires that you first determine how many calories, how much protein, and how much fluid is needed by the client. Refer to Chapter 8 for methods of estimating needs for these nutrients. Also be aware that your own institution or the dietitian may provide alternate methodologies. Calculation schemes may also be part of policies and procedures, nutrition care protocols, standards of practice, and/or regulations with which you must comply. **Standards of practice** are documents that define what constitutes quality in practice. They are standards for doing what you do. Typically, a standard of practice relates to the work of members of one profession. For example, a standard of practice might outline how a dietary manager ensures that food is wholesome and safe. **Care protocols** are documents that outline a care process related to a specific medical condition. For example, an institution may have a care protocol for pressure ulcers that lists some standard steps that must be taken and describes how each member of the healthcare team will contribute. Standards of practice and care protocols are quite similar. You will need to become familiar with the standards that apply in your place of employment, and apply them consistently.

Also keep in mind that disease states can affect needs for calories, protein, and fluid. For example, a client experiencing renal failure or congestive heart failure may need to curtail fluid intake. In these scenarios, the physician should stipulate a fluid restriction in the diet order. This fluid order overrides the standard calculations, and you should use it. A client experiencing a fever and/or vomiting may need significantly more fluid and calories. As you apply standards and formulas, be sure to consider unusual factors, and consult with a dietitian as needed to clarify nutrient needs.

Step 3. For each problem, develop goals that are relevant, measurable and realistic. Establish timeframes.

After identifying problems, it is appropriate to start considering client goals. For each problem, there should be at least one goal. When developing goals, ensure the following:

- Each goal identifies the desired outcome in clear and practical terms.
- Each goal includes words that describe how success will be demonstrated and measured.
- Each goal specifies a target date for accomplishment.
- When practical, the client has been asked to react/contribute to the goal.
- Each goal should consider the client's strengths.

For example, a goal might be stated as, "Client will not have a significant weight loss during the next quarter."

Step 4. For each goal, choose appropriate methods or approaches to reach it.

After the first three steps have been completed, we next have to decide on interventions. Interventions are the steps or approaches to take to help the client achieve the stated goals. Interventions should describe the specific action(s) to be taken, and who is responsible for taking each action. Here are some examples of interventions:

> "Diet as ordered" (nursing/dietary)
>
> "Supplement as ordered" (nursing/dietary)
>
> "Client fed by staff" (all)
>
> "Encourage activities with food" (all)
>
> "Weekly weight with RD notified if > 2 lb weight loss" (nursing/dietary)

Care plans are documented on forms such as the one in Figure 13.1. Figure 13.2 shows a sample care plan. Note that it is not enough to develop a great plan and document it. Each caregiver needs to communicate with other members of the team—including the client—and implement the plan. In particular, when a care plan involves the help of others in your department or in related departments, you need to talk with those involved and ask for their commitment. Be clear and specific, explaining what needs to be done. Offer to answer questions and provide support as needed. In the next chapter, we will follow through with the next steps in the nutrition care process—re-assessing and revising the plan.

Figure 13.1

SAMPLE CARE PLAN FORM

PATIENT NAME: _____ PATIENT NUMBER: _____

ADMISSION DATE: _____ DISCHARGE PLAN: _____

Date	Problem	Goal	Approach/Plan	Progress	Service/Signature

Figure 13.2

SAMPLE CARE PLAN

PATIENT NAME: _Jane Sanchez_   PATIENT NUMBER: _0326179_
ADMISSION DATE: _3/1/04_   DISCHARGE PLAN: _N/A_

Date	Problem	Goal	Approach/Plan	Progress	Service/Signature
3/3/04	dentition- can't chew	consume at least 70% of meals by 3/10	mech. soft diet	3/6/04- consuming 90% of meals	Molly Went, CDM, CFPP
3/3/04	wt. loss	stabilize- no wt. loss by 3/10	mech. soft diet per preferences	3/8/04- wt. stable at 131 lbs	Greg Walters, RN
3/3/04	anemia	increase Hgb/Hct WNL by 4/2/04	adequate protein; Fe suppl.	deferred	Molly Went, CDM, CFPP Greg Walters, RN
3/3/04	pressure ulcer stg. I	no progression; no new ulcers by 4/2/04	ntrn. support; re-position client	3/8/04- no change	Greg Walters, RN

Key Points

- A care plan charts the course for actions that members of the healthcare team will take to support and improve an individual's well-being.

- The care plan assures that team members' actions contribute toward established clinical needs.

- Healthcare standards call for interdisciplinary contributions to the care planning process, as well as coordination and communication among members of the team.

- Steps in developing a nutrition care plan are to: identify nutrition problems; determine calorie, protein, and fluid needs; develop goals that are relevant, measurable and realistic; and choose approaches to reach the goals, with associated timeframes.

- Each caregiver needs to communicate with other members of the team—including the client— and implement the plan.

Key Terms

Care plan: A written plan for medical care. It identifies objectives for helping a client reach the best possible physical, mental, social, and/or spiritual well-being.

Care protocols: documents that outline a care process related to a specific medical condition

Comprehensive care plan: a care plan developed by members of a coordinated healthcare team and that addresses the multi-faceted needs of a client

Standards of practice: documents that define what constitutes quality in practice

1. Which of the following is NOT true about a care plan?

   A. It identifies objectives for helping a client reach the best possible physical, mental, social, and/or spiritual well-being.
   B. It assures that team members' actions contribute toward established clinical needs.
   C. It assures that only the expertise of qualified professionals will be used in the planning process, such that clients will not need to become involved.
   D. It makes the work that each team member performs more effective.

2. A care plan developed by members of a coordinated healthcare team that addresses the multi-faceted needs of a client is called a:

   A. Comprehensive care plan
   B. Problem-oriented care plan
   C. Resident Assessment Instrument
   D. Minimum Data Set

3. CMS regulations about care planning stipulate that:

   A. Members of each discipline set their own care plans independently of each other.
   B. Appropriate staff members contribute to the comprehensive care plan as determined by the resident's needs.
   C. Care plans be developed and maintained on computerized systems.
   D. A comprehensive care plan be developed within 14 days after the completion of a comprehensive assessment.

4. A resident, resident's family member, or resident's legal representative should:

   A. Never participate in care planning
   B. Participate in care planning to whatever extent is practical
   C. Participate in care planning only if they request it
   D. Participate in care planning only if the resident is about to be discharged

5. On a RAP summary in the clinical record, the healthcare team members should show that they:

   A. Considered all RAPs triggered by the MDS as they developed a comprehensive care plan
   B. Are adopting their own standards for triggers
   C. Are planning to develop objectives within 90 days
   D. Are planning to insist that residents will receive all recommended services or treatments, regardless of a resident's wishes

6. In longterm care, how often should the comprehensive care plan be updated?

   A. Every week

   B. Every month

   C. Every three months and whenever the resident's condition changes

   D. Every year and whenever the resident's condition changes

7. You are developing a nutrition care plan. Which of the following is NOT good advice for stating a problem?

   A. Be as specific as possible.

   B. Identify possible reasons for the problem.

   C. Identify client strengths that can help solve the problem.

   D. Be as general as possible.

8. "Client fed by staff" is an example of which step in the nutrition care planning process?

   A. Identify nutrition problems.

   B. Determine calorie, protein and fluid needs.

   C. For each problem, develop goals that are relevant, measurable and realistic.

   D. For each goal, choose appropriate methods or approaches to reach it.

9. Which of the following is an example of an appropriate goal for Step 3 of the nutrition care planning process?

   A. Client will increase weight by at least 5 lbs within 90 days.

   B. Client's serum transferrin level will rise significantly.

   C. Client will eat better.

   D. Client will stop leaving food on the tray.

10. You are determining fluid needs for a resident. When will the standard figures for calculation probably NOT apply?

    A. If the resident usually drinks a lot anyway.

    B. If the resident has congestive heart failure.

    C. If the resident does not like many liquids.

    D. If the resident is on a tube feeding.

To be effective, nutrition care must be dynamic. A dietary manager must routinely assess new information and apply findings to ongoing plans for care.

After completing this chapter, you should be able to:

▶ List examples of information a dietary manager may review in the process of evaluating effectiveness of nutrition care.

▶ Give examples of data to monitor to assess hydration/dehydration.

▶ Give examples of data to monitor to assess management of diabetes mellitus.

▶ Give examples of data to monitor to assess overall protein calorie nutritional status.

▶ Give examples of data to monitor to assess nutritional status as it relates to management of pressure ulcers.

▶ Give examples of data to monitor to assess tolerance of an enteral feeding.

▶ List types of information to include in a follow-up progress note in the medical record.

As you learned in Chapter 13, a nutrition care plan provides the focus for initiating nutrition care. However, care does not end with a plan. The plan is only the beginning. This is particularly true in longterm care environments, in which a client may be receiving care for weeks, months, or years. After documenting and implementing the plan, the final two steps in providing nutrition care are to: re-assess the patient at defined intervals, and (as appropriate), revise the plan. In re-assessing a client, we are answering the question: Is the nutrition care plan working? And of course, we have to consider: How do we know? This requires us to identify specific types of data that will provide answers.

HYDRATION AND DEHYDRATION

Among the most common clinical concerns in a longterm care setting is dehydration, or a lack of water in the body. As you have learned in earlier chapters, water is a nutrient. Inadequate water in the body can lead to a drop in blood volume, with serious consequences. In addition, older individuals may lose some of the sense of thirst, which normally protects us from become dehydrated. Figure 14.1 lists possible signs of dehydration. Remember that thirst itself is not a reliable sign of dehydration. It is possible to becoming dehydrated without experiencing thirst. This situation can also occur under severe heat stress. Other factors that can lead to dehydration include fever, bleeding, severe burns, vomiting, diarrhea, or certain metabolic disorders.

Certain clinical conditions create a different kind of problem—water retention. Unhealthy water retention is called *edema*. This may occur, for example, when the heart is not functioning properly and/or kidneys are not removing excess

Figure 14.1

POSSIBLE SIGNS OF DEHYDRATION

▶ Decrease in urinary output or dark urine

▶ Sudden weight loss (e.g. 5% or more of body weight)

▶ Sunken eyes

▶ Hollow cheekbones

▶ Dry mucous membranes

▶ Cracked lips

▶ Skin turgor (resilience) is poor

▶ Change in state of alertness (in extreme dehydration)

▶ Deep, gasping breathing

Figure 14.2

POSSIBLE SIGNS OF EDEMA

▶ Visible swelling in legs, ankles, feet, and/or abdomen

▶ Elevated blood pressure

▶ Sudden weight gain (e.g. more than 5% of body weight)

water. Signs of edema appear in Figure 14.2. Edema is not a disease; it is a symptom. Fluid retention can make the heart and lungs work harder, and can eventually lead to a medical crisis. To manage diseases in which edema occurs, a physician may order restriction of dietary fluids. For any client following a fluid restriction, part of the follow-up evaluation will be to check on how the edema has changed.

In any situation affecting hydration, be sure to review medications and any changes in medications. A class of drugs called diuretics is often used in reducing edema. Diuretics promote water loss from the body. If new medications are introduced, you will also want to consider possible food-drug interactions and nutrition-related side effects. A potassium-wasting diuretic, for example, makes the body lose potassium. If kidneys are functioning well, a high-potassium diet may be appropriate. You may also want to monitor blood potassium levels. If in doubt, of course, check with a physician. You would not want to change a diet on your own.

MONITORING DIABETES

If one of the problems you are monitoring is diabetes mellitus, there are several indicators that help you understand how well the client is doing. A goal of diabetes management is to maintain blood glucose levels at reasonable levels to prevent complications. What pieces of information will tell you this? One is blood glucose measurements. You can review fasting blood glucose (measured in the morning, before breakfast) for a period of days to find out whether the diabetes is generally well-controlled. The exact standards to apply will depend on your institution and the individual client. If available, you can also review blood glucose values taken at other times of day. These are usually called *random* blood glucose levels. Be sure to note when meals were consumed in relation to these measurements. For some clients, routine measurements may also include a check for glucose and ketones in the urine. Normally, both of these should be zero. Presence of glucose in the urine generally indicates recent high blood glucose values. It occurs as the kidneys remove excess glucose from the bloodstream. Ketones should normally be absent. Ketones can indicate that the body has gone into an abnormal type of metabolism in an attempt to nourish cells.

Ongoing management of blood glucose levels is also measured in glycosylated hemoglobin. This laboratory measurement gives a snapshot of management over time. Depending upon an individual's needs and goals, blood lipid levels and total body weight may also be important.

In monitoring diabetes, it is important to talk to the client regularly, and find out what concerns exist. Check for any symptoms that indicate high glucose levels—such as thirst, excessive hunger, and excessive urination. Also check nursing notes for any reports that the client has experienced hypoglycemia (low blood sugar). In addition, you will want to observe meal intake and menu management. Consider how the client is dong with managing the form of dietary control being used, such as carbohydrate counting, exchange lists, or other system. Is this system proving a good match for the client? Is the client able to apply it? Is the client enjoying meals? Is the client eating any additional foods not on the menu (e.g. gifts from family or visitors)? Is the diet providing an adequate level of control for blood glucose? You would want to review the medication regimen, and note whether medicines and/or dosages have changed as well. As you gather this information and check with other members of the healthcare team, you can develop a solid picture of how the diabetes management plan is working, and make dietary suggestions and/or a referral to the Registered Dietitian as appropriate. For example, a client who is having frequent episodes of hypoglycemia may need liberalization of medications (determined by the physician) and/or of diet. A client whose blood glucose levels run consistently higher than a clinical goal may need a boost or change in medication, a boost in exercise, and/or a more tightly controlled meal plan.

MONITORING NUTRITIONAL STATUS

A variety of clinical conditions relate to nutritional status, especially degree of protein calorie malnutrition. Any time improvement of nutritional status is one of the clinical goals, a dietary manger needs to take an active role in monitoring progress. Here is some objective information to review (as available): weight changes, percent IBW, skinfold thickness, serum transferrin or albumin, prealbumin, and total lymphocyte count. If you have performed a calorie count, review this carefully, too, and compare it with estimated nutrient needs.

Nursing notes can be a helpful source of information about food intake and meal tolerance from day to day. Review them for trends and any notations of concerns or problems related to eating. You can also check intake and output records to find out whether the client is consuming adequate fluids.

Examine the current medication list, and identify any changes. Many medications affect sense of taste. Some cause dry mouth, nausea, or other symptoms that can profoundly affect food intake.

Subjective information is critical too. Questions you want to ask a client may include: How is your appetite? Are you having any problems or concerns with eating? Are you having any problems in chewing? Are you having any problems in swallowing? Are you experiencing any digestive concerns, such as nausea, vomiting, or constipation? Check carefully for tolerance of the current diet. Update food preferences, because they can change. A new medication or other condition may alter how a client tolerates a particular food. In a longterm care environment, repetition of foods may also reduce intake. A client may simply become bored with the same foods. If the client is not able to communicate, look for this same information through observation, the medical record and through consultation with others who are involved in care. Observe mealtime activity, and consider menu tolerance and food intake. You also want to notice any changes in dental health, and any other conditions that may affect a client's ability to feed himself, swallow, and maintain interest and alertness at mealtimes.

If you have implemented special dietary plans to improve nutritional status, review the success of these. You may be including nutritional supplements and/or high-calorie, high-protein foods in the daily menu. If so, consider how well the client is tolerating these. Is the client enjoying these foods? How much is the client consuming? Is there enough variety to keep meals appetizing? The bottom line, of course, is improvement in nutritional status.

MONITORING PRESSURE ULCERS

For a client with pressure ulcers, nutritional monitoring is also essential. Maintaining or improving nutritional status can contribute greatly to solving this clinical problem. Thus, you would want to evaluate changes in nutritional status, weight changes, percent IBW, skinfold thickness, serum transferrin or albumin, prealbumin, and total lymphocyte count. It is also imperative to consider protein, calorie, and fluid intake, and review whether the overall diet provides a reasonable balance of other essential nutrients, including vitamin C and zinc. Furthermore, check on the staging of a pressure ulcer and ask whether it has advanced, stayed the same, or improved. Note whether new pressure ulcers have occurred.

MONITORING AN ENTERAL (TUBE) FEEDING

If a client is receiving part or all of daily nutrients through an enteral feeding, there are some specific complications you want to notice. Nursing notes, flow sheets, and consultation with direct caregivers are critical sources of information about tolerance of a feeding. You would want to know whether the client is experiencing any side effects, such as abdominal cramping, diarrhea, or aspiration. If side effects are occurring, check on how total nutrient intake is affected. Typically, a caregiver stops or reduces the flow of a tube feeding when there is a problem with tolerance. If the client does not build adequate tolerance to a particular regimen, it may be difficult to provide adequate nutrients. If there is an ongoing problem with tolerance, it may be helpful to review the enteral product itself. There may be an alternate product that would be better tolerated.

In an assessment, check the current (actual) feeding with your estimation of nutrient needs. Often, an enteral feeding is part of a plan for maintaining or improving nutritional status. Indicators of nutritional status listed above are important components of a related evaluation.

THE EVALUATION PROCESS

The above sections provide some examples of information to review in evaluating nutrition care. Needless to say, this list does not cover all needs. With each client, you will need to review the problem list carefully, and match all relevant information to determine progress. As part of an evaluation, the dietitian/dietary manager should review or observe the following:

- The client's response to treatment/interventions
- Physician's orders (including any changes in diet order, medications, etc.)
- Flow sheets, such as intake and output records
- Weight records
- Previous nutrition progress notes
- Recent laboratory values
- Other recent additional information in the client's record
- The current problem list

In addition, the dietitian/dietary manager should consult with other members of the healthcare team.

Documenting Progress

As with all professional activity, an evaluation of the effectiveness of care should be documented in the medical record. The purpose of the progress note is to summarize how the client is responding to treatment as well as to document the degree of success in achieving goals identified in the care plan.

Progress notes are written in a specific, accurate, objective, concise and thorough manner. If your institution uses a SOAP charting format, it is appropriate to include information in all four parts: subjective, objective, assessment, and plan. Your progress note may address questions such as the following:

- How has the client responded to treatment?
- Has there been progress in achieving the nutrition goals in the care plan?
- Are there any new nutrition-related problems?
- What has changed since the care plan and previous progress notes were written, such as medications, laboratory values, ability to feed self, etc.?

If progress is satisfactory, you may indicate under "P" that the plan will continue. If progress is not satisfactory, recommend a revision to the plan. Sometimes, this will be a revision you can carry out yourself, such as offering different high-calorie, high-protein foods on the existing high-calorie, high-protein diet. Other times, you may be seeking a change in diet order, as authorized by the physician.

The timing of progress notes you write will depend on the type of facility you work in, as well as the facility's own policies and procedures. Normally, progress notes in longterm care institutions are written quarterly for all clients, monthly for those at risk, and more frequently for those with special circumstances.

Key Points

- After documenting and implementing a nutrition care plan, it is important to re-assess the patient at defined intervals, and (as appropriate), revise the plan.

- Evaluation of the nutrition care process answers questions such as: Is the nutrition care plan working? How do we know?

- Sources for relevant information include the problem list of the medical record, orders listed in the medical record (especially diet order), medication list, laboratory data, weights, calorie counts, nursing notes and other progress notes, meal observation, consultation with the client, and consultation with other caregivers.

- Routine documentation of evaluation follows an institutional procedure. This may be at least quarterly for residents of longterm care facilities or more frequently as appropriate.

1. Which of the following is NOT a sign that a client may be dehydrated?

   A. Client has lost 8 pounds in the past two days.
   B. Client's lips are cracked.
   C. Client has poor skin turgor.
   D. Client shows swelling around the ankles.

2. Which of the following is most likely to indicate edema?

   A. Dry mucous membranes
   B. Extreme thirst
   C. Swelling around the ankles
   D. Excessive hunger

3. The greatest concern with fluid retention is that it:

   A. Makes the heart and lungs work harder
   B. Causes high blood glucose readings
   C. Makes the body retain extra potassium
   D. Makes clients feel hyperactive

4. Which of the following is NOT an indicator of how well diabetes is under control?

   A. Random blood glucose readings
   B. Urinary ketone levels
   C. Blood zinc levels
   D. Fasting blood glucose

5. What is the normal level for glucose in urine?

   A. 0 mg/liter
   B. 0-1 mg/liter
   C. 1-3 mg/liter
   D. 5 mg/liter or higher

6. Which laboratory measurement gives a snapshot of management of blood glucose over time?

   A. Fasting blood glucose
   B. Glycosylated hemoglobin
   C. Serum potassium
   D. Serum albumin

7. You are re-assessing a client who has a pressure ulcer. It has advanced from Stage I to Stage II. Which of the following laboratory values is most likely to help you evaluate effectiveness of the care plan?

   A. Prealbumin
   B. Serum potassium
   C. Serum glucose
   D. Serum iron

8. In talking with the client described in Question #7, you find that a low-sodium diet order is making meals less enjoyable. You find the client was placed on this diet to manage hypertension. Currently, blood pressure readings are normal. Based on this information, what would be the best revision to the plan?

A. Tell the client to use pepper to replace the salt in foods.
B. Suggest no change; just re-evaluate in three months.
C. Suggest liberalization of the diet to "General" to improve intake.
D. Just ignore the diet order.

9. A client has been assessed as having protein calorie malnutrition and is on a high-calorie, high-protein diet. After one month on the regimen, you note that weight has declined by 5 lbs and serum transferrin has also dropped. Which of the following information is NOT relevant to your review?

A. The current medication list
B. Mealtime observations and intake
C. Medical insurance plan
D. Food preferences

10. You are re-assessing a client who is receiving nutrition through an enteral tube feeding. Which of the following is a concern?

A. Serum albumin has increased.
B. Nursing notes indicate frequent aspiration.
C. Body weight has increased.
D. Two pressure ulcers have gone from Stage III to Stage II.

Nutrition education enables clients to participate in caring for themselves. By developing basic skills in this area, a dietary manager can provide valuable resources to clients.

After completing this chapter, you should be able to:

- List reasons for educating clients about their own nutrition care plans.
- Describe what makes a meaningful learning objective for nutrition education.
- Describe methods of teaching clients about nutrition.
- Identify resources for providing nutrition education.

As explained in Chapter 12, the client is active as part of the healthcare team. When it comes to nutrition and diet, the client's role is crucial to success. Nutrition-related care occurs every day—and at every meal. A client has a right to understand the plan of care, as well as to have personal participation in the day-to-day effectiveness of a diet whenever possible. Often, a client takes part in the fine details of managing a diet. The client may choose particular foods, based on a diet order and a menu. With knowledge, the client can choose foods that make meals truly enjoyable. The client can make decisions and exert control over this aspect of clinical treatment. The client can contribute tremendously to the care planning process.

According to The American Dietetic Association, nutrition education is: "a process that assists the public in applying knowledge from nutrition science and the relationship between diet and health to their food practices. It is a deliberate effort to improve the nutritional well-being of people by assessing the multiple factors that affect food choices, tailoring educational methodologies and messages to the public being reached, and evaluating results. It can help individuals develop a knowledge base, make a commitment to good nutrition, select nutritionally adequate diets, and develop decision-making skills." According to this definition, nutrition educators can enhance knowledge, encourage skills to make decisions and select nutritious diets, and help clients develop a positive attitude toward nutrition. Nutrition education is often part of the nutrition care plan.

DEVELOPING OBJECTIVES

Before beginning any type of nutrition education, we first need to answer a simple, direct question: What do I want the client to learn? Our answer to this is one or more learning objectives. A **learning objective** is a specific, measurable statement of the outcome of education. To develop a learning objective, think about what the client will be able to do when you have successfully competed nutrition education. An effective learning objective includes key elements, described in the acronym, RUMBAS.

RUMBAS stands for:

R- Relevant

U- Understandable

M- Measurable

B- Behavioral

A- Attainable

S- Specific

Each learning objective should be relevant to the overall purpose of the instruction. For example, if you want to educate a client about managing hypertension, there is no need to toss in nutrition information about diverticulitis. You want to focus on what the client needs, and address this in an objective. Next, you want the objective to make sense. In addition, you want the outcome you specify to be measurable. Why? So that you will be able to assess whether the education has been successful. Figure 15.1 lists examples of objectives that are and are not measurable. An effective objective is also behavioral. This means it describes what a client will do. Figure 15.2 lists examples of objectives that do and do not describe behavior. Needless to say, an objective must be attainable and realistic. It should also be specific.

Figure 15.1

MEASURABLE OBJECTIVES

Not Measurable: Client will do better with choosing foods on the daily menu.

Measurable: Client will choose foods on the daily menu that meet his 200-gram carbohydrate diet, within 10%.

Not Measurable: Client will eat more calories.

Measurable: Client will select foods that bring intake up to at least 1600 cal/day.

Figure 15.2

BEHAVIORAL OBJECTIVES

Not Behavioral: Client will understand his renal diet.

Behavioral: Client will follow his fluid restriction accurately.

Not Behavioral: Client will note why nutritional status is important.

Behavioral: Client will consume at least 80% of nutritional supplements provided.

GROUP INSTRUCTION

Formal education of clients is most often accomplished through group instruction. An advantage of group instruction is that it allows clients to share experiences and develop a sense of group motivation. If the clients will continue to have contact after an educational session, they can encourage and support each other. A group may include clients, as well as family members and others involved in care. In any institution where a group of clients has common educational needs, this can be an excellent option. A dietary manager may also combine group instruction with individual nutrition counseling (discussed later in this chapter).

After developing learning objectives, a dietary manager planning group instruction needs to develop a class outline that includes an introduction to the topic, organized detail, some form of practice or application, and a closing. Here are some tips for developing these sections of an outline:

Introduction. The class introduction can serve various functions. It orients learners to the subject. It gives the dietitian/dietary manager an opportunity to learn more about the clients. It can also be used to create client involvement and interest, by, for example, tasting a new low fat food. When choosing an introduction, pick an opening that will quickly engage participants' attention. It may be a question, such as: *What do you find most confusing (or annoying) about your _____ diet?* Sometimes, a statistic can capture attention. An example is: *Ninety percent of people who go on weight loss diets end up heavier than when they started. Why is that?* Some introductions allow participants to introduce themselves, and then state one fact about themselves. An introduction needs to feel non-threatening. For example, you can ask each participant to state a favorite food. Make the opening relevant to the group, and design it to put people at ease. As clients share information about themselves, avoid making judgments. You want to encourage open communication, which requires absolute acceptance of each person in the group. If the client is doing something undesirable, your approach should be to present information and help the client draw personal conclusions. During the introduction, you also want to briefly describe the learning objectives. You may or may not include every detail you have used in planning. You may say something like: *When we are finished with this class, you will be able to total carbohydrates in your daily diet.*

Organized Detail. This part of the class outline describes the content, or what you teach; and the teaching methods, or how you teach it. For each learning objective, you must sketch out what you will say, and choose an appropriate teaching method. When choosing your teaching material, pick information that is relevant and significant to the group. Be specific, and use examples.

Practice or Application. When choosing your teaching methods, choose some that allow for participation. Research demonstrates that people remember only 20% of what they hear, 30% of what they see, but 50% of what they hear and see. By having clients actively participate in training, you can expect them to remember 90% of what they say and do. Activities may include checking sample food labels and deciding how they fit into a diet, or marking a selective menu according to a meal plan. They may include practice in modifying recipes to fit special dietary needs, or even simple food preparation.

Closing. Your session needs to end with a closing. The closing may fill several functions: to answer questions, reinforce key points, and evaluate whether learning objectives have been met.

Figure 15.3 shows a sample outline for group instruction. Figure 15.4 lists some ideas for achieving effective communication.

Figure 15.3

SAMPLE OUTLINE: FOOD PYRAMID POWER

INTRODUCTION
Introduce yourself. Tell participants that today we will try to answer the questions: How do we know what to eat? What makes a balanced diet?

Ask each participant to state his/her name, and a favorite food.

DETAIL
Explain that nutrition advice can seem confusing and contradictory. Yet nutrition is important to health, as we hear in the news almost daily.

A tool for making food choices is The Food Guide Pyramid (show visual). Explain shape of the Pyramid—wide at bottom, narrow at top.

Explain each group of the Pyramid, and note that there are no "good" foods or "bad" foods. All foods can fit into a healthy diet. Give each person a copy of the Pyramid. (See copy on CD-ROM with this textbook.) Note the idea of variety. Ask participants to tell where their own favorite foods (named in the Introduction) fit in the Pyramid. Now, ask each to name another favorite food and tell where it fits.

PRACTICE
Divide into groups. Give each group a bin full of food models and/or empty food packages. Give each group a sign representing a food group (e.g. milk group, vegetable group, etc.). Now, ask participants to "trade" foods with each other until all food models/packages are sorted into their respective groups. Ask one person from each group to name the group and all the foods they have.

Now, ask participants what would be a "serving" of some of these foods; discuss.

CLOSING
Thank participants for their activity. Ask for questions and reactions. Summarize key points: The Food Guide Pyramid is a tool for healthy eating. Every food has a place here. Briefly review the groups, number of servings, and serving sizes. The Pyramid is an easy guide!

Give session evaluation.

Figure 15.4

KEYS TO EFFECTIVE COMMUNICATION

RESPECT PERSONAL SPACE

When you first sit down to speak with clients, ask them to sit where they feel the most comfortable or let them tell you where to sit. This will allow people to choose the distance that feels right to them. Comfortable distance varies by culture and individual.

LEARN THE CULTURAL RULES ABOUT TOUCHING

Find out the cultural rules regarding touch for the ethnic groups with whom you work, including differences based on gender. In some Asian cultures, the head should not be touched because it is the seat of wisdom. In many Hispanic cultures, the head of a child should be touched when you admire the child. A vigorous handshake may be considered a sign of aggression by Native Americans.

ESTABLISH RAPPORT

Take time to establish common ground through sharing experiences and exchanging information.

ASK QUESTIONS

Do not be afraid to ask someone about something with which you are unfamiliar or uncomfortable. Nutrition educators suggest open-ended, honest questions that show an interest in the person, a respect for his culture, and a willingness to learn.

LISTEN TO THE ANSWERS

Really listen. Do not interrupt your client or try to put words in her mouth. Let her tell her own story. Appreciate AND USE SILENCE. Observe your client to get a feel for how he or she uses silence. Do not feel that silence has to be filled in with small talk. Give people a chance to formulate their thoughts, especially if they are trying to speak in a language that is not their native tongue. Cultures that value silence learn to distinguish varying qualities of silence, which may be hard for others to discern. "Pause time" is different for different cultures.

NOTICE EYE CONTACT

Notice the kind of eye contact your client is making with family members or your coworkers. Many cultures consider it impolite to look directly at the person speaking.

PAY ATTENTION TO BODY MOVEMENTS

Movements such as upturned palms of the hands, waving one's hand, and pointing with fingers or feet convey varying messages. Observe your clients for clues.

NOTE CLIENT RESPONSES

Note that a "yes" response does not necessarily indicate that a client has understood or is willing to do what is being discussed. It may simply be an offering of respect for the health professional's status. Some clients may not ask questions because this would indicate a lack of clear communication by the provider. In some cultures, smiling and laughing may mask other emotions or prevent conflict.

Here are some additional ideas to enhance your success in teaching groups:

- Start on time.
- Use a seating arrangement such as a circle that enhances communication and vision.
- Make eye contact. Smile and nod to show positive reinforcement.
- Pay attention to the pace, volume, and tone of your voice. Don't talk too fast, and be sure everyone can hear you.
- Ask clients what they already know about the topic to be discussed.
- Actively listen.
- Encourage and facilitate client participation.
- Ask open-ended questions.
- Praise and give encouragement.
- Use visual aids effectively.

VISUAL AIDS

You can reinforce your points with visual aids, such as simple handouts, posters, models, slides, or transparencies. Visual aids keep clients' attention, reinforce main ideas, save time, and increase understanding and retention. Visual aids are also useful in making comparisons. Videotapes may also be useful, but do not use a videotape to replace your teaching. Make sure you use terms that your audience will know and understand, avoiding medical jargon. Make key points simple, and design handouts to be readable, especially for anyone with a vision impairment. The most effective visual aid is limited to one idea that can be communicated within three to five seconds. If you have more ideas, use more aids! Special visual aids for nutrition education include food models, which are synthetic replicas of food; measuring cups and spoons; food packages; and nutrition facts labels from foods.

NUTRITION COUNSELING

Nutrition counseling is the process of helping a client achieve healthful changes in dietary habits, based on an assessment of the client's nutritional needs. Counseling involves exchanges between a client and a counselor (such as a dietary manager). Typically, nutrition counseling is one-on-one education. Alternately, it may be education involving a client and one or two other people who are close to her, such as family members.

Nutrition counseling follows the same basic steps as the nutrition care process, beginning with an assessment followed by development that includes a complete diet history. This is the foundation of personalized diet planning and education. For example, if you learn in a diet history that a client frequently chooses fast foods, then you want to help the client learn to choose foods from a fast food menu as part of the nutrition counseling process. If you discover that a client is a vegetarian, you will need to be sure your recommendations are consistent with this dietary choice. An effective counselor acts as a facilitator, helping a client reach positive goals. A session in which a professional simply rattles off a list of Dos and Don'ts to a client is not actually effective nutrition education. Instead, a counselor needs to relate pieces of information and discuss them with the client. A counselor can ask questions to help the client apply information. An example is: *Now that you know what foods contain potassium, what will you choose?* Figure 15.5 presents some competency criteria for nutrition counselors. This outlines many of the specific behaviors that make counseling effective.

In counseling, as in group education, it is important to be non-judgmental. Respect for clients means that we relate information, help them focus and understand it, and then allow them to apply this information. In addition, The American Dietetic Association has taken the position that "all foods can fit into a healthful eating style". They recommend emphasizing healthy foods, rather than emphasizing a list of "bad foods" or foods to avoid.

Visual aids can be very useful in nutrition counseling, just as in group sessions. Practice and application are likewise helpful. In addition, a client usually appreciates having a printed reference to use after a session. While some institutions develop their own teaching materials, this is a time-consuming proposition. Many high-quality materials are available either free or at low cost from government agencies, industry groups, health organizations, food manufacturers, cooperative extension services, and educational institutions. Sources of free or low-cost food and nutrition materials appear in Appendix D. Many materials are available in various languages. Matching language to your client/audience is very important to support education. An extensive listing of resources is available on the Food and Nutrition Information Center—Foreign Languages Resources list (Appendix D). Note that not only language, but cultural food practices must be addressed when you work with any individual or group. Use relevant food examples, and be sure your suggestions fit with cultural and religious practices. When you are evaluating materials for use, consider the source and be sure you trust its reliability. When you apply printed materials, be sure to help a client use them. Chat about the information, and coach the client in applying this information personally. A checklist to critique written nutrition education materials appears in Figure 15.6.

If you are counseling someone who will be preparing meals at home, help develop a plan for meal preparation. You may want to develop a sample grocery list together, emphasizing choices that meet dietary needs. Explore preparation methods and offer sources for recipes if appropriate. Be sure your suggestions are practical for the client's abilities and lifestyle. Finally, recommend additional resources as relevant, such as a local Meals-on-Wheels program. Make yourself available by phone for questions and follow-up.

Figure 15.5

COMPETENCY CHECKLIST FOR NUTRITION COUNSELORS

NUTRITION INFORMATION FOR PARTICULAR CLIENT

1. Counselor knows the essential elements and rationale behind client's prescribed diet (e.g., low fat, low sodium, etc.).

   ▶ Is familiar with all the food categories of the diet.

   ▶ Is comfortable with substitutions and rationale for selection of food.

   ▶ Is prepared to help client adapt diet to his needs.

2. Counselor has knowledge of local eating patterns.

   ▶ Has some grasp of regional customs and of what foods are available in the area.

   ▶ Is familiar with frequently patronized restaurants and food chains and will ask client his favorites.

3. At the outset, counselor makes reasonably sure that client's knowledge of prescribed diet is adequate.

   ▶ Takes a history to find out client's dietary background.

   ▶ At first session, discusses long-term goals and explains diet thoroughly, making sure client understands.

   ▶ Eliminates client's knowledge gaps (by discussing diet further, giving examples, using visuals, etc.) so following sessions can concentrate on goal-setting.

   ▶ Analyzes diet history with client to assess current diet and eating behavior.

COMMUNICATION SKILLS

4. Counselor sets appropriate tone for counseling sessions through preparation, manner, and physical setting.

   ▶ Makes appointment with client, allowing enough time for comfortable, thorough discussion.

   ▶ Arranges for private, quiet setting.

   ▶ Establishes client's ability to see and to read and speak English. Adapts counseling if necessary.

   ▶ If using a translator, counselor looks at and speaks to the client (not the translator).

   ▶ Shows interest in client as an individual; looks for his particular needs and preferences.

   ▶ Maintains relaxed, comfortable manner. Makes client feel at ease.

   ▶ Indicates intentions to talk and to listen.

5. Counselor prepares self and client for continuing relationship over a specified period.

   ▶ Explains the necessity of follow-up over time.

   ▶ Outlines plans for working with client—a certain number of sessions over a certain period of time with occasional contact by phone or mail.

6. Counselor uses principles of good communication.

   ▶ Uses primarily open-ended questions (rather than those answered by yes or no).

   ▶ Guards against doing most of the talking. Shows ability to listen.

   ▶ Is able to tolerate periods of silence.

   ▶ Shows non-judgmental, noncritical attitude toward client's eating pattern and chosen lifestyle.

   ▶ Uses words the client can understand.

7. Counselor communicates interest and confidence nonverbally as well as verbally.

- Shows poise and interest through posture and "body language".
- Has frequent eye contact with client.
- Uses gestures and words to encourage client to communicate freely, without putting words in client's mouth.

COUNSELING APPROACHES

8. Counselor is aware that the change process is the responsibility of the client.

- Does not assume responsibility for changes or consequences.
- Does not become too ego-involved in the client's eventual success or failure.

9. Counselor is aware of need for client to recognize manageable goals.

- Helps client choose initial goal that is easily achieved.
- Helps client set specific and short-term goals that are progressively more challenging.
- Is able to help client evaluate goals.
- Helps client avoid failure by setting realistic goals.

10. Counselor is able to help client set up record-keeping and/or tally systems.

- Can help client verbalize a method appropriate to the task.
- Can suggest alternate methods for client's consideration without dictating choice.
- Emphasizes need for accurate records.
- Is able to help the client review food records.

11. Counselor is aware of the need to examine and anticipate obstacles that will interfere with progress.

- Can review with client potential obstacles in social, personal and physical environments.
- Can help client identify actual or potential problems and deal with these by encouraging him to restructure environment, and by role-playing problem situations with him.
- Discusses how client will deal with possible failure (accept and keep going).

12. Counselor is able to define own role in giving support and feedback.

- Can avoid taking the major responsibility.
- Can place the responsibility for change on the client.
- Is aware of own biases and belief systems, and is able to ignore them.

13. Counselor is able to evaluate progress toward the stated goal.

- Is able to give client feedback about progress.
- Keeps notes in sufficient detail to depict client's responsibilities and progress.
- Measures progress by a combination of biological measures, food intake evaluation, and subjective judgments, with an emphasis on changing behavior.

14. Counselor encourages client to get family and friends involved.

- Helps client recognize the influence of others; suggests that he ask openly for their support.
- Suggests that client ask them to participate in some way: sharing new tastes and habits; helping with food selection; limiting inappropriate foods.
- Can help client cope with negative feedback by anticipating and rehearsing problem situations.
- Can evaluate whether others are potentially supportive or destructive.
- Can utilize others as a support without losing sight of the primary responsibility resting with client.

15. Counselor is able to understand that his or her role is not simply that of information-giver or instructor.

- Acts as facilitator for client.
- Is appropriately assertive.
- Is able to resist "lecturing".

16. Counselor is aware of the need to keep the client task-oriented.

- Recognizes delaying tactics and distractions.
- Is able to redirect the session toward specifics.
- Responds pleasantly to client's attempts at humor.

Figure 15.6

CHECKLIST FOR EVALUATING PRINTED NUTRITION EDUCATION MATERIALS

- The cover is attractive and clearly identifies the topic.
- The writing style is conversational and in an active voice.
- Technical jargon is not used. In cases when a technical term must be used, it is defined.
- The text is interesting to read and lively.
- The emphasis is on "what to do," or specific behavioral changes.
- The illustrations are simple and relevant to the content.
- The print size is large enough and the font is plain enough to be easily read.
- There is contrast between the color of the print and the color of the paper so the words are easily read.
- The pages are not cluttered with too much information.
- The material is appropriate for the intended audience (gender, culture, age, level of education).
- The publication invites reader thought and/or participation, e.g. through a questionnaire, a recipe, a worksheet, or other techniques.

▶ Educating a client about nutrition promotes client involvement in the plan of care.

▶ Education should begin with learning objectives that are relevant, understandable, measurable, behavioral, attainable, and specific (summarized by the acronym RUMBAS).

▶ Group instruction should include an introduction to the topic, organized detail, some form of practice or application, and a closing.

▶ Research demonstrates that we remember only 20% of what we hear, 30% of what we see, and 50% of what we hear and see. By having clients actively participate in training, you can have them remember 90% of what they say and do.

▶ Special visual aids for nutrition education include food models, which are synthetic replicas of food; measuring cups and spoons; food packages; and nutrition facts labels from foods.

▶ Nutrition counseling involves exchanges between a client and a counselor, and is based on an assessment of the client.

▶ An effective counselor acts as a facilitator, helping a client reach positive goals.

▶ In counseling, as in group education, it is important to be non-judgmental and to emphasize positive food choices.

▶ Many high-quality materials are available either free or at low cost from government agencies, industry groups, health organizations, food manufacturers, cooperative extension services, and educational institutions.

Nutrition counseling: the process of helping a client achieve healthful changes in dietary habits, based on an assessment of the client's nutritional needs

Learning objective: a specific, measurable statement of the intended outcome of education

1. According to the American Dietetic Association, effective nutrition education does all of the following EXCEPT:
    A. Help clients make decisions about foods
    B. Help clients make a commitment to nutrition
    C. Encourage skills for choosing foods
    D. Help clients identify which foods are bad

2. Which of the following learning objectives contains all the elements of RUMBAS?

A. Client will stop eating fatty foods.
B. Client will choose low fat milk and yogurt products at lunch every day for two weeks.
C. Client will avoid visible fat.
D. Client will eat better.

3. Which of the following ideas will help you create an effective introduction for group education?

A. Skip the objectives; they are only for the group leader.
B. Lecture as quickly as possible.
C. Tell participants everything they are doing wrong immediately.
D. Encourage participation and put people at ease.

4. If you ask participants to check food labels and decide how to use particular foods in a meal plan, they are likely to remember:

A. 2% of what you have taught them
B. 5% of what you have taught them
C. 20% of what you have taught them
D. 90% of what you have taught them

5. Which of the following is NOT an example of an appropriate question to ask during a nutrition education session?

A. What do you find most challenging about carbohydrate counting?
B. Why do you keep eating bad foods?
C. What fruits and vegetables do you find most appealing?
D. Does anyone have a favorite dessert idea?

6. If you ask a client whether he understands something, and he says "yes," you can conclude:

A. He may understand it or he may be offering respect or masking emotions.
B. He definitely understands the information, but probably won't use it.
C. He definitely understands the information and will definitely use it.
D. He will most certainly change his eating habits.

7. A very effective visual aid communicates:

A. Three to five ideas in 1 second
B. One idea in 3-5 seconds
C. Three ideas in 60 seconds
D. Five ideas in about 5 minutes

8. Nutrition counseling is a personalized exchange based upon:

   A. Educational videotapes
   B. A list of foods to avoid
   C. A review of common eating habits among other people
   D. A nutrition assessment, including diet history

9. Listening is important during nutrition education because it:

   A. Gives the dietary manager a break
   B. Gives the client time to voice questions and reactions
   C. Makes the time pass more quickly
   D. Gives the dietary manager time to write progress notes

10. Which of the following behaviors is characteristic of an effective nutrition counselor?

   A. Lectures to the client
   B. Takes most of the responsibility for the client's healthful diet
   C. Helps the client practice or rehearse diet-related situation
   D. Avoids eye contact

A dietary manager needs to assess how effective education has been in order to understand a client's ongoing needs better. A dietary manager also incorporates feedback to increase skills as an educator.

After completing this chapter, you should be able to:

- ▶ List reasons for evaluating the effectiveness of nutrition education.
- ▶ Suggest tools and methods for evaluating the effectiveness of nutrition education.
- ▶ Name possible reasons for ineffectiveness, and suggest approaches for dealing with them.
- ▶ Recommend ways of reinforcing nutrition education.

The final, but very important, component of any nutrition education program is evaluation. The key purpose of evaluation is to determine whether you have met the learning objectives. This is, in fact, one of the reasons we insist that learning objectives be measurable. A description of how to measure behavior, as written in an objective, gives us a solid gauge for evaluating the results of education. As we determine how well the nutrition education has worked for a particular client, we can then revise a plan for education accordingly. Much like any other aspect of a nutrition care plan, education requires follow-up assessment, and sometimes, a change in plan.

A second reason for evaluating nutrition education is to obtain feedback about the educational approach itself. Particularly for group education, good practice dictates that we gather feedback from participants at the end. This information helps us refine educational techniques and related materials. Sometimes, it provides feedback to us as professionals to help us focus on how to work with a particular group or tackle a particular topic.

Following an educational session, three levels of evaluation may apply—client reaction, actual learning, and behavioral change. Here is more information about each:

Client reaction. Evaluation focused on client reaction answers the question: *How did the client(s) respond to the education sessions?* To evaluate client reaction for a group class, use a rating sheet such as a class evaluation form, shown in Figure 16.1. Client reaction often provides feedback to group leaders, too. For example, we may find out which techniques worked best, or what questions we may not have addressed. We can use this information to revise outlines for future classes. Following a one-on-one nutrition counseling session, we also solicit the client's reaction. Usually, this is done informally, by asking questions such as:

- ▶ Was this session helpful to you?
- ▶ What questions have we left unanswered?
- ▶ Would you like to meet again to discuss your diet? If so, what would you like to talk about?

Actual learning. The second level of evaluation answers the question: *How much did clients learn?* To evaluate learning, you can use written and verbal

SAMPLE CLASS EVALUATION FORM

Instructions: Please circle your answers to the following questions. Add any comments you'd like. Your feedback is very important to us. Thank you!

1. How well did this session match your interests about nutrition?

   excellent match   fair match   poor match

2. Was this material:

   too complex   too simple   just right

3. Please rate the activities [name them specifically on your form]:

   excellent   good   fair

4. Please rate the handouts:

   excellent   good   fair

5. Please rate the group leader's skills:

   excellent   good   fair

6. What did you like most about this session?

7. What did you like least about this session?

8. Is there anything you will do differently after attending this session?

   no   yes   If yes, what? _____

9. What other topics would you like to see in future classes?

Comments:

questions, often given as a post-test. This is a test about facts and information presented. Some educational strategies require a pre-test before a session begins, and the same test at the end given as the post-test. This allows you to measure how much participants have learned. A drawback, however, is that many people feel intimidated by a formal test. Many people associate a test with uncomfortable situations in school and feel anxious. Two tests in one session can be even worse. Often, it helps to make a test a "quiz" and transform it into a fun, light-hearted activity. Written tests also require language competency and reading and writing skills of your clients. Sometimes this is not practical. An alternative to written tests is a friendly question-and-answer session. Another alternative is to set up a game show, in which participants ask and answer questions. In one-on-one counseling, the process of evaluating learning is typically informal. You may ask a few questions to see what the client knows and remembers so far. It's best to ask small questions as you go along, rather than wait until the end. Or, you may give the client an opportunity to practice applying information. This way, you can obtain feedback during the session and use it immediately to gear your counseling to the client's understanding. You can also provide reinforcement as the session moves along.

Behavioral change. The third level of evaluation answers the question: *Have dietary habits changed?* Refer back to the learning objectives, and observe how behavior corresponds to the objectives themselves. In some cases, a food diary is useful. If clients are using a selective menu in a hospital or nursing facility, you can monitor how they make choices on menus. Likewise, if a client is choosing foods in a dining room, you can evaluate change by visiting the client at mealtime and making observations. If you give a client an activity during a session, you can evaluate effectiveness by watching what the client does. For example, you may ask yourself: Can the client decide which foods to use, and in what portion sizes? Can the client plan a menu that meets fluid restrictions?

REFINING PLANS

If you find that education has not been as effective as you'd like, you need to try to identify reasons. A feedback tool such as the evaluation form may help with this process. If you have already developed rapport with clients, you can discover many reasons simply by asking in a friendly, low-key manner. For example, three days after counseling a client about how to implement a high-calorie diet, you may say: *We are aiming to keep your daily calories up to 1500. Your calorie count for yesterday shows 900 calories. What do you think might be holding you back?* Keeping your responses non-judgmental makes it easier for clients to trust you. In turn, this helps you help them more effectively.

Consider all possible barriers to communication. These may include differences in language, ability to read (if you rely on printed materials), use of terminology a client does not understand, state of alertness, and many others. If any of these barriers exists, you may need to re-evaluate how best to communicate with a client. Also keep in mind that individual learning styles vary. One person may learn best by reading words. Another may learn best by glancing at images and graphics. One needs to hear information. Another needs to do things. Each of these styles is valid, and each requires different educational techniques. If you discover that a client has not understood information, try using a different educational approach.

As you evaluate progress, it's important to be flexible. Do not expect perfection from clients, especially if they are striving to change longstanding dietary habits. Try to notice every positive step towards achieving objectives. Encouragement reassures a client about putting information into practice, and tends to bring about more of the same behaviors.

In addition, it's critical to recognize the distinction between knowledge and behavior. This distinction crops up continually when we examine any type of health education. I might know the information that will make me healthy. However, that doesn't mean I will automatically put it all into practice! Often, the challenge a nutrition counselor faces is not limited to explaining diets or relating information. The real challenge is to help motivate and support an individual in making subtle improvements in habits. This may hinge on much more than nutrition knowledge. In fact, dietary habits have many cultural and psychological undertones, as explained in Chapter 1. Values, emotional needs, and other life priorities may easily affect the final outcomes of nutrition counseling. As possible, try to understand these factors, and help clients address them. As needed, mold your suggestions to the client's preferences, customs, and concerns. You may need to weave nutrition ideas into specialized plans creatively in order to match a client's needs.

Also consider the big picture. Nutrition counseling is only one component of a health plan. Consider the other components, and ask yourself how these fit together for the client. Is the client overwhelmed? Is nutrition high or low on a priority list? If there are many health-related objectives and regimens, it may help to show the client how nutrition can support other needs. For example, a client who has hypertension and is also obese may appreciate discovering how weight loss will likely help reduce hypertension, too. The bottom line is to articulate a payoff. Explain to the client how he will benefit, how he will feel, or what other desirable health effects he may expect from implementing dietary advice.

Furthermore, it is easy for a client to believe that sound nutrition is an all-or-nothing endeavor. This is key to the culture of dieting, and tends to affect our thinking as a culture when it comes to nutrition. Effective counseling depends on our ability to transform dietary advice into a series of small steps and to praise all positive changes. Any time a client experiences difficulty following a restrictive diet, we can provide reassurance and encouragement.

Sometimes, implementing dietary advice simply isn't practical for a client, due to one of various obstacles. As part of any re-assessment, be alert to problems that may interfere with meeting nutrition-related objectives. Factors such as medications, dental changes, or changes in swallowing ability can easily affect how a person eats. If obstacles exist, try to help remove them. If that is not possible, refine the plan and the counseling to make them realistic for the client.

DOCUMENTING EVALUATION

Like any aspect of a nutrition care plan, nutrition education requires evaluation and documentation. If you provide nutrition counseling, include this information in a progress note. You want to tell who was involved (e.g. client and/or family members), what you covered together, and what objectives you have set. You should also name any handout(s) you have provided. You should assess a client's understanding of the educational content. As possible, state what you have seen that shows how the client can meet behavioral objectives. For example, you may write: *Client accurately selected foods to total 160 grams of carbohydrates on tomorrow's menu.* You should state your recommended follow-up. As you re-assess educational objectives, gather new information and provide your assessment. If you revise the plan for education, indicate this in the progress note.

REINFORCING EDUCATION

Typically, one nutrition education session does not change a person's dietary habits. The most effective education is delivered in manageable chunks, over a period of time. Education of any type requires reinforcement. If you have ongoing contact with clients, as in a school, retirement community, or longterm care facility, you have an excellent opportunity to provide intermittent education and reinforcement. Reinforcement can be as simple as:

- Providing a nutrition tip on a menu
- Preparing a bulletin board in your facility to highlight a nutrition topic
- Labeling foods in a group dining area with nutrition facts
- Chatting with a client about daily food choices
- Noticing when a client implements a dietary change at any meal, and providing praise
- Giving a client an opportunity to ask a follow-up question a day or two after an educational session
- Highlighting a special item on a menu and noting how it meets particular needs

Clearly, nutrition education is more than a one-shot endeavor. Quite often, dietary managers are in roles where they can have a tremendous impact on clients' individual dietary choices.

▶ The key purpose of evaluation is to determine whether you have met the learning objectives.

▶ A second reason for evaluating nutrition education is to obtain feedback about the educational approach itself.

▶ Following an educational session, three levels of evaluation may apply—client reaction, actual learning, and behavioral change.

▶ If objectives are not yet met, a dietary manager may seek more feedback from a client, consider barriers to communication, recognize the distinction between knowledge and behavior, consider the big picture, and remove any obstacles. With careful thought, it is often possible to revise a plan of education.

▶ Sound nutrition is not an all-or-nothing endeavor.

▶ A dietary manager should document nutrition education and follow-up as part of the nutrition care process.

▶ The most effective education is delivered in manageable chunks, over a period of time.

▶ Education of any type requires reinforcement.

1. Which of the following is an effective way to obtain client reactions to a nutrition education class?

   A. Use a class evaluation form.
   B. Give a pre-test.
   C. Give a post-test.
   D. Ask another dietary manager what he or she noticed.

2. Which of the following is an effective way to assess actual learning at the end of a nutrition education class?

   A. Use a class evaluation form.
   B. Give a pre-test.
   C. Give a post-test.
   D. Ask another dietary manager what he or she noticed.

3. Which of the following is NOT a drawback of a written post-test?

   A. It may intimidate participants.
   B. It may measure what participants have learned.
   C. It requires language competency.
   D. It requires reading and writing skills.

4. How is behavioral change different from knowledge?

   A. Behavioral change describes what people know; knowledge describes what people do.
   B. Behavioral change describes what people want to do; knowledge describes what people know.
   C. Behavioral change describes what people do; knowledge describes what prevents people from putting information into practice.
   D. Behavioral change describes what people do; knowledge describes what people know.

5. What is the best way to assess behavioral change?

   A. Observe behavior and compare it with learning objectives.
   B. Give a pre-test.
   C. Give a post-test.
   D. Ask participants to complete a class evaluation form.

6. What word best describes an effective nutrition counselor?

   A. Lecturer
   B. Facilitator
   C. Perfectionist
   D. Judge

7. You have given a client a written brochure about her low-sodium diet. In follow-up, you determine she does not understand. What alternate approach could you try?

   A. Ask her to read the brochure again.
   B. Give her a different written brochure.
   C. Ask her to read an article about hypertension.
   D. Go through food packages with her, and ask her to evaluate sodium in these foods.

8. In follow-up to a nutrition counseling session about increasing calorie intake, you find a client is not eating much. Which of the following is NOT a possible obstacle?

   A. The client has little appetite.
   B. The client has started a new medication that makes her nauseous.
   C. The client is alert and hungry at mealtimes.
   D. The client has lost her dentures and can't chew foods well.

9. The most effective education is delivered:

   A. In small chunks, over time
   B. In a lengthy session, all at once
   C. In writing only
   D. On bulletin boards

10. Which of the following is a good way to reinforce dietary change?
    A. Post a list of unhealthy foods.
    B. Disregard cultural and emotional factors that influence diet.
    C. Notice when a client implements a dietary change at any meal, and provide praise.
    D. Point out mistakes as often as possible.

Continuous quality improvement (CQI) is a customized approach to quality management. By understanding concepts and principles, a dietary manager can then implement CQI on the job.

After completing this chapter, you should be able to:

- Define terms related to quality management.
- Explain how regulations influence the quality management process.
- List the steps in continuous quality improvement.
- Identify the role of a dietary manager in the quality management process.

As a manager of a variety of food services and/or clinical care, a dietary manager needs to be concerned with quality. **Quality** is quite simply excellence in services and care. High-quality care meets or exceeds client expectations. It results in the best possible outcomes in a healthcare environment.

A popular approach to quality management is called **continuous quality improvement (CQI)**. The CQI approach has several characteristics:

- CQI focuses on clients and what they need, rather than on workers or departments and what they do.

- CQI uses the *systems approach* to understanding how services are provided. A systems approach defines a series of tasks that connect to make something happen. Connections tend to cross departments, involving many people. In other words, CQI proceeds on the assumption that the work of many individuals and/or departments comes together to create a system for accomplishing something the client needs. An example would be serving a meal tray, or obtaining laboratory blood tests.

- Another premise of CQI is that the process of accomplishing a task can be flawed, and usually can be improved.

- CQI also assumes that because of the systems and process focus, interdisciplinary teamwork is required to accomplish results. Furthermore, teamwork is required to test and manage quality.

- CQI emphasizes using data that can be defined and measured. It is objective and scientific.

- CQI is a proactive, ongoing activity. In other words, we do not wait for a problem to occur. Instead, we analyze our processes for serving clients *continuously*, and look for ways to improve these processes.

CQI uses some key terminology. One term is outcome. An **outcome** is the end result of work. In a healthcare environment, a health outcome describes the consequences of clinical interventions. For instance, if members of the healthcare team work together to improve a client's nutritional status, what happens to that client's nutritional status is the outcome of the clinical care plan. **Quality indicators (QIs)** are measures of outcomes. According to CMS, an indicator is "a key clinical value or quality characteristic used to measure, over time, the performance, processes, and outcomes of an organization or some component of healthcare delivery." As you can see by this definition, indicators are designed to facilitate collection and analysis of data. They are objective and measurable.

A general process for implementing CQI in healthcare uses two acronyms: FOCUS and PDCA. FOCUS means:

> **F**- Find a process to improve
>
> **O**- Organize to improve a process
>
> **C**- Clarify what is known
>
> **U**- Understand variation
>
> **S**- Select a process improvement

Once you have selected a process to improve, the next acronym relates to the plan itself. PDCA means:

> **P**- Plan: Decide what you will do to improve the process. Decide what information you will collect, and how you will measure outcomes.
>
> **D**- Do: Make the improvements.
>
> **C**- Check: Collect and review data, and evaluate how the plan is working.
>
> **A**- Act: Act on what you have learned. If you have made a successful improvement, make sure it becomes part of your policies and procedures. If not, try an alternate plan.

REGULATORY INFLUENCES ON QUALITY INDICATORS

Any institution subject to CMS regulations is concerned with many aspects of quality management as defined by these regulations. CMS lists specific quality indicators for use in ongoing monitoring, as shown in Figure 17.1. The regulations standardize these QIs as a quality evaluation tool for individual institutions, as well as for regulatory surveillance. Surveyors use a Resident Level QI Summary and a Facility QI Summary in reviews of longterm care facilities. The *Resident Level QI Summary* identifies current and past residents and shows applicable quality indicators. This Resident Summary can help managers in an institution focus on residents who need intervention. It may also help surveyors decide where to focus their attention. Based on QIs present, surveyors may pursue specific investigations to understand whether quality issues exist.

Figure 17.1

QUALITY INDICATORS USED BY CMS

Incidence of new fractures

Prevalence of falls

Prevalence of behavioral symptoms affecting others

Prevalence of symptoms of depression

Prevalence of symptoms of depression without antidepressant therapy

Use of nine or more different medications

Incidence of cognitive impairment

Prevalence of bladder or bowel incontinences

Prevalence of occasional or frequent bladder or bowel incontinence without a toileting plan

Prevalence of indwelling catheter

Prevalence of fecal impaction

Prevalence of urinary tract infections

Prevalence of weight loss

Prevalence of tube feeding

Prevalence of dehydration

Prevalence of bedfast residents

Incidence of decline in activities of daily living

Incidence of decline in range of motion

Prevalence of antipsychotic use, in the absence of psychotic or related conditions

Prevalence of antianxiety/hypnotic use

Prevalence of hypnotic use more than two times in the last week

Prevalence of daily physical restraints

Prevalence of little or no activity

Likewise, facility managers can investigate these. For example, if there are many residents experiencing weight loss, a dietary manager should be one of the individuals asking why this is occurring. CMS has designed investigative protocols for unintended weight loss, which appear in Figure 17.2. Another protocol, for hydration, appears in Figure 17.3. Yet another protocol, for the investigation of dining and food service, appears in Figure 17.4. If pressure ulcers are prevalent, another investigative protocol specifically for pressure ulcers may be used. (Figures mentioned begin on page 382.)

An *investgative protocol* is a guide to examining quality as it relates to a specific quality indicator. The presence of a quality indicator is not necessarily problematic in and of itself. For example, tube feeding is a quality indicator. Tube feeding can be a positive step towards improving a client's nutritional status. However, it is a red flag for investigation because we want to be sure the feeding is appropriate and necessary, and that it is being managed effectively. The investigative protocol helps managers evaluate these aspects of feeding. Investigative protocols are used by surveyors evaluating a facility, but should also be used by managers within the faculty.

A *Facility QI Summary* provides a sense of the overall quality of care in an institution. Statistical analysis also compares these results from one institution to another and assigns percentile rankings. Consumers may review this type of information when evaluating longterm care facilities. For example, Medicare maintains a public listing of quality findings for longterm care facilities nationwide, which members of the public may search on the Medicare website (see Appendix A for the address).

The first section of the CMS Quality of Care regulations looks at what are called **activities of daily living (ADL)**, which are routine tasks for self-care, such as getting dressed or eating. The regulations place much emphasis on enabling the resident to maintain or improve these abilities, and preventing decline. The dietitian/dietary manager must identify risk factors for a decline in residents' eating skills and show how these risk factors are being addressed. For example, enough staff time and assistance must be given to monitor residents' eating abilities. Additionally, the use of appropriate assistive devices and seating arrangements/setting must be addressed. When appropriate, treatment and services must be provided to improve a resident's eating skills.

Regulations appear in a document called *Survey Procedures for Long Term Care Facilities*. Besides providing investigative protocols such as those in Figures 17.2 through 17.4, this document provides a detailed investigative protocol for surveying dining services. CMS guidelines use "**F-tag**" numbers to identify specific guidance. For example, tags F321 and F322 address tube feeding. These appear in Figure 17.5. Tags F325 and F326 address nutrition, as shown in Figure 17.6. Tags F360 through F372 address dietary services, including staffing, menus, therapeutic diets, frequency of meals, and sanitation. These appear in Figure 17.7. Survey procedures are subject to revision, so please check with your facility administrator and/or the CMS website for current standards. (Figures 17.2 through 17.7 appear at the end of this chapter.)

A dietary manager is involved in many quality management issues. Remember that interdisciplinary effort is a strong focus of quality management. Thus, neither surveyors nor administrators divide up CMS regulations and hand a section to each manager. Instead, dietary managers can expect to work closely with nursing and other personnel to assure that a facility meets regulations and manages quality.

THE SURVEY PROCESS

As part of its enforcement effort, CMS and its contracted state agencies conduct on-site surveys of healthcare institutions. Each time a team of surveyors arrives to evaluate compliance of a healthcare facility with CMS regulations, all managers become involved. A survey is typically unannounced, and may occur on any day of the week. A standard survey is designed to review compliance with CMS regulations, including all the detail of the various F-tags. According to guidance from CMS, surveyors are examining:

- Compliance with residents' rights and quality of life requirements
- The accuracy of residents' comprehensive assessments and the adequacy of care plans based on these assessments

- The quality of care and services furnished, as measured by indicators of medical, nursing, rehabilitative care and drug therapy, dietary and nutrition services, activities and social participation, sanitation and infection control
- The effectiveness of the physical environment to empower residents, accommodate resident needs, and maintain resident safety, including whether requested room variances meet health, safety, and quality of life needs for the affected residents

Because a survey could occur at any time, a dietary manager in a longterm care facility should always be prepared for a survey. In other words, a dietary manager needs to manage the entire quality process from day to day, and assure that standards are being met. A dietary manager needs to become very familiar with regulations that apply in the workplace, and monitor compliance and quality indicators. It is also important to keep up-to-date with changes in relevant regulations.

At the time of a survey, a dietary manager may be asked to provide documentation and information pertinent to the survey. Surveyors will focus on quality indicators. They will review medical records and interview residents. Part of the survey will include a detailed tour of dietary areas. A dietary manager should accompany a surveyor and cooperate fully. When the survey concludes, the survey team will state any deficiencies noted and reference F-tag numbers. If a problem is identified, the dietary manager and other members of the interdisciplinary team need to follow up promptly and effectively to correct them. In all, a dietary manager plays a critical role in assuring that quality of dietary services meets the needs of clients, and that the end results of care are excellent.

Figure 17.2

CMS INVESTIGATIVE PROTOCOL FOR UNINTENDED WEIGHT LOSS

OBJECTIVES:

▶ To determine if the identified weight loss is avoidable or unavoidable; and

▶ To determine the adequacy of the facility's response to the weight loss.

USE:

Utilize this protocol for a sampled resident with unintended weight loss.

PROCEDURES:

▶ Observations/interviews conducted as part of this procedure should be recorded on the HCFA-805 if they pertain to a specific sampled resident and on the HCFA-807 if they relate to general observations of the dining service/dining room.

▶ Determine if the resident was assessed for conditions that may have put the resident at risk for unintended weight loss such as the following:

> Cancer, renal disease, diabetes, depression, chronic obstructive pulmonary disease, Parkinson's disease, Alzheimer's disease, malnutrition, infection, dehydration, constipation, diarrhea, Body Mass Index (BMI) below 19, dysphagia, chewing and swallowing problems, edentulous, ill fitting dentures, mouth pain, taste/sensory changes, bedfast, totally dependent for eating, pressure ulcer, abnormal laboratory values (review in accordance with the facility's laboratory norms) associated with malnutrition (serum albumin, plasma transferrin, magnesium, hct/hgb, BUN/creatinine ratio, potassium, cholesterol), and use of medications such as diuretics, laxatives, and cardiovascular agents.

NOTE: Amputation of a body part will contribute to a significant decrease in previously targeted weight range. Once the new weight goals are established the resident should be assessed within the parameters of the unintended weight loss investigative protocol.

NOTE: Body Mass Index (BMI) estimates total body mass and is highly correlated with the amount of body fat. It provides important information about body composition, making it a useful indicator of nutritional status. BMI is easy to calculate because only information about height and weight are needed.

BMI = weight (lbs.)/height (inches squared) x 705

▶ Determine if the facility has assessed the resident's nutritive and fluid requirements, dining assistance needs, such as assistive devices, food cultural/religious preferences, food allergies, and frequency of meals.

▶ Review all related information and documentation to look for evidence of identified causes of the condition or problem. This inquiry should include interviews with appropriate facility staff and healthcare practitioners, who by level of training and knowledge of the resident should know of, or be able to provide information about the causes of a resident's condition or problem.

▶ Determine if the care plan was developed utilizing the clinical conditions and risk factors identified in the assessment for unintended weight loss. Were the care plan interventions, such as oral supplements, enteral feeding, alternative eating schedule, liberalized diet, nutrient supplements, adaptive utensils, assistance and/or increased time to eat developed to provide an aggressive program of consistent intervention by all appropriate staff?

▶ Determine if the care plan was evaluated and revised based on the response, outcomes, and needs of the resident.

NOTE: If a resident is at an end of life stage and has an advance directive according to State law, (or a decision has been made by the resident's surrogate or representative in accordance with State law) or the resident has reached an end of life stage in which minimal amounts of nutrients are being consumed or intake has ceased, and all appropriate efforts have been made to encourage and provide intake, then the weight loss may be an expected outcome and may not constitute non-compliance with the requirement for maintaining nutritional parameters. Conduct observations to verify that palliative interventions, as described in the plan of care, are being implemented and revised as necessary, to meet the needs/choices of the resident in order to maintain the resident's comfort and quality of life.

FIGURE 17.2 CONT'D... INVESTIGATIVE PROTOCOL FOR UNINTENDED WEIGHT LOSS

If the facility has failed to provide the palliative care, cite non-compliance with 42 CFR 483.25, F309, Quality of Care.

▶ Observe the delivery of care as described in the care plan (such as staff providing assistance and/or encouragement during dining; serving food as planned with attention to portion sizes, preferences, nutritional supplements, and/or between-meal snacks) to determine if the interventions identified in the care plan have been implemented. Use the Dining and Food Service Investigative Protocol to make this determination.

DETERMINATION OF COMPLIANCE:

▶ Compliance with 42 CFR 483.25 (I), F325, Nutrition

> For this resident, the unintended weight loss is unavoidable if the facility properly assessed, care planned, implemented the care plan, evaluated the resident outcome, and revised the care plan as needed. If not, the weight loss is avoidable; cite at F325.

▶ Compliance with 42 CFR 483.25, F309, Quality of Care:

> For the resident who is in an end-of-life stage and palliative interventions, as described in the plan of care, are being implemented and revised as necessary, to meet the needs/choices of the resident in order to maintain the resident's comfort and quality of life, then for this resident, in the area of palliative care,

the facility is compliant with this requirement. If not, cite at F309.

▶ Compliance with 42 CFR 483.20(b)(1) and (2), F272, Comprehensive Assessments:

> For this resident in the area of unintended weight loss, the facility is compliant with this requirement if they assessed the factors that put the resident at risk for weight loss. If not, cite at F272.

▶ Compliance with 42 CFR 483.20(k)(1), F279, Comprehensive Care Plans:

> For this resident in the area of unintended weight loss, the facility is compliant with this requirement if they developed a care plan that includes measurable objectives and timetables to meet the resident's needs as identified in the resident's assessment. If not, cite at F279.

▶ Compliance with 42 CFR 483.20(k)(3)(ii), F 282, Provision of care in accordance with the care plan:

> For this resident in the area of unintended weight loss, the facility is compliant with this requirement if qualified persons implemented the resident's care plan. If not, cite at F282.

Source: CMS. Survey Procedures for Long Term Care Facilities

Figure 17.3

CMS INVESTIGATIVE PROTOCOL FOR HYDRATION

OBJECTIVES:
- To determine if the facility identified risk factors which lead to dehydration and developed an appropriate preventative care plan; and

- To determine if the facility provided the resident with sufficient fluid intake to maintain proper hydration and health.

USE:
Use this protocol for the following situations:

- A sampled resident who flagged for the sentinel event of dehydration on the Resident Level Summary;

- A sampled resident who has one or more QI conditions identified on the Resident Level Summary, such as:

  #11 - Fecal impaction;
  #12 - Urinary tract infections;
  #13 - Weight loss;
  #14 - Tube feeding;
  #17 - Decline in ADLs;
  #24 - Pressure Ulcer

- A sampled resident who was discovered to have any of the following risk factors: vomiting/diarrhea resulting in fluid loss, elevated temperatures and/or infectious processes, dependence on staff for the provision of fluid intake, use of medications including diuretics, laxatives, and cardiovascular agents, renal disease, dysphagia, a history of refusing fluids, limited fluid intake or lacking the sensation of thirst.

PROCEDURES:
- Observations/interviews conducted as part of this procedure should be recorded on the HCFA-805 and/or the HCFA-807.

- Determine if the resident was assessed to identify risk factors that can lead to dehydration, such as those listed above and also whether there were abnormal laboratory test values which may be an indicator of dehydration.

NOTE: A general guideline for determining baseline daily fluid needs is to multiply the resident's body weight in kilograms (kg) x 30 ml (2.2 lbs = 1 kg), except for residents with renal or cardiac distress, or other restrictions based on physician orders. An excess of fluids can be detrimental for these residents.

- Determine if an interdisciplinary care plan was developed utilizing the clinical conditions and risk factors identified, taking into account the amount of fluid that the resident requires. If the resident is receiving enteral nutritional support, determine if the tube feeding orders included a sufficient amount of free water, and whether the water and feeding are being administered in accordance with physician orders?

- Observe the care delivery to determine if the interventions identified in the care plan have been implemented as described.

   What is the resident's response to the interventions? Do staff provide the necessary fluids as described in the plan? (Do the fluids provided contribute to dehydration, for example, caffeinated beverages, alcohol?) Was the correct type of fluid provided with a resident with dysphagia?

   Is the resident able to reach, pour and drink fluids without assistance and is the resident consuming sufficient fluids? If not, are staff providing the fluids according to the care plan?

   Is the resident's room temperature (heating mechanism) contributing to dehydration? If so, how is the facility addressing this issue?

   If the resident refuses water, are alternative fluids offered that are tolerable to the resident?

   Are the resident's beverage preferences identified and honored at meals?

   Do staff encourage the resident to drink? Are they aware of the resident's fluid needs? Are staff providing fluids during and between meals?

   Determine how the facility monitors to assure that the resident maintains fluid parameters as planned. If the facility is monitoring the intake and output of the resident, review the record to determine if the fluid goals or calculated fluid needs were met consistently.

- Review all related information and documentation to look for evidence of identified causes of the condition or

---

FIGURE 17.3 CONT'D... INVESTIGATIVE PROTOCOL FOR HYDRATION

problem. This inquiry should include interviews with appropriate facility staff and healthcare practitioners, who by level of training and knowledge of the resident, should know of, or be able to provide information about the causes of a resident's condition or problem.

NOTE: If a resident is at an end of life stage and has an advance directive, according to State law, (or a decision has been made by the resident's surrogate or representative, in accordance with State law) or the resident has reached an end of life stage in which minimal amounts of fluids are being consumed or intake has ceased, and all appropriate efforts have been made to encourage and provide intake, then dehydration may be an expected outcome and does not constitute non-compliance with the requirement for hydration. Conduct observations to verify that palliative interventions, as described in the plan of care, are being implemented and revised as necessary, to meet the needs/choices of the resident in order to maintain the resident's comfort and quality of life. If the facility has failed to provide the palliative care, cite non-compliance with 42 CFR 483.25, F309, Quality of Care.

▶ Determine if the care plan is evaluated and revised based on the response, outcomes, and needs of the resident.

DETERMINATION OF COMPLIANCE:

▶ Compliance with 42 CFR 483.25(j), F327, Hydration:

For this resident, the facility is compliant with this requirement to maintain proper hydration if they properly assessed, care planned, implemented the care plan, evaluated the resident outcome, and revised the care plan as needed. If not, cite at F327.

▶ Compliance with 42 CFR 483.20(b)(1) & (2), F272, Comprehensive Assessments:

For this resident in the area of hydration, the facility is compliant with this requirement if they assessed factors that put the resident at risk for dehydration, whether chronic or acute. If not, cite at F272.

▶ Compliance with 42 CFR 483.20(k)(1), F279, Comprehensive Care Plans:

For this resident in the area of hydration, the facility is compliant with this requirement if they developed a care plan that includes measurable objectives and timetables to meet the resident's needs as identified in the resident's assessment. If not, cite at F279.

▶ Compliance with 483.20(k)(3)(ii), F 282, Provision of care in accordance with the care plan:

For this resident in the area of hydration, the facility is compliant with this requirement if qualified persons implemented the resident's care plan. If not, cite at F282.

Source: CMS. Survey Procedures for Long Term Care Facilities

Figure 17.4

CMS INVESTIGATIVE PROTOCOL FOR DINING AND FOOD SERVICE

OBJECTIVES:

- To determine if each resident is provided with nourishing, palatable, attractive meals that meet the resident's daily nutritional and special dietary needs;

- To determine if each resident is provided services to maintain or improve eating skills; and

- To determine if the dining experience enhances the resident's quality of life and is supportive of the resident's needs, including food service and staff support during dining.

USE:

This protocol will be used for:

- All sampled residents identified with malnutrition, unintended weight loss, mechanically altered diet, pressure sores/ulcers, and hydration concerns; and

- Food complaints received from residents, families and others.

GENERAL CONSIDERATIONS:

- Use this protocol at two meals during the survey, preferably the noon and evening meals.

- Record information on the HCFA-805 if it pertains to a specific sampled resident, or on the HCFA-807 if it relates to the general observations of the dining service/dining room.. Discretely observe all residents, including sampled residents, during meals keeping questions to a minimum to prevent disruption in the meal service.

- Identify for each sampled resident being observed, any special needs and the interventions planned to meet their needs. Using the facility's menu, record what is planned in writing to be served to the resident at the meal observed.

- Conduct observations of food preparation and quality of meals.

PROCEDURES:

1. During the meal service, observe the dining room and/or resident's room for the following:

    - Comfortable sound levels;

    - Adequate illumination, furnishings, ventilation; absence of odors; and sufficient space;

    - Tables adjusted to accommodate wheelchairs, etc.; and

    - Appropriate hygiene provided prior to meals.

2. Observe whether each resident is properly prepared for meals, for example:

    - Resident's eyeglasses, dentures, and/or hearing aids are in place;

    - Proper positioning in chair, wheelchair, gerichair, etc. at an appropriate distance from the table (tray table and bed at appropriate height and position); and

    - Assistive devices/utensils identified in care plans provided and used as planned.

3. Observe the food service for:

    - Appropriateness of dishes and flatware for each resident. (Single use disposable dining ware is not used except in an emergency and, other appropriate dining activities.) Each resident (except those with fluid restriction) has an appropriate place setting with water and napkin;

    - Whether meals are attractive, palatable, served at appropriate temperatures and are delivered to residents in a timely fashion.

        Did the meals arrive 30 minutes or more past the scheduled meal time?

        If a substitute was needed, did it arrive more than 15 minutes after the request for a substitute?

    - Are diet cards, portion sizes, preferences, and condiment requests being honored?

4. Determine whether residents are being promptly assisted to eat or provided necessary assistance/cueing in a timely manner after their meal is served.

    - Note whether residents at the same table (or in resident room's) are being served and assisted concurrently.

FIGURE 17.4 CONT'D... INVESTIGATIVE PROTOCOL FOR DINING AND FOOD SERVICE

5. Determine if the meals served were palatable, attractive, nutritious and met the needs of the resident. Note the following:

   ▶ Whether the resident voiced concerns regarding the taste, temperature, quality, quantity and appearance of the meal served;

   ▶ Whether mechanically altered diets, such as pureed, were prepared and served as separate entree items (except when combined food: such as stews, casseroles, etc.);

   ▶ Whether attempts to determine the reason(s) for the refusal and a substitute of equal nutritive value was provided, if the resident refused/rejected food served; and

   ▶ Whether food placement, colors, and textures were in keeping with the resident's needs or deficits (e.g., residents with vision or swallowing deficits).

   Sample Tray Procedure

   If residents complain about the palatability/temperature of food served, the survey team coordinator may request a test meal to obtain quantitative data to assess the complaints. Send the meal to the unit that is the greatest distance from the kitchen or to the affected unit or dining room. Check food temperature and palatability of the test meal at about the time the last resident on the unit is served and begins eating.

6. Observe for institutional medication pass practices that interfere with the quality of the residents' dining experience. This does not prohibit the administration of medications during meal service for medications that are necessary to be given at a meal, nor does this prohibit a medication to be given during a meal upon request of a resident who is accustomed to taking the medication with the meal, as long as it has been determined that this practice does not interfere with the effectiveness of the medication.

   ▶ Has the facility attempted to provide medications at times and in a manner to support the dining experience of the resident, such as:

   Pain medications being given prior to meals so that meals could be eaten in comfort;

   Foods served are not routinely or unnecessarily used as a vehicle to administer medications (mixing the medications with potatoes or other entrees).

7. Determine if the sampled resident consumed adequate amounts of food as planned.

   ▶ Determine if the facility is monitoring the foods/fluids consumed. You may use procedures used by the facility to determine percentage of food consumed, if available, otherwise, determine the percentage of food consumed using the following point system:

   Each food item served except for water, coffee, tea, or condiments equals one point. Example: Breakfast: juice, cereal, milk, bread and butter, coffee (no points) equals four points. If the resident consumes all four items in the amount served, the resident consumes 100% of breakfast. If the resident consumes two of the four food items served, then 50% of the breakfast would have been consumed. If three-fourths of a food item is consumed, give one point; for one half consumed, give .5 points; for one- fourth or less, give no points. Total the points consumed x 100 and divide by the number of points given for that meal to give the percentage of meal consumed. Use these measurements when determining the amount of liquids consumed: Liquid measurements: 8 oz. cup = 240 cc, 6 oz. cup = 180 cc, 4 oz. cup = 120 cc, 1 oz. cup = 30 cc.

   Compare your findings with the facility's documentation to determine if the facility has accurately recorded the intake. Ask the staff if these findings are consistent with the resident's usual intake; and

   Note whether plates are being returned to the kitchen with 75% or more of food not eaten.

FIGURE 17.4 CONT'D... INVESTIGATIVE PROTOCOL FOR DINING AND FOOD SERVICE

8. If concerns are noted with meal service, preparation, quality of meals, etc., interview the person(s) responsible for dietary services to determine how the staff are assigned and monitored to assure meals are prepared according to the menu, that the meals are delivered to residents in a timely fashion, and at proper temperature, both in the dining rooms/areas and in resident rooms.

NOTE: If concerns are identified in providing monitoring by supervisory staff during dining or concerns with assistance for residents to eat, evaluate nursing staffing in accord with 42 CFR 483.30(a), F353, and quality of care at 42 CFR 483.25(a)(2) & (3).

DETERMINATION OF COMPLIANCE:

▶ Compliance with 42 CFR 483.35(d)(1)(2), F364, Food

> The facility is compliant with this requirement when each resident receives food prepared by methods that conserve nutritive value, palatable, attractive and at the proper temperatures. If not, cite F364.

▶ Compliance with 42 CFR 483.35(b), F362, Dietary services, sufficient staff

> The facility is compliant with this requirement if they have sufficient staff to prepare and serve palatable and attractive, nutritionally adequate meals at proper temperatures. If not, cite F362.

NOTE: If serving food is a function of the nursing service, rather than dietary, refer to 42 CFR 483.30(a) F353.

▶ Compliance with 42 CFR 483.15(h)(1), F252, Environment

> The facility is compliant with this requirement if they provide a homelike environment during the dining services that enhances the resident's quality of life. If not, cite F252.

▶ Compliance with 42 CFR 483.70(g)(1)(2)(3)(4), F464, Dining and Resident Activities

> The facility is compliant with this requirement if they provide adequate lighting, ventilation, furnishings and space during the dining services. If not, cite F464.

Source: CMS. Survey Procedures for Long Term Care Facilities

CMS F-Tags Addressing Tube Feeding

F321 and **F322** (g) Naso-gastric tubes

Based on the comprehensive assessment of a resident, the facility must ensure that—

(1) A resident who has been able to eat enough alone or with assistance is not fed by naso-gastric tube unless the resident's clinical condition demonstrates that use of a naso-gastric tube was unavoidable and

(2) A resident who is fed by a naso-gastric or gastrostomy tube receives the appropriate treatment and services to prevent aspiration pneumonia, diarrhea, vomiting, dehydration, metabolic abnormalities, and nasalpharyngeal ulcers and to restore, if possible, normal eating skills.

INTENT: §483.25(G)

The intent of this regulation is that a naso-gastric tube feeding is utilized only after adequate assessment, and the resident's clinical condition makes this treatment necessary.

GUIDELINES: §483.25(G)

This corresponds to MDS, section L; MDS 2.0 sections G, K, P when specified for use by the State.

This requirement is also intended to prevent the use of tube feeding when ordered over the objection of the resident. Decisions about the appropriateness of tube feeding for a resident are developed with the resident or his/her family, surrogate or representative as part of determining the care plan.

Complications in tube feeding are not necessarily the result of improper care, but assessment for the potential for complications and care and treatment are provided to prevent complications in tube feeding by the facility.

Clinical conditions demonstrating that nourishment via an naso-gastric tube is unavoidable include:

- The inability to swallow without choking or aspiration, i.e., in cases of Parkinson's disease, pseudobulbar palsy, or esophageal diverticulum;

- Lack of sufficient alertness for oral nutrition (e.g., resident comatose); and

- Malnutrition not attributable to a single cause or causes that can be isolated and reversed. There is documented evidence that the facility has not been able to maintain or improve the resident's nutritional status through oral intake.

PROBES: §483.25(G)

For sampled residents who, upon admission to the facility, were not tube fed and now have a feeding tube, was tube feeding unavoidable? To determine if the tube feeding was unavoidable, assess the following:

- Did the facility identify the resident at risk for malnutrition?

- What did the facility do to maintain oral feeding, prior to inserting a feeding tube? Did staff provide enough assistance in eating? Did staff cue resident as needed, assist with the use of assistive devices, or feed the resident, if necessary?

- Is the resident receiving therapy to improve or enhance swallowing skills, as need is identified in the comprehensive assessment?

- Was an assessment done to determine the cause of decreased oral intake/weight loss or malnutrition?

- If there was a dietitian consultation, were recommendations followed?

For all sampled residents who are tube fed:

- Is the NG tube properly placed?

- Are staff responsibilities for providing enteral feedings clearly assigned (i.e., who administers the feeding, formula, amount, feeding intervals, flow rate)?

- Do staff monitor feeding complications (e.g., diarrhea, gastric distension, aspiration) and administer corrective actions to allay complications (e.g., changing rate of formula administration)?

FIGURE 17.5 CONT'D... CMS F-TAGS ADDRESSING TUBE FEEDING

▶ Are there negative consequences of tube use (e.g., agitation, depression, self-extubation, infections, aspiration and restraint use without a medical reason for the restraint)?

▶ When long term use is anticipated, is G tube placement considered?

Is the potential for complications from feedings minimized by:

▶ Use of a small bore, flexible naso-gastric tube, unless contraindicated;

▶ Securely attached the tube to the nose/face;

▶ Checking for correct tube placement prior to beginning a feeding or administering medications and after episodes of vomiting or suctioning;

▶ Checking a resident with a newly inserted gastric tube for gastric residual volume every 2-4 hours until the resident has demonstrated an ability to empty his/her stomach;

▶ Properly elevating the resident's head;

▶ Providing the type, rate and volume of the feeding as ordered;

▶ Using universal precautions and clean technique and as per facility/manufacturer's directions when stopping, starting, flushing, and giving medications through the tube;

▶ Using hang time recommendations by the manufacturer to prevent excessive microbial growth;

▶ Implement the procedures to ensure cleanliness of supplies, e.g. irrigating syringes changed on a regular bases as per facility policy. It is not necessary to change the irrigating syringe each time it is used;

▶ Using a pump equipped with a functional alarm (if pump used);

▶ The facility's criteria for determining that a resident may be able to return to eating by mouth (e.g., a resident whose Parkinson's symptoms have been controlled);

▶ There are sampled residents meet these criteria;

▶ If so, the facility has assisted them in returning to normal eating; and

▶ Identify if resident triggers RAPs for feeding tubes, nutritional status, and dehydration/fluid maintenance. Consider whether the RAPs were used to assess causal factors for decline, potential for decline and lack of improvement.

Source: CMS. Survey Procedures for Long Term Care Facilities

Figure 17.6

CMS F-Tags Addressing Nutrition

(i) Nutrition.

Based on a resident's comprehensive assessment, the facility must ensure that a resident—

F325 (1) Maintains acceptable parameters of nutritional status, such as body weight and protein levels, unless the resident's clinical condition demonstrates that this is not possible; and

F326 (2) Receives a therapeutic diet when there is a nutritional problem

INTENT §483.25(I)

The intent of this regulation is to assure that the resident maintains acceptable parameters of nutritional status, taking into account the resident's clinical condition or other appropriate intervention, when there is a nutritional problem.

GUIDELINES: §483.25(I)

This corresponds to MDS, section L; MDS 2.0 sections G, I, J, K and L when specified for use by the State.

Parameters of nutritional status which are unacceptable include unplanned weight loss as well as other indices such as peripheral edema, cachexia and laboratory tests indicating malnourishment (e.g., serum albumin levels).

Weight: Since ideal body weight charts have not yet been validated for the institutionalized elderly, weight loss (or gain) is a guide in determining nutritional status. An analysis of weight loss or gain should be examined in light of the individual's former life style as well as the current diagnosis.

Suggested parameters for evaluating significance of unplanned and undesired weight loss are:

Interval	Significant Loss	Severe Loss
1 month	5%	Greater than 5%
3 months	7.5%	Greater than 7.5%
6 months	10%	Greater than 10%

The following formula determines percentage of loss:

$$\% \text{ of body weight loss} = \frac{\text{usual weight - actual weight}}{\text{usual weight}} \times 100$$

In evaluating weight loss, consider the resident's usual weight through adult life; the assessment of potential for weight loss; and care plan for weight management. Also, was the resident on a calorie restricted diet, or if newly admitted and obese, and on a normal diet, are fewer calories provided than prior to admission? Was the resident edematous when initially weighed, and with treatment, no longer has edema? Has the resident refused food?

Suggested laboratory values are:

Albumin >60 yr.: 3.4 - 4.8 g/dl (good for examining marginal protein depletion)

Plasma Transferrin >60 yr.:180-380 g/dl. (Rises with iron deficiency anemia. More persistent indicator of protein status.)

Hemoglobin	Males: 14-17 g/dl
	Females: 12-15 g/dl
Hematocrit	Males: 41 - 53
	Females: 36 - 46
Potassium	3.5 - 5.0 mEq/l
Magnesium	1.3 - 2.0 mEg/l

Some laboratories may have different "normals". Determine range for the specific laboratory.

Because some healthy elderly people have abnormal laboratory values, and because abnormal values can be expected in some disease processes, do not expect laboratory values to be within normal ranges for all residents. Consider abnormal values in conjunction with the resident's clinical condition and baseline normal values.

NOTE: There is no requirement that facilities order the tests referenced above.

Clinical Observations: Potential indicators of malnutrition are pale skin, dull eyes, swollen lips, swollen gums, swollen and/or

FIGURE 17.6 CONT'D... F-TAGS ADDRESSING NUTRITION

dry tongue with scarlet or magenta hue, poor skin turgor, cachexia, bilateral edema, and muscle wasting.

Risk factors for malnutrition are:

1. Drug therapy that may contribute to nutritional deficiencies such as:

   a. Cardiac glycosides;
   b. Diuretics;
   c. Anti-inflammatory drugs;
   d. Antacids (antacid overuse);
   e. Laxatives (laxative overuse);
   f. Psychotropic drug overuse;
   g. Anticonvulsants;
   h. Antineoplastic drugs;
   i. Phenothiazines;
   j. Oral hypoglycemics;

2. Poor oral health status or hygiene, eyesight, motor coordination, or taste alterations;
3. Depression or dementia;
4. Therapeutic or mechanically altered diet;
5. Lack of access to culturally acceptable foods;
6. Slow eating pace resulting in food becoming unpalatable, or in staff removing the tray before resident has finished eating; and
7. Cancer.

Clinical conditions demonstrating that the maintenance of acceptable nutritional status may not be possible to include, but are not limited to:

▶ Refusal to eat and refusal of other methods of nourishment;

▶ Advanced disease (e.g., cancer, malabsorption syndrome);

▶ Increased nutritional/caloric needs associated with pressure sores and wound healing (e.g., fractures, burns);

▶ Radiation or chemotherapy;

▶ Kidney disease, alcohol/drug abuse, chronic blood loss, hyperthyroidism;

▶ Gastrointestinal surgery; and

▶ Prolonged nausea, vomiting, diarrhea not relieved by treatment given according to accepted standards of practice.

"Therapeutic diet" means a diet ordered by a physician as part of treatment for a disease or clinical condition, to eliminate or decrease certain substances in the diet, (e.g., sodium) or to increase certain substances in the diet (e.g., potassium), or to provide food the resident is able to eat (e.g., a mechanically altered diet).

PROCEDURES: §483.25(I)

Determine if residents selected for a comprehensive review or focused review as appropriate, have maintained acceptable parameters of nutritional status. Where indicated by the resident's medical status, have clinically appropriate therapeutic diets been prescribed?

PROBES: §483.25(I)

For sampled residents whose nutritional status is inadequate, do clinical conditions demonstrate that maintenance of inadequate nutritional status was unavoidable:

▶ Did the facility identify factors that put the resident at risk for malnutrition?

▶ Identify if resident triggered RAPs for nutritional status, ADL functional/rehabilitation potential, feeding tubes, psychotropic drug use, and dehydration/fluid balance. Consider whether the RAPs were used to assess the causal factors for decline, potential for decline or lack of improvement.

▶ What routine preventive measures and care did the resident receive to address unique risk factors for malnutrition (e.g., provision of an adequate diet with supplements or modifications as indicated by nutrient needs)?

FIGURE 17.6 CONT'D... F-TAGS ADDRESSING NUTRITION

▶ Were staff responsibilities for maintaining nutritional status clear, including monitoring the amount of food the resident is eating at each meal and offering substitutes?

▶ Was this care provided consistently?

▶ Were individual goals of the plan of care periodically evaluated and if not met, were alternative approaches considered or attempted?

Source: CMS. Survey Procedures for Long Term Care Facilities

Figure 17.7

F-Tags Addressing Dietary Services

F360 §483.35 DIETARY SERVICES.
The facility must provide each resident with a nourishing, palatable, well-balanced diet that meets the daily nutritional and special dietary needs of each resident.

F361 (A) STAFFING.
The facility must employ a qualified dietitian either full-time, part-time, or on a consultant basis.

(1) If a qualified dietitian is not employed full-time, the facility must designate a person to serve as the director of food service who receives frequently scheduled consultation from a qualified dietitian.

(2) A qualified dietitian is one who is qualified based upon either registration by the Commission on Dietetic Registration of the American Dietetic Association, or on the basis of education, training, or experience in identification of dietary needs, planning, and implementation of dietary programs.

Intent: §483.35(a)
The intent of this regulation is to ensure that a qualified dietitian is utilized in planning, managing and implementing dietary service activities in order to assure that the residents receive adequate nutrition. A director of food services has no required minimum qualifications, but must be able to function collaboratively with a qualified dietitian in meeting the nutritional needs of the residents.

Guidelines: §483.35(a)
A dietitian qualified on the basis of education, training, or experience in identification of dietary needs, planning and implementation of dietary programs has experience or training which includes:

- Assessing special nutritional needs of geriatric and physically impaired persons;

- Developing therapeutic diets;

- Developing "regular diets" to meet the specialized needs of geriatric and physically impaired persons;

- Developing and implementing continuing education programs for dietary services and nursing personnel;

- Participating in interdisciplinary care planning;

- Budgeting and purchasing food and supplies; and

- Supervising institutional food preparation, service and storage.

Procedures: §483.35(a)
If resident reviews determine that residents have nutritional problems, determine if these nutritional problems relate to inadequate or inappropriate diet nutrition/assessment and monitoring. Determine if these are related to dietitian qualifications.

Probes: §483.35(a)
If the survey team finds problems in resident nutritional status:

- Do practices of the dietitian or food services director contribute to the identified problems in residents' nutritional status? If yes, what are they?

- What are the educational, training, and experience qualifications of the facility's dietitian?

F362 (B) SUFFICIENT STAFF.
The facility must employ sufficient support personnel competent to carry out the functions of the dietary service.

Guidelines: §483.35(b)
"Sufficient support personnel" is defined as enough staff to prepare and serve palatable, attractive, nutritionally adequate meals at proper temperatures and appropriate times and support proper sanitary techniques being utilized.

Procedures: §483.35(b)
For residents who have been triggered for a dining review, do they report that meals are palatable, attractive, served at the proper temperatures and at appropriate times?

Probes: §483.35(b)
Is food prepared in scheduled timeframes in accordance with established professional practices?

FIGURE 17.7 CONT'D... F-TAGS ADDRESSING DIETARY SERVICES

Observe food service:

Does food leave kitchen in scheduled timeframes? Is food served to residents in scheduled timeframes?

F563 (c) Menus and nutritional adequacy.

Menus must:

(1) Meet the nutritional needs of residents in accordance with the Recommended Dietary Allowances of the Food and Nutrition Board of the National Research Council, National Academy of Sciences;

(2) Be prepared in advance; and

(3) Be followed.

Intent: §483.35(c)(1)(2)(3)

The intent of this regulation is to assure that the meals served meet the nutritional needs of the resident in accordance with the recommended dietary allowances (RDAs) of the Food and Nutrition Board of the National Research Council, of the National Academy of Sciences. This regulation also assures that there is a prepared menu by which nutritionally adequate meals have been planned for the resident and followed.

Procedures: §483.35(c)(1)

▶ For sampled residents who have a comprehensive review or a focused review, as appropriate, observe if meals served are consistent with the planned menu and care plan in the amounts, types and consistency of foods served.

If the survey team observes deviation from the planned menu, review appropriate documentation from diet card, record review, and interviews with food service manager or dietitian to support reason(s) for deviation from the written menu.

Probes: §483.35(c)(1)

▶ Are residents receiving food in the amount, type, consistency and frequency to maintain normal body weight and acceptable nutritional values?

▶ If food intake appears inadequate based on meal observations, or resident's nutritional status is poor based on

resident review, determine if menus have been adjusted to meet the caloric and nutrient-intake needs of each resident.

▶ If a food group is missing from the resident's daily diet, does the facility have an alternative means of satisfying the resident's nutrient needs? If so, does the facility perform a follow-up?

Does the menu meet basic nutritional needs by providing daily food in the groups of the food pyramid system and based on individual nutritional assessment taking into account current nutritional recommendations?

NOTE: A standard meal planning guide (e.g., food pyramid) is used primarily for menu planning and food purchasing. It is not intended to meet the nutritional needs of all residents. This guide must be adjusted to consider individual differences. Some residents will need more due to age, size, gender, physical activity, and state of health. There are many meal planning guides from reputable sources, i.e., American Diabetes Association, American Dietetic Association, American Medical Association, or U.S. Department of Agriculture, that are available and appropriate for use when adjusted to meet each resident's needs.

Probes: §483.35(c)(2)

Are there preplanned menus for both regular and therapeutic diets?

Probes: §483.35(c)(3)

Is food served as planned? If not, why? There may be legitimate and extenuating circumstances why food may not be available on the day of the survey and must be considered before a concern is noted.

(d) Food.

Each resident receives and the facility provides:

F364 (1) Food prepared by methods that conserve nutritive value, flavor, and appearance;

(2) Food that is palatable, attractive, and at the proper temperature;

Figure 17.7 cont'd... F-Tags Addressing Dietary Services

F365 (3) Food prepared in a form designed to meet individual needs; and

F366 (4) Substitutes offered of similar nutritive value to residents who refuse food served.

Intent: §483.35(d)(1)(2)

The intent of this regulation is to assure that the nutritive value of food is not compromised and destroyed because of prolonged food storage, light, and air exposure; prolonged cooking of foods in a large volume of water and prolong holding on steam table, and the addition of baking soda. Food should be palatable, attractive, and at the proper temperature as determined by the type of food to ensure resident's satisfaction. Refer to §483.15(e) and/or §483.15(a).

Guidelines: §483.35(d)(1)

"Food-palatability" refers to the taste and/or flavor of the food.

"Food attractiveness" refers to the appearance of the food when served to residents.

Procedures: §483.35(d)(1)

Evidence for palatability and attractiveness of food, from day to day and meal to meal, may be strengthened through sources such as: additional observation, resident and staff interviews, and review of resident council minutes. Review nutritional adequacy in §483.25(i)(l).

Probes: §483.35(d)(1)(2)

Does food have a distinctly appetizing aroma and appearance, which is varied in color and texture?

Is food generally well seasoned (use of spices, herbs, etc.) and acceptable to residents?

Is food prepared in a way to preserve vitamins? Method of storage and preparation should cause minimum loss of nutrients.

Is food served at preferable temperature (hot foods are served hot and cold foods are served cold) as discerned by the resident and customary practice? Not to be confused with the proper holding temperature.

Intent: §483.35(d)(3)(4)

The intent of this regulation is to assure that food is served in a form that meets the resident's needs and satisfaction; and that the resident receives appropriate nutrition when a substitute is offered.

Procedures: §483.35(d)(3)(4)

Observe trays to assure that food is appropriate to resident according to assessment and care plan. Ask the resident how well the food meets their taste needs. Ask if the resident is offered or is given the opportunity to receive substitutes when refusing food on the original menu.

Probes: §483.35(d)(3)(4)

Is food cut, chopped, or ground for individual resident's needs?

Are residents who refuse food offered substitutes of similar nutritive value?

Guidelines: §483.35(d)(4)

A food substitute should be consistent with the usual and ordinary food items provided by the facility. For example, if a facility never serves smoked salmon, they would not be required to serve this as a food substitute; or the facility may, instead of grapefruit juice, substitute another citrus juice or vitamin C rich juice that the resident likes.

F367 (E) THERAPEUTIC DIETS.

Therapeutic diets must be prescribed by the attending physician.

Intent: §483.35(e)

The intent of this regulation is to assure that the resident receives and consumes foods in the appropriate form and/or the appropriate nutritive content as prescribed by a physician and/or assessed by the interdisciplinary team to support the treatment and plan of care.

Guidelines: §483.35(e)

"Therapeutic Diet" is defined as a diet ordered by a physician as part of treatment for a disease or clinical condition, or to eliminate or decrease specific nutrients in the diet, (e.g., sodium) or to increase specific nutrients in the diet (e.g., potassium), or to provide food the resident is able to eat (e.g., a mechanically altered diet).

FIGURE 17.7 CONT'D... F-TAGS ADDRESSING DIETARY SERVICES

"Mechanically altered diet" is one in which the texture of a diet is altered. When the texture is modified, the type of texture modification must be specific and part of the physicians' order.

Procedures: §483.35(e)

If the resident has inadequate nutrition or nutritional deficits that manifests into and/or are a product of weight loss or other medical problems, determine if there is a therapeutic diet that is medically prescribed.

Probes: §483.35(e)

Is the therapeutic diet that the resident receives prescribed by the physician?

Also, see §483.25(i), Nutritional Status.

F368 (F) FREQUENCY OF MEALS.

(1) Each resident receives and the facility provides at least three meals daily, at regular times comparable to normal mealtimes in the community.

(2) There must be no more than 14 hours between a substantial evening meal and breakfast the following day, except as provided in (4) below.

(3) The facility must offer snacks at bedtime daily.

(4) When a nourishing snack is provided at bedtime, up to 16 hours may elapse between a substantial evening meal and breakfast the following day if a resident group agrees to this meal span, and a nourishing snack is served.

Intent: §483.35(f)(1)(2)(3)(4)

The intent of this regulation is to assure that the resident receives his/her meals at times most accepted by the community and that there are not extensive time lapses between meals. This assures that the resident receives adequate and frequent meals.

Guidelines: §483.35(f)(1)(2)(3)(4)

A "substantial evening meal" is defined as an offering of three or more menu items at one time, one of which includes a

high-quality protein such as meat, fish, eggs, or cheese. The meal should represent no less than 20 percent of the day's total nutritional requirements.

"Nourishing snack" is defined as a verbal offering of items, single or in combination, from the basic food groups. Adequacy of the "nourishing snack" will be determined both by resident interviews and by evaluation of the overall nutritional status of residents in the facility, (e.g., Is the offered snack usually satisfying?)

Procedures: §483.35(f)(1)(2)(3)(4)

Observe meal times and schedules and determine if there is a lapse in time between meals. Ask for resident input on meal service schedules, to verify if there are extensive lapses in time between meals.

F369 (G) ASSISTIVE DEVICES.

The facility must provide special eating equipment and utensils for residents who need them.

Intent: §483.35(g)

The intent of this regulation is to provide residents with assistive devices to maintain or improve their ability to eat independently. For example, improving poor grasp by enlarging silverware handles with foam padding, aiding residents with impaired coordination or tremor by installing plate guards, or providing postural supports for head, trunk, and arms.

Procedures: §483.35(g)

Review sampled residents comprehensive assessment for eating ability. Determine if recommendations were made for adaptive utensils and if they were, determine if these utensils are available and utilized by resident. If recommended but not used, determine if this is by resident's choice. If utensils are not being utilized, determine when these were recommended and how their use is being monitored by the facility and if the staff is developing alternative recommendations.

Source: CMS. Survey Procedures for Long Term Care Facilities

Key Terms

Activities of daily living (ADL): routine tasks for self-care, such as getting dressed or eating

Continuous quality improvement (CQI): a popular approach to quality management that focuses on systems and processes and emphasizes teamwork

F-tags: labels for components of the CMS regulations

Outcome: the end result of work

Quality: excellence in services and care

Quality indicators (QIs): measures of outcomes

Key Points

- High-quality care meets or exceeds client expectations. It results in the best possible outcomes in a healthcare environment.

- CQI focuses on clients and what they need, rather than on workers or departments and what they do. It uses a systems approach. It emphasizes using data that can be defined and measured.

- A general process for implementing CQI in healthcare uses two acronyms: FOCUS and PDCA.

- Quality indicators (QIs) are measures of outcomes. CMS defines specific quality indicators for monitoring and investigating.

- A Facility QI Summary provides a sense of the overall quality of care in an institution.

- In CMS regulations, F-tags identify standards for nutrition, tube feeding, and dietary services.

- As part of its enforcement effort, CMS and its contracted state agencies conduct on-site surveys of healthcare institutions.

- A dietary manager needs to manage the entire quality process from day to day, and assure that standards are being met.

1. Which of the following is true of continuous quality improvement (CQI)?

   A. It emphasizes having each department take care of its own quality issues.
   B. It uses data that can be defined and measured.
   C. It is an occasional process, triggered when there is a problem.
   D. It focuses only on dietary services.

2. Which of the following is NOT an example of an outcome?

   A. Improved nutritional status as measured by serum tranferrin
   B. Weight gain
   C. Reduction in number of pressure ulcers
   D. A care plan for monitoring tube feeding

3. A Facility QI Summary:

   A. Provides a sense of the overall quality of care in an institution
   B. Lists F-tags a facility should comply with
   C. Lists F-tags a facility has not complied with
   D. Lists activities of daily living

4. Which of the following is an objective of the CMS investigative protocol for unintended weight loss (Figure 17.2)?

   A. To find out if the weight loss was greater than 10%
   B. To find out what the IBW is for each resident
   C. To find out how many calories a resident is consuming
   D. To find out whether the weight loss could have been avoided

5. Surveyors may use a point system to determine how much residents are consuming (Figure 17.4). In this system, if a resident eats two out of four items served at breakfast, we conclude that the resident has eaten:

   A. 10% of the meal
   B. 20% of the meal
   C. 50% of the meal
   D. 100% of the meal

6. According to CMS regulations (Figure 17.6), a significant amount of weight loss over three months is:

   A. 1% of body weight
   B. 2% of body weight
   C. 3% of body weight
   D. 7.5% of body weight

7. What do CMS regulations say about staffing for a dietary department (Figure 17.7)?
    A. Staff must all wear attractive uniforms
    B. Staff must work weekdays only
    C. Staffing must be adequate to provide palatable, nutritious meals at appropriate times
    D. Staffing must consist only of dietary managers

8. What do CMS regulations say about the dining environment (Figure 17.7)?
    A. It should be homelike and enhance the resident's quality of life
    B. It should be sterile to prevent foodborne illness
    C. It should be designed by an interior decorator
    D. It is irrelevant to dietary care

9. Which of the following is an example of an activity of daily living (ADL)?
    A. Feeding oneself
    B. Taking physical therapy
    C. Having a blood sample drawn
    D. Seeing the doctor

10. What do CMS regulations say about a resident who refuses a food (Figure 17.7)?
    A. Dietary services should weigh the food and record the refusal
    B. Dietary services should offer a substitute of similar nutritive value
    C. Dietary services should tell the resident to eat better
    D. Dietary services should recommend a tube feeding

Planning menus both for client groups and for individuals requires a synthesis of much of the information learned in this course. A dietary manager needs to be able to apply menu planning principles to a variety of needs.

After completing this chapter, you should be able to:

▶ Describe ways in which a menu must meet the needs of clients.

▶ List standards that may be used for assuring nutritional adequacy of menus.

▶ Explain how a variety of therapeutic diets can be served through a common menu.

▶ Explain how dietary staff may make modifications of individual menus.

▶ List and explain criteria for making a menu aesthetically pleasing.

▶ Describe the influence of regulations on menu planning.

In any institution, a menu is the fundamental tool for planning diets. It becomes the blueprint for what clients will eat. Knowing that many clients may have special therapeutic needs, a dietary manager needs to plan and manage a master menu in such a way that it meets the diet order of each client. Consider this example. Let's say that you plan to serve tuna noodle casserole at lunch tomorrow. Some of your clients need to follow sodium restrictions. Others are following diets that are controlled for saturated fat and cholesterol. Others are following portion-controlled diets for management of diabetes. Yet others are eating pureed foods. How can you manage this product in a way that you will be able to serve it to all these clients and meet their unique needs?

This is the type of question a manager must consider during the menu planning process. In quantity food production, it's important to offer food that will meet the needs of all clients. Besides having various therapeutic dietary needs, each client presents a unique cultural background and a personal set of food preferences. A dietary manager strives to serve these interests with a versatile and appealing menu.

Furthermore, an institutional menu is typically serving the same clients over and over again. Each of us has a strong need for variety in meals. A **cycle menu** is one that repeats itself over a defined period of time. For example, a menu that spans three weeks and then repeats itself is a three-week cycle menu. The first day of the cycle is called Cycle Day 1, which corresponds to a designated date. A cycle menu must offer variety.

Along with these considerations, a menu must meet the nutritional needs of clients. It must supply adequate calories, protein, carbohydrate, fat, vitamins, minerals, and fluid. Depending on the setting, specific nutritional standards may apply. For example, in a school participating in the USDA School Lunch

Program, a dietary manager needs to serve a menu that complies with USDA standards for this program (Chapter 5). In many healthcare institutions, a common standard for nutritional evaluation is the Recommended Dietary Allowances (RDAs). An analysis of RDAs is most effective when it spans a period of days. For example, if there is a seven-day cycle menu, we can analyze the percent of RDAs met for key nutrients, including vitamins and minerals, as averaged over seven days. This is a cumbersome task, and is best accomplished with the help of computer software designed for nutrient analysis. RDAs are designed for application to groups. However, RDA values vary based on age and sex. In addition, calorie needs can vary widely. In performing an RDA analysis, it's best to select the standards most representative of the group being served. For example, a menu for a preschool child care center can use the RDA standards for this age group. In another example, in a correctional facility, a special menu for a boot camp group involved in heavy physical activity may require very high calorie levels to be considered nutritionally adequate. When we offer variety, there tend to be certain days or meals that offer greater amounts of particular vitamins and minerals over time, and a composite RDA analysis reflects this. On the other hand, an analysis of school lunch menus must address the nutrients in menus for each individual meal. A typical standard uses one-third of daily nutrient needs. For detailed options in school menu planning, check the USDA Healthy Schools Meal Resource System listed in Appendix A.

Many menus also comply with the Dietary Guidelines for Americans, limiting total fat and saturated fat, for example. Another nutritional standard for use in menu planning is the Food Guide Pyramid. To verify compliance, simply total the number of servings in each group and compare it with the Food Pyramid recommendations. With certain therapeutic diets, it is not always possible to meet all nutritional needs. For example, a typical clear liquid diet is lacking in protein and calories, as well as major vitamins and minerals. A diet such as this one is not usually intended for long-term use. Its nutritional inadequacy is also noted in an institution's diet manual. Unless liquid nutritional supplements are incorporated, a full liquid menu is likewise inadequate in key nutrients.

DIET SPREADSHEETS

In an institution serving clients who follow a variety of therapeutic diets, a menu must be versatile enough to provide nutritious, satisfying meals on every diet. This detail is mapped out on a diet spreadsheet. A **diet spreadsheet** displays the menu offerings and portion sizes for each diet, for each meal, for each day of the cycle menu (if applicable). Figure 18.1 shows a segment of a diet spreadsheet for a lunch meal. Note that with the trend in liberalization of therapeutic diets in healthcare, diet spreadsheets are developed to be as simple as possible, with no more restriction than is therapeutically necessary. At the same time, the strategy of making all menus "healthy" means that menu planners strive to limit total fat, saturated fat, cholesterol, and sodium in even a general

Figure 18.1

SEGMENT OF A DIET SPREADSHEET – LUNCH FOR CYCLE DAY 3

General Diet	Sodium-Controlled Diet	Diabetic Diet	Renal Diet	Pureed Diet	Full Liquid Diet
Tossed salad w/ lowfat dressing	Tossed salad w/ lowfat dressing	Tossed salad w/ lowfat dressing	Tossed salad w/ low sodium dressing X 2	½ c. Pureed vegetable medley	1 c. Strained cream of chicken soup
Roast turkey sandwich: 3 oz turkey on wheat bun, with lettuce and tomato	Roast turkey sandwich: 3 oz turkey on wheat bun, with lettuce and tomato	Roast turkey sandwich: 3 oz turkey on wheat bun, with lettuce and tomato	Roast turkey 2 oz. turkey sandwich on wheat bun, with lettuce and low sodium mayo	Pureed turkey and rice portion with garnish	
Assorted fresh fruit	Assorted fresh fruit	Assorted fresh fruit	Fresh apple	½ c. Applesauce	1 c. Strained fruit juice
Fresh cookie	Fresh cookie	½ c. Sugar-free gelatin	½ c. Regular gelatin [count in fluid restriction]	½ c. Regular gelatin	½ c. Regular gelatin
Coffee, tea, or beverage of choice	Coffee, tea, or beverage of choice	Coffee, tea, or beverage of choice	½ c. Fruit punch [count in fluid restriction]	Coffee, tea, or beverage of choice	Coffee, tea, or beverage of choice
Skim or lowfat milk	Skim or lowfat milk	Skim or lowfat milk	Potassium and sodium free candy as desired, e.g. gum drops	Skim or lowfat milk	1 c. Milkshake
Condiments as desired	Mayo, sugar, pepper, herb-based sodium-free seasoning as desired (No potassium-based salt substitute without a physician's order.)	Sugar substitute, salt, pepper as desired	Low sodium mayo, herb-based sodium-free seasoning, sugar, pepper as desired (No potassium-based salt substitute without a physician's order.)	Condiments as desired	Condiments as desired
NOTES	Note that if a fresh, roast turkey product low in sodium is used, the same meat is appropriate on sodium-controlled menus	Adjust portion sizes of bread, fruit, and milk if needed for specific meal pattern or carbohydrate count	Mayo is not reduced for fat, as fat is an important source of calories in a renal diet. Omit tomato because it is high in potassium; add low-sodium mayo for extra fat calories	Adjust thickness of products as needed to meet individualized orders for National Dysphagia Diet	

(unrestricted) diet. Implementing healthful guidelines may also mean providing a variety of fruits and vegetables, including high-fiber foods in a menu, and more. Thus, a healthy "general" diet emerges that may be suitable for certain therapeutic needs as well.

In all, the goal is to keep a list of therapeutic diets reasonably short. This can lead to optimal health for all clients, while providing the best possible range of choices for each client. Management considerations apply, too. It is ideal to plan a menu in which many products are common to all diets. This minimizes the need to produce many different products at once, and also minimizes food waste. Sometimes, portion sizes vary among diets. Unique portion sizes are specified on the menus. A foodservice operation must be able to produce foods on a given menu in a manner that meets standards for quality and budget, while accommodating the unique therapeutic and nutritional needs of each client.

INDIVIDUAL MENUS

The menu-related needs of clients can vary, and are often quite specific. One client may be following a 150-gram carbohydrate controlled diet. Another may be combining a diet for diabetes with sodium restriction to help manage hypertension. Yet another may be following a specific diet for dysphagia, combined with a sodium restriction. One client may follow a general diet, but need to avoid citrus fruits due to an allergy. Another may be on a full liquid diet, with a lactose restriction due to a lactose intolerance. The possibilities are endless. Thus, it becomes clear that there is no such thing as a one-size-fits-all therapeutic menu. In fact, dietary caregivers need to adapt menus to clients' actual diet orders. At the same time, it is also important to tailor a menu to food preferences. How do we accomplish this? There are several solutions. Each interplays with the system devised for providing dietary services. One way of doing this is through a selective menu. A **selective menu** is one in which clients have the opportunity to make choices or selections in advance of meal service. For example, a selective menu usually offers at least two choices for an entrée, and multiple choices for most items on the menu. Selective menus are becoming increasingly popular in longterm care institutions, because they provide a way for residents to exert choice over daily meals. Typically, a selective menu is distributed to clients in advance of the meal (about a day or half a day before service, depending on the system). Clients note their selections, which are retrieved and used in the kitchen as trays or meals are prepared. Computer-based selective menu systems may use handheld computers and/or telephone systems for entry of choices into an automated system. A planned selective menu also has standard default selections, used in the event that a client does not make any choices. A **non-selective menu** is one in which clients do not have the opportunity to make choices. Instead, they receive a standard, pre-defined menu. In some service models, it is not necessary to work out all menu selections in advance. For example, if clients eat from a buffet, they can choose their own foods at the time of service.

In healthcare institutions, or in any environment where the dietary department is responsible for honoring therapeutic diets, it is standard practice to review menu choices before they are served. If clients make choices on a selective menu, a member of the dietary staff then reviews these choices against a nutrition kardex card, and makes minor adjustments if needed. What might need to be adjusted? Here are some examples:

- Portion sizes of products that count as fluid, for a fluid-restricted diet
- Portion sizes of high-carbohydrate foods, for a carbohydrate counting diet
- Number of servings of items that count as various exchanges, for an exchange system diet
- Consistency of foods and liquids for specific dysphagia diets
- Special adjustments for diets with multiple restrictions
- Adjustments to incorporate a standing order, such as the addition of a liquid nutritional supplement to meals

In addition, a client may not request enough food on a selective menu. One may mark only soup and coffee, for example. This could be due to a low appetite, or it could reflect confusion. A member of the dietary staff may need to mark additional choices to provide an adequate meal. Follow-up with the client is wise, to pinpoint any problems and needs. Clients may also overlook marking condiments, such as a salad dressing choice to accompany a salad, or may forget to choose a beverage. A dietary staff member should add key items to assure the meal will be complete and satisfying. On a selective menu, there may also be items a client writes in as special requests. How this is handled depends on institutional policy. In general, healthcare institutions attempt to honor write-in requests as practical. Many institutions develop a standardized list of write-in options to provide greater choice for clients.

In a non-selective menu system, it is also important to review and modify standard menu choices to accommodate specific diet orders. A member of the dietary staff needs to review the standard menu and make individual adjustments according to the diet order. In addition, it is important to review any food preferences and/or standing food requests on file, and adjust the menu to reflect these. In some longterm care institutions, individual menu adjustments are made during the tray assembly process, with employees referring to a tray card as they place foods on a tray. This is not ideal, as it is difficult to make accurate adjustments in this process. Many computerized systems track preferences and individual meal plans, and then produce individual tray tickets for use in tray assembly. Most computerized diet office software also has the ability to make many of the individual modifications needed to make menus comply with individual diet orders, as well. No matter what the mechanics are, key objectives in menu management are to: 1) create a master menu or diet spreadsheet that is capable of accommodating the needs of clients, and 2) use a procedure that allows flexibility and accuracy in adapting master menus to the unique needs of each client.

AESTHETIC CONCERNS

As we know, nutrition is not just a matter of nutrients. Thus, engineering menus to meet diet orders alone is not enough. A dietary manager also needs to ensure that menus as planned and served are enjoyable, appealing, and satisfying to clients. Ultimately, the appeal of a menu can have a great effect on nutritional well-being of clients. Many therapeutic diet restrictions make this a special challenge. One example is a pureed diet. Simply puréeing foods and spooning them into dishes does not make for an appealing meal. Dietary managers can use a number of approaches to improve the aesthetic value of pureed foods. For example, we can puree whole entrees (rather than individual components), to provide appealing flavors. We can form pureed foods into molds so they retain attractive shapes. We can add garnishes, gravies, and sauces to make them look pleasing and interesting. A mechanical soft diet is another in which modified consistency may require attention to look attractive. Some foods appropriate for this diet are easy to handle, such as a tuna noodle casserole or ground beef pie. However, a roast meat that is chopped for a mechanical soft diet may need a sauce, a gravy, and/or a garnish. Another diet that presents challenges is a sodium-controlled diet. Anyone who is accustomed to high-sodium foods and table salt may have difficulty adjusting to the blandness of this diet. Once again, it is not enough to simply prepare recipes without salt. For flavor, other seasonings need to take the place of salt. A dietary manager can incorporate seasonings such as herbal blends, spices, lemon juice, low sodium sauces, and other low sodium seasonings to improve enjoyment. Garnishes, such as the simple parsley sprig, lemon wedge, or carved vegetable can cast a very positive impression of food. Furthermore, all menus should provide variety in color, shapes, and texture (as possible), to create a positive presentation on a tray. Theme meals, special events involving food, and the dining environment itself contribute greatly to enjoyment of meals. It is up to a dietary manager to think creatively and apply culinary skills to assure that special diets do not look and feel like deprivation to clients. Instead, all meals should be able to hold their own with respect to aesthetic value.

REGULATORY ISSUES

In longterm care institutions subject to CMS regulations, some specific advice applies to menu planning. As noted in Chapter 17, the menu planning considerations include the following:

> ▶ Each resident receives, and facility provides, at least three meals daily, at regular times comparable to normal mealtimes in the community.

- There must be no more than 14 hours between a substantial evening meal and breakfast the following day (or 16 hours if a nourishing snack is provided at bedtime.)
- An evening meal should provide at least 20% of the day's total nutritional requirements.
- The facility must offer snacks at bedtime daily.
- Food is attractive and palatable, incorporating needs as identified through observation, resident and staff interviews, and review of resident council minutes.
- If a food group is missing from the resident's daily diet, the facility has an alternative means of satisfying the resident's nutrient needs.
- Substitutes of similar nutritive value are offered to residents who refuse food served.

CMS regulations emphasize residents' rights—their options to exert control over their own care. This certainly extends to meals and menus. Both the menu as planned and the manner in which dietary managers implement it must address these rights. If a resident specifically refuses a food or requests a substitute, it is up to the dietary manager to be of service in every way that is practical. If the institution uses a non-selective menu, it is especially important to make alternates available upon request. A resident also has the right to refuse treatment, including a therapeutic diet. In making choices, a resident should also be well informed. It is up to the dietary manager to work with other members of the healthcare team as needed to review any diet-related concerns and assure that residents' rights are being honored. In longterm care, a *resident council* is a committee composed of residents who provide feedback and suggestions about care—including dietary services. In other institutional settings, there may be a similar body of clients. In a university, for example, there may be a council of students and/or other patrons who provide comments and suggestions for menu planning. A dietary manager must solicit and respond to input from client groups such as these when planning menus and serving meals.

▶ Besides having various therapeutic dietary needs, each client presents a unique cultural background and a personal set of food preferences. A dietary manager strives to serve these interests with a versatile and appealing menu.

▶ A menu must be nutritionally adequate. It may be compared with standards such as Recommended Dietary Allowances (RDAs), Dietary Guidelines for Americans, the Food Guide Pyramid, or others.

▶ In an institution serving clients who follow a variety of therapeutic diets, a menu must be flexible enough to provide nutritious, satisfying meals on every diet. This detail is mapped out on a diet spreadsheet.

▶ Together, the two strategies of making menus healthy and liberalizing therapeutic diets tend to generate streamlined diet spreadsheets.

▶ A standardized menu must be adapted to meet dietary requirements, food preferences, and other specific needs of each client through an established procedure.

▶ It is up to a dietary manger to think creatively and apply culinary skills to assure that all diets present aesthetic appeal.

▶ CMS regulations emphasize residents' rights with respect to menus. A dietary manager working in longterm care needs to be familiar with CMS regulations that affect menu planning and menu management.

Cycle menu: one that repeats itself over a defined period of time

Diet spreadsheet: a document that displays the offerings for each diet, for each meal, for each day of the cycle menu (if applicable)

Non-selective menu: one in which clients do not have the opportunity to make choices

Selective menu: one in which clients have the opportunity to make choices or selections in advance of meal service

1. A cycle menu is one that:

    A. Repeats itself over a defined period of time
    B. Offers a variety of fruits at each meal
    C. Follows trends in eating habits
    D. Offers no selection for clients

2. In an institution where clients eat for weeks or months, a chief concern with menu planning is:

    A. Avoiding any deviations from the standard menu
    B. Minimizing write-in items
    C. Offering variety to prevent boredom with meals
    D. Meeting government guidelines for providing fiber

3. If you want to compare the nutrient content of menus with RDAs, it's best to:

    A. Select only calories and protein for comparison
    B. Average menus over a period of days for comparison
    C. Use only the RDA levels for women as the standard
    D. Avoid using a computer

4. Which of the following therapeutic diets is unlikely to meet nutritional needs?

    A. Puree diet
    B. Low sodium diet
    C. Dysphagia diet
    D. Clear liquid diet

5. Due to recent surgery, a client has to remain on a full liquid diet for at least two weeks. How can you improve nutritional adequacy?

    A. Add a liquid nutritional supplement that provides key nutrients
    B. Add applesauce
    C. Add milk
    D. Add cream soups

6. How can you enhance the appeal of a pureed menu?

    A. Avoid placing pureed products into molds
    B. Add a sauce and garnish
    C. Avoid gravies
    D. Stick with plain foods, not mixed dishes

7. Which of the following is NOT an appropriate condiment to include in a diet spreadsheet for a sodium-controlled diet? (see Figure 18.1)

    A. High potassium salt substitute
    B. Pepper
    C. Herb blend for seasoning
    D. Sugar

8. You are using a sodium-controlled menu for a patient who also has a very low fluid restriction and is lactose intolerant. Which of the following changes might you need to make to the standard menu?

A. Remove milk
B. Add soda pop
C. Add soup
D. Remove carrot sticks

9. You are reviewing selective menus in the computer before meal service, and notice that a patient has selected only cottage cheese for lunch. You should:

A. Let it go as marked to honor his rights
B. Document his choice in the medical record and take no further action
C. Call a care planning conference immediately
D. Add more food to the menu, and follow up with the patient

10. In a longterm care setting, which of the following is NOT a good source for feedback you can use to assure menus are appealing?

A. Resident interviews
B. Staff interviews
C. RDAs
D. A resident council

CHAPTER 19 MEAL SERVICE AND NUTRITIONAL SUPPLEMENTS

Providing nutritional care goes hand-in-hand with meal service systems. In specialized cases, a unique set of procedures and service mechanisms is required for nutritional support. A dietary manager needs to understand how these concepts interplay.

After completing this chapter, you should be able to:

- Describe methods of providing client/resident meal service.
- List factors that influence the choice of meal service systems.
- Describe the role of the dietary manager in providing nutritional supplements and nourishments.
- Name factors to consider when selecting or recommending an enteral product.
- Describe the role of a dietary manager in provision of enteral tube feeding and parenteral nutrition.

By now, it is no doubt clear that clients' health-related needs, personal dietary patterns, nutritional requirements, regulatory influences, menus, and institutional procedures all converge in the provision of meal service in any institution. A dietary manager is in the unique position of managing all these factors, bringing them together to achieve excellent dietary services. One significant piece of the dietary services puzzle is the system for providing meals. Some of the options include a trayline system, a cafeteria system, and group dining.

A *trayline system* is one in which trays move through an assembly line, and workers place both hot and cold foods on trays. Designated employees then distribute trays to clients. Alternately, trays are assembled in a chilled state and held for later rethermalization at the time of service. A trayline system can work in conjunction with either a selective or a non-selective menu. Disadvantages of a trayline system include the advanced preparation required; difficulties involved in making last minute changes to accommodate new diet orders or changes in census; challenges in satisfying clients' choices and expectations; food temperature maintenance; and labor intensity. On the other hand, tray service is an expedient way to deliver controlled meals to clients in controlled locations, such as hospitalized patients who are not well enough to leave their rooms, or confined inmates in a correctional institution.

A *cafeteria system* allows clients to walk through serving areas and select foods, placing them on a tray. This is very popular in schools, universities, and business dining. Most food is prepared in bulk, and served from steamtables or chilled holding units. Dietary employees may serve food or even prepare certain items to order (such as on a grill). Some cafeterias also incorporate many self-service features, such as salad bars. An advantage of a cafeteria system is that it allows each client to select foods that look appealing. It allows for a broad range of choices at every meal. It requires minimal advance work with individual menus. However, for clients following specialized diets, it requires some form of monitoring to assure that diet orders are met. Clients may need to be equipped with written menus to follow, or a qualified staff member may need to review menu choices with the client at the time of service.

In *group dining*, clients assemble in a common dining area. From here, several options exist. Dietary staff may wait on tables, as in a restaurant, allowing clients to choose from a restaurant style menu. A common alternative in assisted living and other longterm care institutions is buffet dining. Here, clients serve themselves from serving areas where they pick up a plate or bowl and fill it with whatever looks good. Clients may return to serving areas to pick up clean plates and choose more food at any time. Sometimes, table service and buffet service are combined, such that a client may pick and choose. As needed, dietary staff may visit buffet areas for clients who cannot ambulate easily. Like cafeteria service, a group dining system can provide choice for clients at the point of service. Dietary monitoring and assistance may be required. An advantage of group dining is the environment itself. People enjoy eating in a social environment, where they can enjoy the company of others. A dining room offers ambiance and a change of pace from a hospital or nursing home room. In this scenario, it is also practical to offer a wide variety of choices at every meal, which can lead to greater satisfaction among clients.

A popular meal service method in healthcare facilities is *room service*, modeled after hotel meal service, in which a client can order from a menu on demand. This provides great flexibility in accommodating client needs and minimizing food waste. However, it may challenge production and forecasting systems, and may also be labor-intensive.

Any service model that gives clients freedom to choose foods and dine much as they would at home is likely to support overall well-being and encourage adequate nutrition for clients. Choosing a meal service system requires evaluating the clients themselves. Decisions may hinge on the frequency and complexity of therapeutic diets, which have to be managed in any service model. They may also hinge on the ability of clients to move about freely. The degree of feeding assistance clients need may also influence decisions, as staffing must be provided in a timely manner wherever clients are served. Physical layout and equipment available in an institution also affect the choice of service models. In some institutions, several dining options exist to meet the varying needs of clients. Some may eat in a group dining area, while clients requiring intensive assistance may eat in their own rooms. Based on the service model, an institution needs to devise procedures and provide adequate staffing to assist with individual dietary needs. In any scenario, dietary staff work with other team members to make the dining experience enjoyable. For more detail about meal service options, please refer to *Managing Foodservice Opertions*, fourth edition (DMA, 2002), Chapter 4.

NUTRITION SUPPORT

Some degree of protein and calorie malnutrition is strikingly prevalent in today's healthcare institutions. Experts estimate that in nursing homes, 17-65% of residents are affected. Medical conditions, surgery, and many other factors contribute to loss of body mass. Medical experts now recognize that supporting sound nutrition can reduce complications and improve outcomes for nearly every medical treatment imaginable—from surgery to cancer treatment to healing of fractures and more. **Nutrition support** is a general term describing proactive techniques to improve nutritional status and support good medicine. Often, caregivers think of nutrition support as being either enteral—provided through the gastrointestinal tract—or parenteral—provided by vein.

In the hospital or nursing facility, there are always some clients in poor nutritional status, or with high nutrient needs, whose diets simply do not meet their nutritional requirements. These clients are often in need of concentrated sources of nutrition. **Enteral nutrition** refers to the feeding, by mouth or by tube, of formulas that contain essential nutrients. It requires that the gastrointestinal tract be functioning. The most simple form of nutritional support is a high protein, high calorie diet. Generally, there are two approaches to providing added protein and calories. One is to use conventional foods, selecting those that are particularly nutrient-dense. Another is to add commercial nutritional supplements to menus. Each has its pros and cons. Conventional foods have the advantage of familiarity, and are often readily accepted by clients. To make effective dietary recommendations, it is important to complete a diet history and discuss food tastes, preferences, and tolerances with a client. This helps to identify good candidates for menu enhancements. Figure 19.1 lists examples of simple menu modifications that can add calories to foods. When there is a nutritional problem, there may also be changes in appetite, taste sensation, or chewing ability. There may be mouth sores or other factors that affect nutrient intake. Consider these together to devise a workable solution. For example, a client undergoing cancer therapy may find the aromas of hot foods distressing. Here, it may be helpful to substitute chilled items for hot entrees. One client may enjoy a cottage cheese and fruit plate more than a hot meatloaf sandwich. Very large serving sizes and packed meal trays can be overwhelming to a person whose appetite or ability to eat is limited. The visual impact of a tray should feel comfortable to a client. If appetites are limited, some clients may eat best with six small meals, rather than three large ones. Nibbling or "grazing" can be an effective way to add calories to the diet throughout the day. Appropriate choices may include items such as celery sticks with peanut butter, egg salad, tuna salad, cheese and crackers, nuts, puddings, and milkshakes. Also consider lactose tolerance when using conventional foods to boost protein and calories. Many typical choices involve dairy products. If a client is not accustomed to these or has lactose intolerance, discomfort may ensue. Increase dairy products in the diet slowly, and monitor tolerance. If lactose creates concerns, consider lactose-free alternatives, or incorporate a commercial supplement.

Figure 19.1

INCREASING CALORIES AND PROTEIN

▸ Use margarine liberally on bread, toast, vegetables, rice, pasta, and in sandwiches.

▸ Add gravies or sauces to entrees and side dishes.

▸ Add sour cream to potatoes, casseroles, and fruits.

▸ Use whipped cream on top of desserts and fruits.

▸ Add 2 tablespoons dried milk powder to each cup of whole milk. Use for drinking and when making cream soups, hot cereal, pudding, custard, hot chocolate, mashed potatoes, casseroles, milkshakes, and creamed dishes.

▸ Add dried milk powder to scrambled eggs, gravies, casseroles, meatloaf, and meatballs.

▸ Spread peanut butter on toast or English muffins, on crackers and cookies, and on apple slices and celery sticks.

▸ Add cheese to sandwiches, scrambled eggs, casseroles, vegetables, and sauces.

▸ Add chopped eggs and diced or ground meat to salads, sauces, casseroles, and sandwiches.

▸ Use mayonnaise liberally on sandwiches.

▸ Choose desserts such as custard, bread pudding, rice pudding, and fruited yogurt. Serve with whipped cream or ice cream.

▸ Offer whole milk products or cream in place of skim milk. Or, offer milkshakes as beverages.

▸ Cook cream soups or hot cereal with whole milk; add margarine or butter.

Specialized commercial products exist for providing nutrition support. A standard enteral formula provides one calorie per milliliter (ml). (About 240 ml equal one cup.) A *complete* enteral product contains a nutritional balance of protein, carbohydrates, fat, vitamins, and minerals. Some products are modified in carbohydrate content for routine use by individuals with diabetes. Highly specialized enteral formulas exist for patients in liver failure, renal failure, or pancreatic illness, as well.

Many enteral formulas are flavored so they can be taken orally, as oral supplements to supplement intake of ordinary food. This is helpful for an individual who needs a high calorie, high protein diet and is not able to eat enough food to provide these nutrients. Commercial nutritional supplements offer several advantages over conventional foods. Complete nutritional supplements provide controlled and measured amounts of nutrients. When a client is not able to consume a variety of foods, these products offer one means of assuring adequate nutrition. In addition, they are available with key dietary modifications, such as lactose-free formulations, high fiber formulations, and so forth. Commercial products are available in calorically dense concentrations, in ranges from 1-2 calories per ml of liquid product. This means an eight-ounce glass of a supplement may provide about 240-480 calories—a significant nutritional addition to a diet.

Disadvantages to commercial supplements include acceptance and cost. Client acceptance may vary, as clients may perceive a flavor described as "medicinal" or tasting "like vitamin supplements". On the other hand, these products are available in a variety of flavors and textures that may help to overcome this drawback. When offering commercial supplements, it's helpful to allow a client to taste several products and choose what seems most enjoyable. A client may also need variety in supplement flavors and textures, just as with conventional foods. Many commercial supplements taste best when chilled, rather than served at room temperature. It is also possible to combine commercial products with conventional foods. For example, a client who does not enjoy a liquid supplement may enjoy a milkshake made from the supplement plus ice cream. For clients who prefer it—or for certain dysphagia diets—specialized nutritional pudding products represent another choice. Pudding supplements that are nutritionally similar to liquid products are available. A garnish of whipped cream, chocolate shavings, or fruit may also make these products more appealing.

Incomplete nutritional supplements offer another way to boost nutritional intake. For example, a product of carbohydrate powder with minimal flavor can be stirred into beverages, soups, applesauce, and other foods to add almost invisible calories. This type of product does not provide protein. Therefore, it can be added to foods on a renal diet to boost calories without breaching a protein restriction. Yet another commercial product is a protein powder, which may be added to mashed potatoes, hot cereal, soup, or other products to boost protein content. If a client has developed an aversion or intolerance to meats and other high protein foods, this can be a means of boosting protein content in the diet. As compared with a conventional dry milk powder, a commercial protein additive can be low in lactose.

A disadvantage of commercial nutritional supplements is that they tend to be more expensive than conventional foods. In many healthcare situations, though, third-party insurers reimburse for nutritional supplements if they are specified in physicians' diet orders.

TUBE FEEDING
When drinking an enteral feeding is not possible or practical, enteral feedings may be given through a tube. This type of enteral feeding is called a **tube feeding**. Tube feedings are given through a pliable tube, most often inserted through the nose in a nonsurgical procedure. A common tube enters from the nasal cavity directly into the stomach. This is called a *nasogastric (NG)* tube. If the tube is passed to the intestine, it may be either a *nasoduodenal (ND)* tube (the tube ends at the duodenum) or a *nasojejunal (NJ)* tube (the tube ends at the jejunum). Feeding tubes can also be inserted when necessary through surgically created openings in the esophagus (esophagostomy), stomach (gastrostomy), or jejunum (jejunostomy). These types of tube feedings may be necessary for clients who will need to be fed enterally for long periods of time,

Figure 19.2

SITES OF TUBE FEEDINGS

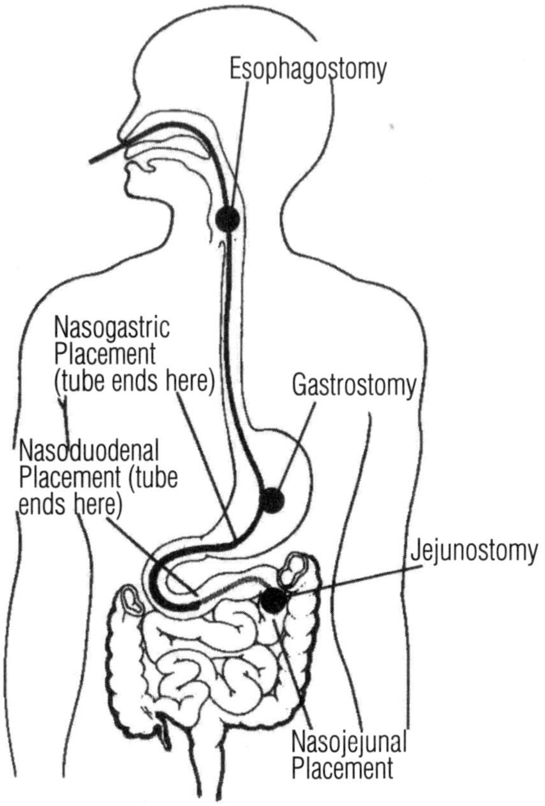

Esophagostomy

Nasogastric Placement (tube ends here)

Gastrostomy

Nasoduodenal Placement (tube ends here)

Jejunostomy

Nasojejunal Placement

such as three to six months. Figure 19.2 shows sites of feeding tubes and these semi-permanent openings for tubes.

Tube feedings may be used in clients:

- Who are not able to swallow or take food by mouth, such as after head/neck surgery, stroke, trauma; or due to inflammation
- Whose caloric and protein needs are greater than can be ingested orally (such as with cancer or burns), and attempts to provide adequate nutrition through food and oral supplements have been unsuccessful
- Who have medical conditions that require modified diets the client can't tolerate orally (e.g. an elemental diet in which proteins are provided as amino acids, such as for treatment of Crohn's disease or pancreatitis)
- Who will not eat (such as anorexia nervosa)
- Who are in a coma (NG feeding not used)

In cases where the gastrointestinal tract is not functioning, enteral nutrition is not an appropriate choice.

Tube feedings can be administered continuously or intermittently. A pump is often used to administer continuous drip feedings over a 12-24 hour period. This type of feeding allows more formula to be given and decreases the chances of diarrhea. Once tube feeding tolerance is well established, a feeding may be changed to an intermittent schedule. *Intermittent feedings* are usually given four to six times each day by gravity drip for a period of 30 to 60 minutes. One advantage of intermittent feedings is that they give the client freedom of movement between feedings. For jejunal feedings, which enter low in the gastrointestinal tract, intermittent feedings usually aren't practical, as they are quite likely to cause diarrhea. A typical jejunal feeding remains on a continuous drip regimen.

There are three types of complications that can occur in tube fed clients: gastrointestinal disturbances, metabolic complications, and mechanical complications. The most common gastrointestinal disturbance is diarrhea, due to the fact that enteral products are concentrated. Concentrated components tend to pull water into the intestines. Sometimes this is a function of how healthy the gastrointestinal tract is, as well as how quickly the feeding is administered. Fiber content of formulas may also play a role. To prevent diarrhea, it is usually necessary to begin a tube feeding at low concentrations (i.e. diluted with water) and a slow rate of administration, building up gradually as the feeding is tolerated. If diarrhea occurs, it may respond to drug therapy or a change in formula. Sanitation is essential during the preparation, storage, and administration of the enteral formula. This will prevent bacterial contamination that could cause foodborne illness. Feeding containers and tubing must be changed daily.

When enteral feedings are initiated, the client may complain of a mild feeling of fullness. If the client is monitored and the complaints diminish, tube feedings should continue. More severe symptoms—such as vomiting, swelling of the abdomen, or elevated gastric residual—increase the risk of aspiration (inhaling fluid into the lungs). If these symptoms occur, it may be time to stop the tube feeding. The **gastric residual** is the amount of formula in the stomach at any given point in time. Nursing staff normally check the residual every four to eight hours (in a continuously fed client) to make sure it does not exceed the amount of formula given during the last two hours. This is a way of assuring that the stomach is "keeping up" with the rate of feeding. If the residual is more than the suggested amount, the feeding may be stopped or slowed down. Frequent gastric residual checks are a major preventive measure for avoiding aspiration. Another preventive measure is to have the head of the bed elevated to a 45-degree angle at all times if the client is on continuous feeding.

Metabolic complications of tube feeding, such as electrolyte imbalance, frequently occur due to inadequate fluid intake, diarrhea, and/or vomiting. Tube feeding frequently serves as a client's sole source of fluid, so careful attention must be paid to fluid requirements. Fluid intake should be adequate to make up for normal losses. There is about a 500 ml difference between input and output over 24 hours. Fluid intake should accommodate unusual losses associated with increased body temperature, vomiting, and diarrhea.

Mechanical complications may be caused by improper feeding tube placement, tube malfunction, clogging due to improper flushing, or improper administration of drugs. Monitoring the condition and placement of the feeding tube itself must be an ongoing process. Clogged tubes interfere with adequate delivery of nutrients and are particularly common if small bore feeding tubes are used. Administration of medication via the feeding tube is the most common cause of clogged tubes. To keep the tube clear, it must be periodically flushed with water. Flushing is also a means of providing the needed fluid to the client. No formula provides enough free water to meet a client's fluid requirements.

Note that nursing personnel typically bear most of the responsibility for administering and managing tube feedings. However, a dietary manager is often involved in recommending a product, concentration, and rate of administration that will provide adequate nutrients. Like a menu, a tube-feeding regimen is a type of diet that must be matched to estimated nutrient needs and specific therapeutic needs. As a feeding progresses, a dietary manager often assists in monitoring tolerance and re-assessing nutritional status. If a client is going to make a transition from tube feeding to conventional foods, the dietary manager may be involved in planning a gradual transition and monitoring dietary intake.

There are many different enteral formulas on the market that can be used orally or by tube. Each institution buys certain formulas and maintains a list of formulas available for use, which is called an **enteral formulary**. Each institution also maintains its own policy and procedure for preparation and delivery of enteral feedings.

One type of enteral formula that is used for tube feeding but rarely for oral supplementation is a *chemically defined formula*. Whereas usual formulas require some digestion, chemically defined formulas (also called elemental or hydrolyzed formulas) are almost completely digested so they require only minimal digestion. These formulas are absorbed quickly and are useful for clients with severe digestive problems, such as pancreatitis. Chemically defined formulas generally cost more than other types of formulas, and are less palatable.

In selecting an enteral product for oral or tube feeding, a nutrition caregiver should consider the product concentration; the need for a nutritionally complete formulation; needs for modification in carbohydrate, fat, or protein composition; tolerance of lactose; location of the feeding tube; and whether or not to include fiber. In selecting an enteral product for oral feeding, a dietary manager should consider taste, texture, and individual client acceptance as well.

PARENTERAL NUTRITION

Parenteral nutrition is the administration of simple essential nutrients into a vein. Parenteral solutions may contain dextrose, lipids, amino acids, electrolytes, vitamins, and trace elements. They may be used in cases where the client's gastrointestinal tract is no longer able to digest and absorb food properly, or to maintain fluid and electrolyte balance both before and after surgery or when a client is not receiving enough nourishment by other feeding methods. Other examples of situations that may require parenteral feedings include the following:

- Severely malnourished clients with a nonfunctional gastrointestinal tract
- Clients with diseases of the small intestines who are not absorbing nutrients
- Clients with sepsis or burns who have very high nutrient needs

When a client receives his or her total nutrient needs via parenteral nutrition, it is called *total parenteral nutrition (TPN)*. Parenteral nutrition may use a central or peripheral vein. In *central parenteral nutrition (CPN)*, a central vein near the heart is used because these veins are large in diameter. At other times, a peripheral vein (a vein in the arm or leg) is chosen, and this is called *peripheral parenteral nutrition (PPN)*. PPN is used when only short-term support is needed and the client is not severely malnourished. PPN may be used to supplement ordinary eating. CPN is used in more severely malnourished clients who may also need more long-term nutrition support.

Although parenteral nutrition is very helpful to certain clients, it has its disadvantages. Inserting a catheter (tube) for parenteral nutrition is a surgical procedure, and once it is inserted, the catheter must be well cared for to prevent infection, a complication of parenteral nutrition. Also, when the gastrointestinal tract is not used for a long time, intestinal cells involved in absorption shrink in size, making a transition back to enteral feeding challenging. Furthermore, clients fed by vein have to forgo the usual satisfaction characteristic of eating, with all its social and emotional meanings. Lastly, parenteral solutions are very costly compared to enteral feedings.

In parenteral nutrition, an evaluation of nutritional status and an estimation of nutrient needs provide useful starting points for planning therapy. A dietary manager may be involved in this groundwork. Later, a dietary manager may play a role in re-assessing nutritional status. If a client is going to make a transition from parenteral feeding to conventional foods, the dietary manager may be involved in the transition.

Key Points

▶ A trayline system is one in which trays move through an assembly line, and workers place both hot and cold foods on trays. It offers a means of controlling diets but may provide a less appealing dining experience, compared with other service models.

▶ A cafeteria system allows clients to walk through serving areas and select foods, placing them on a tray. It permits a broad range of choices for each meal, but requires that clients ambulate and manage dietary choices.

▶ Group dining, through table and/or buffet service, can provide many menu choices and a comfortable environment. It may pose special staffing needs.

▶ Choosing a meal service system requires evaluating the clients and available resources.

▶ Nutrition support describes proactive techniques to improve nutritional status.

▶ The term *enteral nutrition* describes nutrition provided through the gastrointestinal system, and may include oral supplements or tube feeding.

▶ A variety of enteral formulas exist for enteral nutritional support. In an institution, the list of available products is called the *enteral formulary*.

▶ Tube feeding may be used for an individual who cannot swallow, whose nutritional needs exceed what he is able to eat, or who will not eat.

▶ Tube feedings require ongoing monitoring for complications and tolerance.

▶ *Parenteral nutrition* is the provision of nutrients by vein, and is generally necessary when the gastrointestinal tract is not functioning.

Key Terms

Enteral formulary: a list of formulas regularly stocked and available for use in a particular institution

Enteral nutrition: feeding, by mouth or by tube, of formulas that contain essential nutrients

Gastric residual: in tube feeding, the amount of formula in the stomach at any given point in time

Nutrition support: proactive techniques to improve nutritional status and support good medicine

Parenteral nutrition: the administration of simple essential nutrients into a vein

Tube feeding: enteral feeding given through a tube

1. Which of the following is true about a trayline system for meal service?

   A. It always involves group dining.
   B. It is possible only with a non-selective menu.
   C. It can be subject to challenges with last minute changes in diet orders.
   D. It is an expedient way to deliver controlled meals to clients in controlled locations.

2. Which of the following is true about a cafeteria system?

   A. It requires minimal advance work with individual menus.
   B. All food is prepared and pre-portioned in individual serving units.
   C. It cannot allow for self-service.
   D. It is an excellent fit for clients who are not able to walk around easily.

3. A major advantage of group dining is:

   A. It works well for clients who cannot easily leave their rooms.
   B. It provides all food pre-assembled on trays.
   C. It offers an enjoyable dining environment.
   D. It relies upon minimal choices at each meal.

4. A common element to any healthcare meal delivery system is:

   A. The need to assure compliance with therapeutic diets and special needs
   B. The necessity of providing non-selective menus
   C. The necessity of cooking all foods to order, one by one
   D. The need to eliminate assistance from staff members

5. In nursing homes, malnutrition is:

   A. Virtually unheard of
   B. Present in 2-5% of residents
   C. Present in 10-15% of residents
   D. Present in 17-65% of residents

6. Which of the following is NOT an example of enteral nutritional support?

   A. Including pudding between meals as a high protein, high calorie snack
   B. Providing nutrition through a peripheral vein
   C. Implementing a nasogastric tube feeding
   D. Offering a complete liquid nutritional supplement with lunch

7. A client has some malnutrition, and the gastrointestinal tract is not functioning due to severe inflammation. Which of the following is a likely means of providing nutritional support?

   A. A nasogastric tube feeding
   B. A jejunal tube feeding
   C. A complete oral supplement
   D. Total parenteral nutrition

8. An intermittent tube feeding regimen typically provides:

    A. Four to six feedings per day, each lasting up to an hour

    B. Ten to 12 feedings each day, each lasting up to 2 hours

    C. Continuous drip feeding, in which feeding occurs all the time

    D. Continuous drip feeding, in which feeding occurs only during waking hours

9. To help promote tolerance of a tube feeding, it is best to begin with:

    A. Low concentrations of product and a slow rate of administration

    B. High concentrations of product and a slow rate of administration

    C. High concentrations of product and a fast rate of administration

    D. Low concentrations of product and a fast rate of administration

10. To prevent aspiration of tube-feeding products, it is important to:

    A. Assure there is a high gastric residual at all times

    B. Assure that a client lies flat while a feeding is being administered

    C. Assure that the head of the bed is elevated to at least a 45-degree angle while a feeding is being administered

    D. Use only fiber-free enteral formulas

CHAPTER 1

Global Gourmet: http://www.globalgourmet.com/destinations

Smith, David and Robert Margolskee. Making Sense of Taste. *Scientific American*, March 2001: http://www.sciam.com/article.cfm?articleID=000641D5-F855-1C70-84A9809EC588EF21&catID=2

USDA Food and Nutrition Information Center. Ethnic/Cultural Topic Page: http://www.nal.usda.gov/fnic/etext/000010.html#1

CHAPTER 2

American Dietetic Association: http://www.eatright.org

Arbor Nutrition Guide: http://arborcom.com/

Ask the Dietitian: http://www.dietitian.com/

Food Reflections Newsletter (University of Nebraska – Lincoln): http://www.lancaster.unl.edu/food/archives.htm

Food Reference: http://www.foodreference.com

healthfinder®—Gateway to Reliable Consumer Health Information: http://www.healthfinder.gov/

Mayo Clinic Health Information: http://www.mayoclinic.com

Nutrition Navigator: http://www.navigator.tufts.edu/

USDA Center for Nutrition Policy and Promotion: http://www.usda.gov/cnpp

USDA Food and Nutrition Information Center: http://www.nal.usda.gov/fnic/

US Food and Drug Administration: http://www.fda.gov

CHAPTER 3

5 A Day Program Websites:
http://www.5aday.gov/
http://www.cdc.gov/nccdphp/dnpa/5ADay/
http://www.dole5aday.com

American Cancer Society: http://www.cancer.org

American Heart Association. Guidelines on Trans Fatty Acids, Butter and Margarine: http://www.americanheart.org/presenter.jhtml?identifier=4776

American Heart Association. Delicious Decisions: http://www.deliciousdecisions.org

Dietary Guidelines for Americans: http://www.nal.usda.gov/fnic/dga/

Dietary Reference Intakes: http://www.nal.usda.gov/fnic/etext/000105.html

Food Guide Pyramid: http://www.nal.usda.gov/fnic/Fpyr/pyramid.html

Health Benefits of Fruits and Vegetables: http://www.5aday.org/pdfs/research/health_benefits.pdf

Nutrition and Non-Communicable Disease Prevention:
http://www.who.int/hpr/nutrition/ExpertConsultationGE.htm

Obesity Facts: http://www.surgeongeneral.gov/topics/obesity/calltoaction/fact_glance.htm

USDA. Food & Nutrition Information Center Resource List - Food Guide Pyramid:
http://www.nal.usda.gov/fnic/etext/000023.html#xtocid2381818

USDA. Food Guide Pyramid updates and policy information:
http://www.usda.gov/cnpp/pyramid-update/FGP%20docs/Additional%20Info.html

CHAPTER 4
National Digestive Diseases Information Clearinghouse. Your Digestive System and How it Works:
http://digestive.niddk.nih.gov/ddiseases/pubs/yrdd/index.htm

CHAPTER 5
Tufts University Modified Food Pyramid for Older Adults:
http://nutrition.tufts.edu/consumer/pyramid.html

University of Nebraska. Pregnancy and Lactation Information:
http://www.ianr.unl.edu/pubs/foods/g1088.htm

US Administration on Aging: http://www.aoa.gov

USDA. Healthy School Meals Resource System: http://schoolmeals.nal.usda.gov/

USDA. Helping Students Learn to Eat Healthy:
http://www.fns.usda.gov/tn/Resources/sebrochure2.pdf

USDA. National School Lunch Program: http://www.fns.usda.gov/cnd/Lunch/

USDA. Tips for Using the Food Guide Pyramid for Young Children:
http://www.usda.gov/cnpp/KidsPyra/PyrBook.pdf

CHAPTER 6
American Dietetic Association. Liberalized Diets for Older Adults in Longterm Care:
http://www.eatright.org/Public/GovernmentAffairs/92_adar0902.cfm

American Diabetes Association: http://www.diabetes.org

American Diabetes Association. Oral Diabetes Medications:
http://www.diabetes.org/type-2-diabetes/oral-medications.jsp

American Heart Association: http://www.americanheart.org

American Heart Association Heart Profilers:
http://www.americanheart.org/presenter.jhtml?identifier=3000416

Centers for Disease Control and Prevention: http://www.cdc.gov

National Cancer Institute Cancer Information Service: http://cis.nci.nih.gov

National Heart, Lung, and Blood Institute: http://www.nhlbi.nih.gov

National Heart, Lung, and Blood Institute. National Cholesterol Education Program: http://www.nhlbi.nih.gov/about/ncep/

National Heart, Lung, and Blood Institute. DASH Eating Plan: http://www.nhlbi.nih.gov/health/public/heart/hbp/dash/

National Institute of Diabetes & Digestive & Kidney Diseases: http://www.niddk.nih.gov/

National Institute on Alcohol Abuse and Alcoholism: http://www.niaaa.nih.gov

CHAPTER 7
FDA. Dietary Supplement Health And Education Act of 1994: http://vm.cfsan.fda.gov/~dms/dietsupp.html

FDA. Center for Food Safety and Applied Nutrition: http://www.cfsan.fda.gov/

FDA. MedWatch: http://www.fda.gov/medwatch/index.html

FDA. Office of Dietary Supplements: http://vm.cfsan.fda.gov/~dms/supplmnt.html

HerbMed® Database: http://www.herbmed.org/

National Center for Complementary and Alternative Medicine: http://www.nccam.nih.gov

National Institutes of Health Office of Dietary Supplements: http://ods.od.nih.gov

Quackwatch: http://www.quackwatch.com

National Institutes of Health. MedlinePlus Drug Information: http://www.nlm.nih.gov/medlineplus/druginformation.html

CHAPTER 8
American Dietetic Association. White Paper: Public Policy Strategies for Nutrition and Aging: http://www.eatright.org/Public/GovernmentAffairs/98_11128.cfm

BMI: Medical College of Wisconsin, Online Body Mass Index Calculator: http://www.intmed.mcw.edu/clincalc/body.html

BMI: Dietary Guidelines for Americans BMI Chart: http://www.health.gov/dietaryguidelines/dga2000/document/aim.htm#figure1

Etools: Calculate Percent of Ideal Body Weight: http://www.emedicine.com/splash/etools_xml.pl

Nestle Nutrition Services. Mini Nutritional Assessment: http://www.nestleclinicalnutrition.com/images/MNA_Assessment.pdf

Nutrition Screening Initiative. DETERMINE checklists: http://www.aafp.org/x17367.xml

Nutrition Screening Initiative. Malnutrition in the Elderly: http://www.aafp.org/x16093.xml

CHAPTER 9
Daily Values: http://www.fda.gov/fdac/special/foodlabel/dvs.html

FDA Backgrounder: The Food Label: http://www.cfsan.fda.gov/~dms/fdnewlab.html

FDA Consumer Reprint: The New Food Label: Scouting for Sodium:
http://www.fda.gov/fdac/foodlabel/sodium.html

Nutrtiondata.com: http://www.nutritiondata.com/

USDA Nutrient Data Laboratory: http://www.nal.usda.gov/fnic/foodcomp/

USDA Nutrient Data Laboratory. Reports by Single Nutrients:
http://www.nal.usda.gov/fnic/foodcomp/Data/SR16/wtrank/wt_rank.html

Using Food Labels to Reduce Fat and Cholesterol in the Diet:
http://www.cfsan.fda.gov/~dms/qa-lab5.html

CHAPTER 10
Dietary Citations...and how to avoid them. DMA Member Intelligence Report:
http://www.dmaonline.org/resource/member.html

Nestle Clinical Nutrition – Case Studies: http://www.woundnutrition.com/case_studies/index.asp

CHAPTER 11
CMS. MDS 2.0 Information Site: http://www.cms.gov/medicaid/mds20/default.asp

CMS. MDS Draft Revision 3.0: http://www.cms.hhs.gov/quality/mds30

HCPro PPS Resource Center: http://www.snfinfo.com/ppsrc/index.cfm#MDS

State RAI Contacts: http://cms.hhs.gov/medicaid/mds20/state.asp

CHAPTER 12
Care Plans: http://www.careplans.com

CHAPTER 13
DMA Standards of Practice: http://www.dmaonline.org/resource/stds.html

CHAPTER 14
Nutrition Care Alerts. http://www.ahca.org/quality/care-alert/care-alerts.pdf

CHAPTERS 15 AND 16
American Dietetic Association. Good Nutrition Reading List:
http://www.eatright.org/Public/NutritionInformation/92_13216.cfm

American Dietetic Association. Position Paper: Total Diet Approach to Communicating Food and
Nutrition Information: http://www.eatright.org/Public/GovernmentAffairs/92_adar_0102.cfm

International Food Information Council New Nutrition Conversation: http://www.newconversation.org

Society for Nutrition Education: http://www.sne.org

USDA Food and Nutrition Information Center. Foreign Language Resources:
http://www.nal.usda.gov/fnic/etext/000088.html#lang

CHAPTER 17

American Health Care Association. Resources on Quality:
http://www.ahca.org/quality/qf_resources.htm

CMS Nursing Home Quality Initiative: http://www.cms.hhs.gov/quality/nhqi/

CMS Survey Protocol for Long Term Care Facilities:
http://www.cms.hhs.gov/manuals/pub07pdf/AP-P-PP.pdf

Medicare. Nursing Home Compare (online search): http://www.medicare.gov/NHCompare

CHAPTER 18

Dorner, Becky, RD, LD. End of Life Nutrition and Hydration:
http://www.beckydorner.com/pdf/EndofLife2.pdf

Dorner, Becky, RD, LD and Vicki Redovian, MA, RD, LD. Health Care: Making Food Fun:
http://www.beckydorner.com/pdf/hcfun.pdf

Dorner, Becky, RD, LD. Holiday Menus Make Dining Special for Everyone:
http://www.beckydorner.com/pdf/holiday.pdf

Dorner, Becky, RD, LD. When Mrs. Smith Won't Eat: http://www.beckydorner.com/pdf/mrssmith.pdf

CHAPTER 19

American Society for Parenteral and Enteral Nutrition: http://www.nutritioncare.org/

Dorner, Becky, RD, LD. Dignity in Dining: Feeding Techniques for Elderly and Disabled Clients
http://www.beckydorner.com/pdf/dignity.pdf

Manufacturers of Enteral Products:

Hormel Healthlabs: http://www.hormelhealthlabs.com/home.asp

Mead/Johnson: http://www.meadjohnson.com/professional/mjenteralinstitutional.html

Nestle Clinical Nutrition: http://www.nestleclinicalnutrition.com

Novartis: http://www.rxgoodhealth.com/shop/Novartis/NovartisIndex.html

Ross Products: http://www.ross.com

ADDITIONAL REFERENCES - PUBLICATIONS

ADA and DMA. *Dietary Documentation Pocket Guide*. 2002.

Berdanier, Carolyn. *Handbook of Nutrition and Food*. CRC Press, 2002.

Brummit, Pam. What You Should Know About HIPAA, *Dietary Manager* Magazine, February 2003.

Grossbauer, Sue. *Managing Foodservice Operations*, fourth edition. DMA, 2002.

Hisel, Eileen. *Regulatory Readiness in Long Term Care*. DMA, 2002.

Litchford, Mary. Master Track Series: *Alzheimer's Disease*. DMA, 2002.

Litchford, Mary. Master Track Series: *Diabetes and Carbohydrate Counting*. DMA, 2002.

Litchford, Mary. Master Track Series: *Renal Diets*. DMA, 2002.

Pennington, J., A. Bowes, and H. Church. *Bowes & Church's Food Values of Portions Commonly Used*. Lippincott Williams & Wilkins Publishers.

Roth, Ruth and Carolyn Townsend. *Nutrition & Diet Therapy, eighth edition*. Thomson Delmar Learning, 2003.

Russell, Carlene. Master Track Series: *Dining with Dysphagia*. DMA, 2003.

Scott, Michael P. Master Track Series: *Legal Issues in Nutrition Assessment*. DMA, 2002.

Whitney, Eleanor and Sharon Rolfes. *Understanding Nutrition, ninth edition*. Wadsworth/Thomson Learning, 2002.

HEALTHY EATING IS THE FIRST STEP IN TAKING CARE OF YOUR DIABETES

People with diabetes do not need special foods. In fact, the foods that are good for you are good for everyone. You can make a difference in your blood glucose control through your food choices. To keep your blood glucose levels near normal, you need to balance the food you eat with the insulin your body makes or gets by injection and with your physical activities.

Blood glucose monitoring gives you information to help you with this balancing act. Near-normal blood glucose levels help you feel better, and they may reduce or prevent the complications of diabetes.

It is important to eat about the same amount of food at the same time each day. Regardless of what your blood glucose level is, try not to skip meals or snacks. Skipping meals and snacks may lead to low blood glucose levels.

Of course, everyone needs to eat nutritious foods. Our good health depends on eating a variety of foods that contain the right amounts of carbohydrate, protein, fat, vitamins, minerals, fiber, and water. For adolescents and adults, a "healthy" daily meal plan should include at least 3 servings of vegetables, 2 servings of fruits, 6 servings of grains, beans, and starchy vegetables, 2 servings of low-fat or fat-free milk, about 6 oz of meat or meat substitutes, and small amounts of fat and sugar. The actual amounts will depend on the number of calories you need, which in turn depends on your size, age, and activity level. If you are an adult, eating the right number of calories can help you reach and stay at a reasonable weight. Children and adolescents must eat enough calories so they grow and develop normally. Don't limit their calories to try to control blood glucose levels. Instead, for children and adolescents with Type 1 or Type 2 diabetes, encourage healthy eating habits and regular physical activity. For children and adolescents taking insulin, adjustments should be made to cover the calories needed.

What Are Carbohydrate, Protein, and Fat?

Carbohydrate, protein, and fat are found in the food you eat. They supply your body with energy, or calories. Your body needs insulin to use this energy. Insulin is made in the pancreas. If you have diabetes, either your pancreas is no longer making insulin or your body is resistant to the insulin. In either case, your blood glucose levels are too high.

Carbohydrate. Starch and sugar in foods are carbohydrates. Starch is in breads, pasta, cereals, potatoes, beans, peas, and lentils. Naturally present sugars are in fruits, milk, and vegetables. Added sugars are in desserts, candy, jams, and syrups. All of these carbohydrates provide 4 calories per gram and can affect your blood glucose levels.

When you eat carbohydrates, they break down to glucose that travels in your bloodstream. Insulin helps the glucose enter the cells, where it can be used for energy or stored. Eating the same amount of carbohydrate daily at meals and snacks can help you keep your blood glucose levels within your target range.

Protein. Protein is in meats, poultry, fish, milk, and other dairy products, eggs, beans, peas, and lentils. Starches and vegetables also have small amounts of protein.

The body uses protein for growth, maintenance, and energy. Protein has 4 calories of energy per gram. Again, your body needs insulin to use the protein you eat.

Fat. Fat is in margarine, butter, oils, salad dressings, nuts, seeds, milk, cheese, meat, fish, poultry, snack foods, ice cream, and desserts.

There are different types of fat: monounsaturated, polyunsaturated, saturated, and trans. Eat less of the saturated fat found in meats, dairy products, coconut, palm or palm kernel oil, and hardened shortenings. Trans fats are fats that have been "hydrogenated" and are mainly found in hard margarine and baked "dessert-type" foods. Saturated and trans fat can raise your blood levels of cholesterol. The healthiest fat is the monounsaturated fat found in canola oil, olive oil, nuts, and avocado. The polyunsaturated fat found in corn oil, soybean oil, or sunflower oil is also a good choice. Omega-3 fat is a type of polyunsaturated fat that protects the heart. Eat 2-3 servings per week of fish high in Omega-3 fat, such as tuna and salmon.

It is important to limit the total amount of fat you eat. Fat has 9 calories per gram, more than two times the calories you get from carbohydrate and protein. You need insulin to store fat in the cells of your body. Fat is used for energy.

What Else Do I Need to Know?

Vitamins and Minerals. Most foods in the following lists are good sources of vitamins and minerals. If you eat a variety of these foods, you probably do not need a vitamin or mineral supplement.

Salt or Sodium. High blood pressure may be made worse by eating too much sodium (salt and salty foods). Even people who do not have high blood pressure can benefit from using less salt in cooking and at the table. When possible, use less salt in cooking and at the table. Snack foods, processed foods, frozen foods, and restaurant fare all tend to be high in sodium.

In the Exchange Lists, foods that are high in sodium (400 milligrams or more of sodium per exchange) have an asterisk (*).

Alcohol. If you choose to have an alcoholic beverage, men should limit consumption to two or fewer drinks per day and women to one or fewer per day. A 5 oz glass of wine, 12 oz of beer, or 1 1/2 oz of distilled spirits all contain approximately the same amount of alcohol, approximately 15 g, and each is considered to be one alcoholic drink. If you do drink alcohol, do not omit food from your meal plan because alcohol is considered an addition, not a replacement. If you take insulin or a diabetes pill, be sure to eat food containing carbohydrate with your drink. Drinking alcohol on an empty stomach can cause low blood glucose.

How Do I Know What to Eat and When?

You and your dietitian will work out a meal plan to get the right balance between your food, medication, and exercise. This meal plan is based on your usual food intake and your food preferences, including your favorite family recipes or ethnic foods.

The lists of food choices (Exchange Lists) in this booklet can help you make interesting and healthy food choices. Exchange Lists and a meal plan help you know what to eat, how much to eat, and when to eat.

There are three main groups — the carbohydrate group, the meat and meat substitutes group, and the fat group. Starch, fruit, milk, other carbohydrates, and vegetables are in the carbohydrate group. The meat and meat substitutes group is divided into very lean, lean, medium-fat, and high-fat foods. You can see at a glance which choices are lower in fat. Foods in the fat group are grouped into monounsaturated, polyunsaturated, and saturated fats and have very small serving sizes.

What Are Exchange Lists?

Exchange Lists are foods grouped together because they are alike. Each serving of a food has about the same amount of carbohydrate, protein, fat, and calories as the other foods on that list. That is why any food on a list can be "exchanged," or traded, for any other food on the same list. For example, you can trade the slice of bread you might eat for breakfast for one-half cup of cooked cereal. Each of these foods equals one starch choice. A caveat: Each list represents average nutrient and calorie values. If your diabetes goals are not being met, you might want to check the Nutrition Facts panel on food labels or nutrient analyses for specific foods.

Exchange Lists

Foods are listed with their serving sizes, which are usually measured after cooking. When you begin, measuring the size of each serving will help you learn to "eyeball" correct serving sizes.

The following chart shows the amount of nutrients in one serving from each list.

Groups/Lists	Carbohydrate (grams)	Protein (grams)	Fat (grams)	Calories
Carbohydrate Group				
Starch	15	3	0–1	80
Fruit	15	—	—	60
Milk				
Fat-free	12	8	0–3	90
Reduced-fat	12	8	5	120
Whole	12	8	8	150
Other carbohydrates	15	varies	varies	varies
Nonstarchy vegetables	5	2	—	25
Meat and Meat Substitutes Group				
Very lean	—	7	0–1	35
Lean	—	7	3	55
Medium-fat	—	7	5	75
High-fat	—	7	8	100
Fat Group	—	—	5	45

The Exchange Lists provide you with a lot of food choices (foods from the basic food groups, foods with added sugar, free foods, combination foods, and fast foods). Their purpose is to provide you with variety in your meals. Several foods, such as beans, peas, lentils, bacon, and peanut butter, are on two lists. This gives you flexibility in putting your meals together. Whenever you choose new foods or vary your meal plan, monitor your blood glucose to see how these different foods affect your blood glucose level.

Foods on the starch, fruit, and milk lists are similar in that they contain 12-15 grams of carbohydrate per serving. (Foods on the fat and meat lists contain no carbohydrate.) Some vegetables are starchy, such as potatoes, corn, and peas, and contain 15 grams of carbohydrate per serving. Other vegetables are nonstarchy, such as green beans, tomatoes, and carrots and contain 5 grams of carbohydrate per serving.

A Word About Food Labels and Recipes
Exchange information is based on foods found in grocery stores. However, food companies often change the ingredients in their products. That is why you need to check the Nutrition Facts panel of the food label.

The Nutrition Facts tell you the number of calories and grams of carbohydrate, protein, and fat in one serving. Compare these numbers with the exchange information in this booklet to see how many exchanges you will be eating. In this way, food labels can help you add foods to your meal plans. Remember that the serving size on a label is not necessarily the same as an Exchange Lists serving size.

Your home recipes may vary substantially from similar foods listed in this booklet. To determine your recipe nutrients, find the carbohydrate grams, protein grams, fat grams, and calories for each of the recipe ingredients; total each of the nutrients; then divide the totals by the number of servings the recipe yields. Compare these numbers with the exchange information in this booklet.

Ask your dietitian to help you use food label and recipe information to plan your meals, and read the section entitled "Using Food Labels" for more tips on how to use food labels.

Getting Started!
See your dietitian regularly when you are first learning how to use your meal plan and the Exchange Lists. Your meal plan can be adjusted to fit changes in your lifestyle, such as work, school, vacation, or travel. Regular nutrition counseling can help you make positive changes in your eating habits.

Careful eating habits will help you feel better and be healthier, too. Best wishes and good eating with *Exchange Lists for Meal Planning.*

STARCH LIST

Cereals, grains, pasta, breads, crackers, snacks, starchy vegetables, and cooked beans, peas, and lentils are starches. In general, one starch is:

- 1/2 cup of cooked cereal, grain, or starchy vegetable
- 1/3 cup of cooked rice or pasta
- 1 oz of a bread product, such as 1 slice of bread
- 3/4 to 1 oz of most snack foods. (Some snack foods may also have added fat.)

Nutrition Tips

1. Most starch choices are good sources of B vitamins.
2. Foods made from whole grains are good sources of fiber.
   - A serving from the bread list, on average, has 1 gram of fiber.
   - A serving from the cereals and grains list or the crackers and snacks list, on average, has 2 grams of fiber.
   - A serving from the starchy vegetables list, on average, has 3 grams of fiber.
3. Beans, peas, and lentils are good sources of protein and fiber.
   - A serving from this food group, on average, has 6 grams of fiber.

Selection Tips

1. Choose starches made with little fat as often as you can.
2. Starchy vegetables prepared with fat count as one starch and one fat.
3. For many starchy foods (e.g., bagels, muffins, dinner rolls, buns), a general rule of thumb is 1 oz equals 1 carbohydrate serving. However, bagels or muffins range widely in size. Check the size you eat. Also, use the Nutrition Facts on food labels when available.
4. Beans, peas, and lentils are also found on the meat and meat substitutes list.
5. A waffle or pancake is about the size of a compact disc (CD) and about 1/4 inch thick.
6. Because starches often swell in cooking, a small amount of uncooked starch will become a much larger amount of cooked food.
7. Most of the serving sizes are measured or weighed after cooking.
8. For specific information, check Nutrition Facts on the food label.

One starch exchange equals 15 grams of carbohydrate, 3 grams of protein, 0–1 grams of fat, and 80 calories.

Bread

Bagel, 4 oz	1/4 (1 oz)
Bread, reduced-calorie	2 slices (1 1/2 oz)
Bread, white, whole wheat, pumpernickel, rye	1 slice (1 oz)
Bread sticks, crisp, 4 inch x 1/2 inch	4 (2/3 oz)
English muffin	1/2
Hot dog bun or hamburger bun	1/2 (1 oz)
Naan, 8 x 2 inch	1/4
Pancake, 4 inch across, 1/4 inch thick	1
Pita, 6 inch across	1/2
Roll, plain, small	1 (1 oz)
Raisin bread, unfrosted	1 slice (1 oz)
Tortilla, corn, 6 inch across	1
Tortilla, flour, 6 inch across	1
Tortilla, flour, 10 inch across	1/3
Waffle, 4 inch square or across, reduced-fat	1

Cereals and Grains

Bran cereals	1/2 cup
Bulgur	1/2 cup
Cereals, cooked	1/2 cup
Cereals, unsweetened, ready-to-eat	3/4 cup
Cornmeal (dry)	3 Tbsp
Couscous	1/3 cup
Flour (dry)	3 Tbsp
Granola, low-fat	1/4 cup
Grape-Nuts®	1/4 cup
Grits	1/2 cup
Kasha	1/2 cup
Millet	1/3 cup
Muesli	1/4 cup
Oats	1/2 cup
Pasta	1/3 cup
Puffed cereal	1 1/2 cups
Rice, white or brown	1/3 cup
Shredded Wheat®	1/2 cup
Sugar-frosted cereal	1/2 cup
Wheat germ	3 Tbsp

One starch exchange equals 15 grams of carbohydrate, 3 grams of protein, 0–1 grams of fat, and 80 calories.

Starchy Vegetables

Baked beans . . . . .1/3 cup
Corn . . . . .1/2 cup
Corn on cob, large . . . . .1/2 cob (5 oz)
Mixed vegetables with corn, peas, or pasta . . . . .1 cup
Peas, green . . . . .1/2 cup
Plantain . . . . .1/2 cup
Potato, boiled . . . . .1/2 cup or 1/2 medium (3 oz)
Potato, baked with skin . . . . .1/4 large (3 oz)
Potato, mashed . . . . .1/2 cup
Squash, winter (acorn, butternut, pumpkin) . . . . .1 cup
Yam, sweet potato, plain .1/2 cup

Crackers and Snacks

Animal crackers 8
Graham cracker, 2 1/2 inch square 3
Matzoh . . . . .3/4 oz
Melba toast . . . . .4 slices
Oyster crackers 24
Popcorn (popped, no fat added, or low-fat microwave) . . .3 cups
Pretzels . . . . .3/4 oz
Rice cakes, 4 inch across 2
Saltine-type crackers 6
Snack chips, fat-free (tortilla, potato) . . . . .15–20 (3/4 oz)
whole wheat crackers, no fat added . . . . .2–5 (3/4 oz)

Beans, Peas, And Lentils

(Count as 1 starch exchange, plus 1 very lean meat exchange.)
Beans and peas (garbanzo, pinto, kidney, white, split, black-eyed)
. . . . .1/2 cup
Lima beans . . . . .2/3 cup
Lentils . . . . .1/2 cup
Miso * . . . . .3 Tbsp
* = 400 mg or more sodium per exchange.

One starch exchange equals 15 grams of carbohydrate, 3 grams of protein, 0–1 grams of fat, and 80 calories.

Starchy Foods Prepared with Fat

(Count as 1 starch exchange, plus 1 fat exchange.)
Biscuit, 2 1/2 inch across 1
Chow mein noodles . . . . .1/2 cup

Corn bread, 2 inch cube . . . . .1 (2 oz)
Crackers, round butter type 6
Croutons . . . . .1 cup
French-fried potatoes (oven-baked)(see also fast food list) . . . . .
. . . . .1 cup (2 oz)
Granola . . . . .1/4 cup
Hummus . . . . .1/3 cup
Muffin, 5 oz . . . . .1/5 (1 oz)
Popcorn, microwaved . . . . .3 cups
Sandwich crackers, cheese or peanut butter filling 3
Snack chips (potato, tortilla) . . . . .9–13 (3/4 oz)
Stuffing, bread (prepared) . . . . .1/3 cup
Taco shell, 6 inch across 2
Waffle, 4 inch square or across 1
whole wheat crackers, fat added . . . . .4-7 (1 oz)

Common Measurements

3 tsp = 1 Tbsp   4 oz = 1/2 cup
4 Tbsp = 1/4 cup   8 oz = 1 cup
5 1/3 Tbsp = 1/3 cup   1 cup = 1/2 pint

FRUIT LIST

Fresh, frozen, canned, and dried fruits and fruit juices are on this list. In general, one fruit exchange is:

- 1 small fresh fruit (4 oz)
- 1/2 cup of canned or fresh fruit or unsweetened fruit juice
- 1/4 cup of dried fruit

Nutrition Tips

1. Fresh, frozen, and dried fruits have about 2 grams of fiber per choice. Fruit juices contain very little fiber.

2. Citrus fruits, berries, and melons are good sources of vitamin C.

Selection Tips

1. Count 1/2 cup cranberries or rhubarb sweetened with sugar substitutes as free foods.

2. Read the Nutrition Facts on the food label. If one serving has more than 15 grams of carbohydrate, you will need to adjust the size of the serving you eat or drink.

3. Portion sizes for canned fruits are for the fruit and a small amount of juice.

4. Whole fruit is more filling than fruit juice and may be a better choice.

5. Food labels for fruits may contain the words "no sugar added" or "unsweetened." This means that no sucrose (table sugar) has been added.

6. Generally, fruit canned in extra light syrup has the same amount of carbohydrate per serving as the "no sugar added" or the juice pack. All canned fruits on the fruit list are based on one of these three types of pack.

One fruit exchange equals 15 grams of carbohydrate and 60 calories. The weight includes skin, core, seeds, and rind.

Fruit

Apple, unpeeled, small	.1 (4 oz)
Applesauce, unsweetened	.1/2 cup
Apples, dried	.4 rings
Apricots, fresh	.4 whole (5 1/2 oz)
Apricots, dried	.8 halves
Apricots, canned	.1/2 cup
Banana, small	.1 (4 oz)
Blackberries	.3/4 cup
Blueberries	.3/4 cup
Cantaloupe, small	.1/3 melon (11 oz) or 1 cup cubes
Cherries, sweet, fresh	.12 (3 oz)
Cherries, sweet, canned	.1/2 cup
Dates	.3
Figs, fresh	.1 1/2 large or 2 medium (3 1/2 oz)
Figs, dried	.1 1/2
Fruit cocktail	.1/2 cup
Grapefruit, large	.1/2 (11 oz)
Grapefruit sections, canned	.3/4 cup
Grapes, small	.17 (3 oz)
Honeydew melon	.1 slice (10 oz) or 1 cup cubes
Kiwi	.1 (3 1/2 oz)
Mandarin oranges, canned	.3/4 cup
Mango, small	.1/2 fruit (5 1/2 oz) or 1/2 cup
Nectarine, small	.1 (5 oz)
Orange, small	.1 (6 1/2 oz)
Papaya	.1/2 fruit (8 oz) or 1 cup cubes
Peach, medium, fresh	.1 (4 oz)
Peaches, canned	.1/2 cup
Pear, large, fresh	.1/2 (4 oz)
Pears, canned	.1/2 cup
Pineapple, fresh	.3/4 cup
Pineapple, canned	.1/2 cup
Plums, small	.2 (5 oz)
Plums, canned	.1/2 cup
Plums, dried (prunes)	.3
Raisins	.2 Tbsp
Raspberries	.1 cup
Strawberries	.1 1/4 cup whole berries
Tangerines, small	.2 (8 oz)
Watermelon	.1 slice (13 1/2 oz) or 1 1/4 cup cubes

Fruit Juice, Unsweetened

Apple juice/cider	.1/2 cup
Cranberry juice cocktail	.1/3 cup
Cranberry juice cocktail, reduced-calorie	.1 cup
Fruit juice blends, 100% juice	.1/3 cup
Grape juice	.1/3 cup
Grapefruit juice	.1/2 cup
Orange juice	.1/2 cup
Pineapple juice	.1/2 cup
Prune juice	.1/3 cup

MILK LIST

Different types of milk and milk products are on this list. Cheeses are on the meat and meat substitutes list and cream and other dairy fats are on the fat list. Based on the amount of fat they contain, milks are divided into fat-free/low-fat milk, reduced-fat milk, and whole milk. One choice of these includes:

	Carbohydrate (grams)	Protein (grams)	Fat (grams)	Calories
Fat-free/low-fat (1/2% or 1%)				
	12	8	0–3	90
Reduced-fat (2%)				
	12	8	5	120
Whole				
	12	8	8	150

Nutrition Tips

1. Milk and yogurt are good sources of calcium and protein. Check the Nutrition Facts on the food label.

2. The higher the fat content of milk and yogurt, the greater the amount of saturated fat and cholesterol. Choose lower-fat varieties.

3. For those who are lactose intolerant, look for lactose-reduced

or lactose-free varieties of milk. Check the food label for total amount of carbohydrate per serving.

Selection Tips

1. 1 cup equals 8 fluid ounces or 1/2 pint.

2. Look for chocolate milk, rice milk, frozen yogurt, and ice cream on the sweets, desserts, and other carbohydrates list.

3. Nondairy creamers are on the free foods list.

One milk exchange equals 12 grams of carbohydrate and 8 grams of protein.

Fat-free and Low-fat Milk
(0–3 grams fat per serving)

Fat-free milk	1 cup
1/2% milk	1 cup
1% milk	1 cup
Buttermilk, low-fat or fat-free	1 cup
Evaporated fat-free milk	1/2 cup
Fat-free dry milk	1/3 cup dry
Soy milk, low-fat or fat-free	1 cup
Yogurt, fat-free, flavored, sweetened with nonnutritive sweetener and fructose	6 oz
Yogurt, plain fat-free	6 oz

Reduced-fat
(5 grams fat per serving)

2% milk	1 cup
Soy milk	1 cup
Sweet acidophilus milk	1 cup
Yogurt, plain low-fat	6 oz

Whole Milk
(8 grams fat per serving)

Whole milk	1 cup
Evaporated whole milk	1/2 cup
Goat's milk	1 cup
Kefir	1 cup
Yogurt, plain (made from whole milk)	8 oz

SWEETS, DESSERTS, AND OTHER CARBOHYDRATES LIST

You can substitute food choices from this list for a starch, fruit, or milk choice on your meal plan. Some choices will also count as one or more fat choices.

Nutrition Tips

1. These foods can be substituted for other carbohydrate-containing foods in your meal plan, even though they contain added sugars or fat. However, they do not contain as many important vitamins and minerals as the choices on the starch, fruit, or milk list.

2. When planning to include these foods in your meal, be sure to include foods from all the lists to eat a balanced meal.

Selection Tips

1. Because many of these foods are concentrated sources of carbohydrate and fat, saturated fat, and trans fat, the portion sizes are often very small.

2. Look for the words "hydrogenated" or "partially hydrogenated" on the ingredient label. The lower down on the list these words appear, the fewer trans fats there are.

3. Be sure to check the Nutrition Facts on the food label. It will be your most accurate source of information.

4. Many fat-free or reduced-fat products made with fat replacers contain carbohydrate. When eaten in large amounts, they may need to be counted. Talk with your dietitian to determine how to count these in your meal plan.

5. Look for fat-free salad dressings in smaller amounts on the free food list.

One exchange equals 15 grams of carbohydrate, or 1 starch, or 1 fruit, or 1 milk.

FOOD SERVING SIZE	EXCHANGES PER SERVING
Angel food cake, unfrosted 1/12th cake (about 2 oz)	2 carbohydrates
Brownie, small, unfrosted 2 inch square (about 1 oz)	1 carbohydrate, 1 fat
Cake, unfrosted 2 inch square (about 1 oz)	1 carbohydrate, 1 fat
Cake, frosted 2 inch square (about 2 oz)	2 carbohydrates, 1 fat
Cookie or sandwich cookie with creme filling 2 small (about 2/3 oz)	1 carbohydrate, 1 fat
Cookies, sugar-free 3 small or 1 large (3/4–1 oz)	1 carbohydrate, 1–2 fats
Cranberry sauce, jellied 1/4 cup	1 1/2 carbohydrates
Cupcake, frosted 1 small (about 2 oz)	2 carbohydrates, 1 fat

Doughnut, plain cake
1 medium (1 1/2 oz) . . . . .1 1/2 carbohydrates, 2 fats

Doughnut, glazed
3 3/4 inch across (2 oz) . . . . .2 carbohydrates, 2 fats

Energy, sport, or breakfast bar
1 bar (1 1/3 oz) . . . . .1 1/2 carbohydrates, 0–1 fat

Energy, sport, or breakfast bar
1 bar (2 oz) .2 carbohydrates, 1 fat

Fruit cobbler
1/2 cup (3 1/2 oz) . . . . .3 carbohydrates, 1 fat

Fruit juice bars, frozen, 100% juice
1 bar (3 oz) . . . . .1 carbohydrate

Fruit snacks, chewy (pureed fruit concentrate)
1 roll (3/4 oz) . . . . .1 carbohydrate

Fruit spreads, 100% fruit
1 1/2 Tbsp . . . . .1 carbohydrate

Gelatin, regular
1/2 cup . . . . .1 carbohydrate

Gingersnaps
3 . . . . .1 carbohydrate

Granola or snack bar, regular or low-fat
1 bar (1 oz) . . . . .1 1/2 carbohydrates

Honey
1 Tbsp . . . . .1 carbohydrate

Ice cream
1/2 cup . . . . .1 carbohydrate, 2 fats

Ice cream, light
1/2 cup . . . . .1 carbohydrate, 1 fat

Ice cream, low-fat
1/2 cup . . . . .1 1/2 carbohydrates

Ice cream, fat-free, no sugar added
1/2 cup . . . . .1 carbohydrate

Jam or jelly, regular
1 Tbsp . . . . .1 carbohydrate

Milk, chocolate, whole
1 cup . . . . .2 carbohydrates, 1 fat

Pie, fruit, 2 crusts
1/6 of 8 inch commercially prepared pie . . . .
. . . . .3 carbohydrates, 2 fats

Pie, pumpkin or custard
1/8 of 8 inch commercially prepared pie . . . .
. . . . .2 carbohydrates, 2 fats

Pudding, regular (made with reduced-fat milk)
1/2 cup . . . . .2 carbohydrates

Pudding, sugar-free or sugar-free and fat-free (made with fat-free milk)
1/2 cup . . . . .1 carbohydrate

Reduced calorie meal replacement (shake)
1 can (10–11 oz) . . . . .1 1/2 carbohydrates, 0–1 fat

Rice milk, low-fat or fat-free, plain
1 cup . . . . .1 carbohydrate

Rice milk, low-fat, flavored
1 cup . . . . .1 1/2 carbohydrates

Salad dressing, fat-free *
1/4 cup . . . . .1 carbohydrate

Sherbet, sorbet
1/2 cup . . . . .2 carbohydrates

Spaghetti or pasta sauce, canned *
1/2 cup . . . . .1 carbohydrate, 1 fat

Sports drinks
8 oz (about 1 cup) .1 carbohydrate

Sugar
1 Tbsp . . . . .1 carbohydrate

Sweet roll or Danish
1 (2 1/2 oz) . . . . .2 1/2 carbohydrates, 2 fats

Syrup, light
2 Tbsp . . . . .1 carbohydrate

Syrup, regular
1 Tbsp . . . . .1 carbohydrate

Syrup, regular
1/4 cup . . . . .4 carbohydrates

Vanilla wafers
5 . . . . .1 carbohydrate, 1 fat

Yogurt, frozen
1/2 cup . . . . .1 carbohydrate, 0–1 fat

Yogurt, frozen, fat-free
1/3 cup . . . . .1 carbohydrate

Yogurt, low-fat with fruit
1 cup . . . . .3 carbohydrates, 0–1 fat

* = 400 mg or more of sodium per exchange.

NONSTARCHY VEGETABLE LIST

Vegetables that contain small amounts of carbohydrates and calories are on this list. Vegetables contain important nutrients. Try to eat at least 2 or 3 vegetable choices each day. In general, one vegetable exchange is:

- 1/2 cup of cooked vegetables or vegetable juice
- 1 cup of raw vegetables

If you eat 3 cups or more of raw vegetables or 1 1/2 cups of cooked vegetables at one meal, count them as 1 carbohydrate choice.

Nutrition Tips

1. Fresh and frozen vegetables have less added salt than canned vegetables. Drain and rinse canned vegetables if you want to remove some salt.

2. Choose more dark green and dark yellow vegetables, such as spinach, broccoli, romaine, carrots, chilies, and peppers.

3. Broccoli, brussels sprouts, cauliflower, greens, peppers, spinach, and tomatoes are good sources of vitamin C.

4. Vegetables contain 1 to 4 grams of fiber per serving.

Selection Tips

1. A 1-cup portion of broccoli is a portion about the size of a light bulb.

2. Tomato sauce is different from spaghetti sauce, which is on the sweets, desserts, and other carbohydrates list.

3. Canned vegetables and juices are available without added salt.

4. Starchy vegetables such as corn, peas, winter squash, and potatoes that contain larger amounts of calories and carbohydrates are on the Starch list.

One vegetable exchange (1/2 cup cooked or 1 cup raw) equals 5 grams of carbohydrate, 2 grams of protein, 0 grams of fat, and 25 calories.

Artichoke
Artichoke hearts
Asparagus
Beans (green, wax, Italian)
Bean sprouts
Beets
Broccoli
Brussels sprouts
Cabbage
Carrots
Cauliflower
Celery
Cucumber
Eggplant
Green onions or scallions
Greens (collard, kale, mustard, turnip)
Kohlrabi
Leeks
Mixed vegetables (without corn, peas, or pasta)
Mushrooms
Okra
Onions
Pea pods

Peppers (all varieties)
Radishes
Salad greens (endive, escarole, lettuce, romaine, spinach)
Sauerkraut*
Spinach
Summer squash
Tomato
Tomatoes, canned
Tomato sauce*
Tomato/vegetable juice*
Turnips
Water chestnuts
Watercress
Zucchini

* = 400 mg or more sodium per exchange.

MEAT AND MEAT SUBSTITUTES LIST

Meat and meat substitutes that contain both protein and fat are on this list. In general, one meat exchange is:

- 1 oz of meat, fish, poultry, or cheese
- 1/2 cup of beans, peas, or lentils

Based on the amount of fat they contain, meats are divided into very lean, lean, medium-fat, and high-fat lists. This is done so you can see which ones contain the least amount of fat. One ounce (one exchange) of each of these includes:

	Carbohydrate (grams)	Protein (grams)	Fat (grams)	Calories
Very lean	0	7	0–1	35
Lean	0	7	3	55
Medium-fat	0	7	5	75
High-fat	0	7	8	100

Nutrition Tips

1. Choose very lean and lean meat choices whenever possible. Items from the high-fat group are high in saturated fat, cholesterol, and calories and can raise blood cholesterol levels.

2. Beans, peas, and lentils are good sources of fiber, about 3 grams per serving.

3. Some processed meats, seafood, and soy products may contain carbohydrate when consumed in large amounts. Check the Nutrition Facts on the label to see if the amount is close to 15 grams. If so, count it as a carbohydrate choice as well as a meat choice.

Selection Tips

1. Weigh meat after cooking and removing bones and fat. Four ounces of raw meat is equal to 3 ounces of cooked meat. Some examples of meat portions are:

   - ▸ 1 oz cheese = 1 meat choice and is about the size of a 1-inch cube or 4 cubes the size of dice

   - ▸ 2 oz meat = 2 meat choices, such as 1 small chicken leg or thigh, or 1/2 cup cottage cheese or tuna

   - ▸ 3 oz meat = 3 meat choices and is about the size of a deck of cards, such as 1 medium pork chop, 1 small hamburger, 1/2 of a whole chicken breast, or 1 unbreaded fish fillet

2. Limit your choices from the high-fat group to three times per week or less.

3. Most grocery stores stock Select and Choice grades of meat. The Select grades of meat are the leanest. The Choice grades contain a moderate amount of fat, and Prime cuts of meat have the highest amount of fat.

4. "Hamburger" may contain added seasoning and fat, but ground beef does not.

5. Read labels to find products that are low in fat and cholesterol (5 grams of fat or less per serving).

6. Dried beans, peas, and lentils are also found on the starch list.

7. Peanut butter, in smaller amounts, is also found on the fats list.

8. Bacon, in smaller amounts, is also found on the fats list.

9. Don't be fooled by ground beef packages that say X% lean (e.g. 90% lean). This is the percentage of fat by weight, NOT the percentage of calories from fat. A 3.5 oz patty of this raw ground beef has about half of its calories from fat.

10. Meatless burgers in the combination foods list (3 oz of soy based burger = 1/2 carbohydrate + 2 very lean meats; 3 oz of vegetable and starch based burger = 1 carbohydrate + 1 lean meat).

Meal Planning Tips

1. Bake, roast, broil, grill, poach, steam, or boil meat and fish rather than frying.

2. Place meat on a rack so the fat will drain off during cooking.

3. Use a nonstick spray and a nonstick pan to brown or fry foods.

4. Trim off visible fat or skin before or after cooking.

5. If you add flour, bread crumbs, coating mixes, fat, or marinades when cooking, ask your dietitian how to count it in your meal plan.

Very Lean Meat and Substitutes List
One exchange equals 0 grams of carbohydrate, 7 grams of protein, 0–1 grams of fat, and 35 calories.

One very lean meat exchange is equal to any one of the following items:

Poultry: Chicken or turkey (white meat, no skin), Cornish hen (no skin) . . . . .1 oz

Fish: Fresh or frozen cod, flounder, haddock, halibut, trout, lox (smoked salmon)*; tuna fresh or canned in water . . . . .1 oz

Shellfish: Clams, crab, lobster, scallops, shrimp, imitation shellfish . . . . .1 oz

Game: Duck or pheasant (no skin), venison, buffalo, ostrich 1 oz

Cheese with 1 gram of fat or less per ounce: Fat-free or low-fat cottage cheese . . . . .1/4 cup

Fat-free cheese . . . . .1 oz

Other: Processed sandwich meats with 1 gram of fat or less per ounce, such as deli thin, shaved meats, chipped beef*, turkey ham . . . . .1 oz

Egg whites 2

Egg substitutes, plain . . . . .1/4 cup

Hot dogs with 1 gram of fat or less per ounce* . . . . .1 oz

Kidney (high in cholesterol) . . . . .1 oz

Sausage with 1 gram of fat or less per ounce . . . . .1 oz

Count the following items as one very lean meat and one starch exchange.

Beans, peas, lentils (cooked) . . . . .1/2 cup
* = 400 mg or more sodium per exchange.

Lean Meat and Substitutes List
One exchange equals 0 grams of carbohydrate, 7 grams of protein, 3 grams of fat, and 55 calories.

One lean meat exchange is equal to any one of the following items:

Beef: USDA Select or Choice grades of lean beef trimmed of fat, such as round, sirloin, and flank steak; tenderloin; roast (rib, chuck, rump); steak (T-bone, porterhouse, cubed); ground round . . . . .1 oz

Pork: Lean pork, such as fresh ham; canned, cured, or boiled ham; Canadian bacon*; tenderloin, center loin chop . . . . . .1 oz

Lamb: Roast, chop, or leg . . . . .1 oz

Veal: Lean chop, roast . . . . .1 oz

Poultry: Chicken, turkey (dark meat, no skin), chicken (white meat, with skin), domestic duck or goose (well-drained of fat, no skin) . . . . .1 oz

Fish: Herring (uncreamed or smoked) . . . . .1 oz

Oysters . . . . .6 medium

Salmon (fresh or canned), catfish . . . . .1 oz

Sardines (canned) . . . . .2 medium

Tuna (canned in oil, drained) . . . . .1 oz

Game: Goose (no skin), rabbit .1 oz

Cheese: 4.5%-fat cottage cheese . . . . .1/4 cup

Grated Parmesan . . . . .2 Tbsp

Cheeses with 3 grams of fat or less per ounce . . . . .1 oz

Other: Hot dogs with 3 grams of fat or less per ounce* . . . .
. . . . .1 1/2 oz

Processed sandwich meat with 3 grams of fat or less per ounce, such as turkey pastrami or kielbasa . . . . .1 oz

Liver, heart (high in cholesterol) . . . . .1 oz

Medium-Fat Meat and Substitutes List
One exchange equals 0 grams of carbohydrate, 7 grams of protein, 5 grams of fat, and 75 calories.

One medium-fat meat exchange is equal to any one of the following items:

Beef: Most beef products fall into this category (ground beef, meatloaf, corned beef, short ribs, Prime grades of meat trimmed of fat, such as prime rib) . . . . .1 oz

Pork: Top loin, chop, Boston butt, cutlet . . . . .1 oz

Lamb: Rib roast, ground . . . . .1 oz

Veal: Cutlet (ground or cubed, unbreaded) . . . . .1 oz

Poultry: Chicken (dark meat, with skin), ground turkey or ground chicken, fried chicken (with skin) . . . . .1 oz

Fish: Any fried fish product . . . . .1 oz

Cheese with 5 grams or less fat per ounce: Feta . . . .1 oz

Mozzarella . . . . .1 oz

Ricotta . . . . .1/4 cup (2 oz)

Other: Egg (high in cholesterol, limit to 3 per week) 1

Sausage with 5 grams of fat or less per ounce . . . . .1 oz

Tempeh . . . . .1/4 cup

Tofu . . . . .4 oz or 1/2 cup

* = 400 mg or more sodium per exchange.

High-Fat Meat and Substitutes List
One exchange equals 0 grams of carbohydrate, 7 grams of protein, 8 grams of fat, and 100 calories.

Remember these items are high in saturated fat, cholesterol, and calories and may raise blood cholesterol levels if eaten on a regular basis.

One high-fat meat exchange is equal to any one of the following items:

Pork: Spareribs, ground pork, pork sausage . . . . .1 oz

Cheese: All regular cheeses, such as American*, cheddar, Monterey Jack, Swiss . . . . .1 oz

Other: Processed sandwich meats with 8 grams of fat or less per ounce, such as bologna, pimento loaf, salami . . . . .1 oz

Sausage, such as bratwurst, Italian, knockwurst, Polish, smoked . . . . .1 oz

Hot dog (turkey or chicken)* 1 (10/lb)

Bacon . . . . .3 slices (20 slices/lb)

Peanut butter (contains unsaturated fat) . . . . .1 Tbsp

Count the following items as 1 high-fat meat plus 1 fat exchange:

Hot dog (beef, pork, or combination)* 1 (10/lb)

* = 400 mg or more sodium per exchange

Fat List
Fats are divided into three groups, based on the main type of fat they contain: monounsaturated, polyunsaturated, and saturated. Monounsaturated and polyunsaturated fats in the foods we eat are linked with good health benefits. Saturated fats and fats called trans fatty acids (or trans unsaturated fatty acids) are linked with heart disease. In general, one fat exchange is:

- ▶ 1 teaspoon of regular margarine or vegetable oil
- ▶ 1 tablespoon of regular salad dressings

Nutrition Tips
1. All fats are high in calories. Limit serving sizes for good nutrition and health.
2. Nuts and seeds contain small amounts of fiber, protein, and magnesium.
3. If blood pressure is a concern, choose fats in the unsalted form to help lower sodium intake, such as unsalted peanuts.

Selection Tips
1. Check the Nutrition Facts on food labels for serving sizes. One fat exchange is based on a serving size containing 5 grams of fat.

2. The Nutrition Facts on food labels usually list total fat grams and saturated fat grams per serving. When most of the calories come from saturated fat, the food fits into the saturated fats list.

3. Occasionally the Nutrition Facts on food labels will list monounsaturated and/or polyunsaturated fats in addition to total and saturated fats. If more than half the total fat is monounsaturated, the food fits into the monounsaturated fats list; if more than half is polyunsaturated, the food fits into the polyunsaturated fats list.

4. When selecting fats to use with your meal plan, consider replacing saturated fats with monounsaturated fats.

5. When selecting regular margarine, choose those with liquid vegetable oil as the first ingredient. Soft margarines are not as saturated as stick margarines and are healthier choices.

6. Avoid foods on the fat list (such as margarines) listing hydrogenated or partially hydrogenated fat as the first ingredient because these foods will contain higher amounts of trans fatty acids.

7. When selecting reduced-fat or lower-fat margarines, look for liquid vegetable oil as the second ingredient. Water is usually the first ingredient.

8. When used in smaller amounts, bacon and peanut butter are counted as fat choices. When used in larger amounts, they are counted as high-fat meat choices.

9. Fat-free salad dressings are on the sweets, desserts, and other carbohydrates list and the free foods list.

10. See the free foods list for nondairy coffee creamers, whipped topping, and fat-free products, such as margarines, salad dressings, mayonnaise, sour cream, cream cheese, and nonstick cooking spray.

Monounsaturated Fats List
One fat exchange equals 5 grams fat and 45 calories.

Avocado, medium	.2 Tbsp (1 oz)
Oil (canola, olive, peanut)	.1 tsp
Olives: ripe (black)	.8 large
green, stuffed*	.10 large
Nuts: almonds, cashews	.6 nuts
mixed (50% peanuts)	.6 nuts
peanuts	.10 nuts
pecans	.4 halves
Peanut butter, smooth or crunchy	.1/2 Tbsp

Sesame seeds	.1 Tbsp
Tahini or sesame paste	.2 tsp

Polyunsaturated Fats List
One fat exchange equals 5 grams fat and 45 calories.

Margarine: stick, tub, or squeeze	.1 tsp
lower-fat spread (30% to 50% vegetable oil)	.1 Tbsp
Mayonnaise: regular	.1 tsp
reduced-fat	.1 Tbsp
Nuts: walnuts, English	.4 halves
Oil (corn, safflower, soybean)	.1 tsp
Salad dressing: regular*	.1 Tbsp
reduced-fat	.2 Tbsp
Miracle Whip Salad Dressing®: regular	.2 tsp
reduced-fat	.1 Tbsp
Seeds: pumpkin, sunflower	.1 Tbsp

* = 400 mg or more sodium per exchange.

Saturated Fats List
One fat exchange equals 5 grams of fat and 45 calories.

Bacon, cooked	.1 slice (20 slices/lb)
Bacon, grease	.1 tsp
Butter: stick	.1 tsp
whipped	.2 tsp
reduced-fat	.1 Tbsp
Chitterlings, boiled	.2 Tbsp (1/2 oz)
Coconut, sweetened, shredded	.2 Tbsp
Coconut milk	.1 Tbsp
Cream, half and half	.2 Tbsp
Cream cheese: regular	.1 Tbsp (1/2 oz)
reduced-fat	.1 1/2 Tbsp (3/4 oz)
Fatback or salt pork*, see below[a]	
Shortening or lard	.1 tsp
Sour cream: regular	.2 Tbsp
reduced-fat	.3 Tbsp

[a]Use a piece 1 inch x 1 inch x 1/4 inch if you plan to eat the fatback cooked with vegetables. Use a piece 2 inch x 1 inch x 1/2 inch when eating only the vegetables with the fatback removed.

FREE FOODS LIST
A free food is any food or drink that contains less than 20 calories or less than 5 grams of carbohydrate per serving. Foods with a serving size listed should be limited to 3 servings per day. Be sure

to spread them out throughout the day. If you eat all 3 servings at one time, it could raise your blood glucose level. Foods listed without a serving size can be eaten whenever you like.

Fat-free or Reduced-fat Foods

Cream cheese, fat-free . . . . .1 Tbsp (1/2 oz)

Creamers, nondairy, liquid . . . . .1 Tbsp

Creamers, nondairy, powdered . . . . .2 tsp

Mayonnaise, fat-free . . . . .1 Tbsp

Mayonnaise, reduced-fat . . . . .1 tsp

Margarine spread, fat-free . . . . .4 Tbsp

Margarine spread, reduced-fat . . . . .1 tsp

Miracle Whip®, fat-free . . . . .1 Tbsp

Miracle Whip®, reduced-fat . . . . .1 tsp

Nonstick cooking spray

Salad dressing, fat-free or low fat . . . . .1 Tbsp

Salad dressing, fat-free, Italian . . . . .2 Tbsp

Sour cream, fat-free, reduced-fat . . . . .1 Tbsp

Whipped topping, regular . . . . .1 Tbsp

Whipped topping, light or fat-free . . . . .2 Tbsp

Sugar-free Foods

Candy, hard, sugar-free . . . . .1 candy

Gelatin dessert, sugar-free

Gelatin, unflavored

Gum, sugar-free

Jam or jelly, light . . . . .2 tsp

Sugar substitutes[a]

Syrup, sugar-free . . . . .2 Tbsp

[a]Sugar substitutes, alternatives, or replacements that are approved by the Food and Drug Administration (FDA) are safe to use. Common brand names include:

Equal® (aspartame)

Splenda® (sucralose)

Sprinkle Sweet® (saccharin)

Sweet One® (acesulfame K)

Sweet-10® (saccharin)

Sugar Twin® (saccharin)

Sweet 'N Low® (saccharin)

Drinks

Bouillon, broth, consommé*

Bouillon or broth, low-sodium

Carbonated or mineral water

Club soda

Cocoa powder, unsweetened .1 Tbsp

Coffee

Diet soft drinks, sugar-free

Drink mixes, sugar-free

Tea

Tonic water, sugar-free

Condiments

Catsup . . . . .1 Tbsp

Horseradish

Lemon juice

Lime juice

Mustard

Pickle relish . . . . .1 Tbsp

Pickles, sweet (bread and butter) . . . . .2 slices

Pickles, sweet (gherkin) . . . . .3/4 oz

Pickles, dill* . . . . .1 1/2 large

Salsa . . . . .1/4 cup

Soy sauce, regular or light* .1 Tbsp

Taco sauce . . . . .1 Tbsp

Vinegar

Yogurt . . . . .2 Tbsp

Seasonings

Flavoring extracts

Garlic

Herbs, fresh or dried

Pimento

Spices

Tabasco® or hot pepper sauce

Wine, used in cooking

Worcestershire sauce

Be careful with seasonings that contain sodium or are salts, such as garlic or celery salt, and lemon pepper.

* = 400 mg or more of sodium per exchange.

COMBINATION FOODS LIST

Many of the foods we eat are mixed together in various combinations. These combination foods do not fit into any one exchange list. Often it is hard to tell what is in a casserole dish or prepared food item. This is a list of exchanges for some typical combination foods. This list will help you fit these foods into your meal plan. Ask your dietitian for information about any other combination foods you would like to eat.

FOOD

SERVING SIZE . . . . .EXCHANGES PER SERVING

Entrees

Tuna noodle casserole, lasagna, spaghetti with meatballs, chili with beans, macaroni and cheese*

1 cup (8 oz) . . . . .2 carbohydrates, 2 medium-fat meats

Chow mein (without noodles or rice)*

2 cups (16 oz) . . . . .1 carbohydrate, 2 lean meats

Tuna or chicken salad

1/2 cup (3 1/2 oz) . . . . . . .1/2 carbohydrate, 2 lean meats, 1 fat

Frozen entrees and meals

Dinner-type meal*

generally 14–17 oz .3 carbohydrates, 3 medium-fat meats, 3 fats

Meatless burger, soy based

3 oz . . . . .1/2 carbohydrate, 2 lean meats

Meatless burger, vegetable and starch based

3 oz .1 carbohydrate, 1 lean meat

Pizza, cheese, thin crust*

1/4 of 12 inch (6 oz) . . . . .2 carbohydrates, 2 medium-fat meats

Pizza, meat topping, thin crust*

1/4 of 12 inch (6 oz) . . . .

. . . . .2 carbohydrates, 2 medium-fat meats, 1 1/2 fats

Pot pie*

1 (7 oz) . . . . . . .2 1/2 carbohydrates, 1 medium-fat meat, 3 fats

Entree or meal with less than 340 calories*

about 8–11 oz . . . . .2–3 carbohydrates, 1–2 lean meats

Soups

Bean*

1 cup . . . . .1 carbohydrate, 1 very lean meat

Cream (made with water)*

1 cup (8 oz) . . . . .1 carbohydrate, 1 fat

Instant*

6 oz prepared . . . . .1 carbohydrate

Instant with beans/lentils*

8 oz prepared . . . . .2 1/2 carbohydrates, 1 very lean meat

Split pea (made with water)*

1/2 cup (4 oz) . . . . .1 carbohydrate

Tomato (made with water)*

1 cup (8 oz) . . . . .1 carbohydrate

Vegetable beef, chicken noodle, or other broth-type*

1 cup (8 oz) . . . . .1 carbohydrate

* = 400 mg or more sodium per exchange.

FAST FOODS[a]

FOOD

SERVING SIZE . . . . .EXCHANGES PER SERVING

Burrito with beef*

1 (5–7 oz) . . . . .3 carbohydrates, 1 medium-fat meat, 1 fat

Chicken nuggets*

6 . . . . .1 carbohydrate, 2 medium-fat meats, 1 fat

Chicken breast and wing, breaded and fried*

1 each . . . . .1 carbohydrate, 4 medium-fat meats, 2 fats

Chicken sandwich, grilled*

1 .2 carbohydrates, 3 very lean meats

Chicken wings, hot*

6 (5 oz) . . . . .1 carbohydrate, 3 medium-fat meats, 4 fats

Fish sandwich/tartar sauce*

1 . . . . .3 carbohydrates, 1 medium-fat meat, 3 fats

French fries*

1 medium serving (5 oz) . . . . .4 carbohydrates, 4 fats

Hamburger, regular

1 . . . . .2 carbohydrates, 2 medium-fat meats

Hamburger, large*

1 . . . . .2 carbohydrates, 3 medium-fat meats, 1 fat

Hot dog with bun*

1 . . . . .1 carbohydrate, 1 high-fat meat, 1 fat

Individual pan pizza*

1 . . . . .5 carbohydrates, 3 medium-fat meats, 3 fats

Pizza, cheese, thin crust*

1/4 of medium (12 inch round) about 6 oz . . . .

. . . . .1/2 carbohydrates, 2 medium-fat meats, 1 1/2 fats

Pizza, meat, thin crust*

1/4 of medium (12 inch round) about 6 oz . . . .

. . . . .2 1/2 carbohydrates, 2 medium-fat meats, 2 fats

Soft-serve cone

1 small (5 oz) . . . . .2 1/2 carbohydrates, 1 fat

Submarine sandwich (regular)*

1 sub (6 inch)....3 1/2 carbohydrates, 2 medium-fat meats, 1 fat

Submarine sandwich* (less than 6 gm fat)

1 sub (6 inch) . . . . .3 carbohydrates, 2 very lean meats

Taco, hard or soft shell*

1 (3-3 1/2 oz) . . . . . . .1 carbohydrate, 1 medium-fat meat, 1 fat

* = 400 mg or more of sodium per exchange.

[a]Ask at your fast-food restaurant for nutrition information about your favorite fast foods or check web sites.

USING FOOD LABELS

Nutrition Facts on food labels can help you with food choices. These labels are required by law for most foods and are based on standard serving sizes. However, these serving sizes may not always be the same as the serving sizes in this booklet.

- Check the serving size on the label. Is it nearly the same size as the food exchange? You may need to adjust the size of the serving to fit your meal plan.

- Look at the grams of carbohydrate in the serving size. (One starch, fruit, milk, or other carbohydrate has about 15 grams of carbohydrate.) So, if 1 cup of cereal has 30 grams of carbohydrate, it will count as 2 starch choices in your meal plan. You may need to adjust the size of the serving so it contains the number of carbohydrate choices you have for a meal or a snack.

- Look at the grams of protein in the serving size. (One meat choice has 7 grams of protein.) If the food has more than 7 grams of protein in a serving, you can figure out the number of meat choices by dividing the grams of protein by 7. Meats generally contain fat, too.

- Look at the grams of fat in the serving size. (One fat choice has 5 grams of fat.) If one waffle has 15 grams of carbohydrate and 5 grams of fat, it counts as 1 starch choice and 1 fat choice.

- Look at the number of calories in the serving size. If there are less than 20 calories per serving, it is a free food. However, if it has more than 20 calories, follow the steps listed above to count the food choices.

Food labels don't list trans fats. If the Nutrition Facts label lists total, saturated, polyunsaturated, and monounsaturated fats, add the last three and subtract from the total fat. The remainder, if any, is grams of trans fat.

Nutrient content claims that might be found on the label are the following:

Reduced-fat: at least 25% less fat per serving than the original food

Low-fat: 3 grams or less fat per serving

Fat-free: Less than 0.5 grams fat per serving

Light: 1/3 fewer calories or 1/2 the fat (per serving) of the original product (to which it's compared)

Sugar-free (or sugars-free): less than 0.5 grams sugar/serving

Reduced calorie: At least 25% fewer calories

Ask your dietitian for help using information on food labels. Some food labels may also give exchanges. For this food, one serving would count as 1 1/2 carbohydrate and 3 lean meats. These are based on information in this booklet.

CHILI WITH BEANS	
Nutrition Facts	
Serving Size: 1 cup (253 g)	
Servings Per: Container 2	
Amount Per Serving	
Calories 260	Calories from Fat 72
	% Daily Value
Total Fat 8g	13%
Saturated Fat 3g	17%
Cholesterol 130mg	44%
Sodium 1010mg	42%
Total Carbohydrate 22g	7%
Dietary Fiber 9g	36%
Sugars 4g	
Protein 25g	

GLOSSARY

Alcohol – An ingredient in a variety of beverages, including beer, wine, liqueurs, cordials, and mixed or straight drinks. Pure alcohol itself yields about 7 calories per gram.

Calorie – A unit used to express the heat or energy value of food. Calories come from carbohydrate, protein, fat, and alcohol.

Carbohydrate – One of the three major energy sources in foods. The most common carbohydrates are sugars and starches. Carbohydrates yield about 4 calories per gram. Carbohydrates are found in foods from the milk, vegetable, fruit, and starch lists.

Certified Diabetes Educators (CDE) – Health educators who specialize in diabetes and have passed the Certification Examination for Diabetes Educators are certified by the National Certification Board for Diabetes Educators. These educators stay up-to-date on diabetes care and can help you with your diabetes management.

Cholesterol – A fat-like substance normally found in blood. A high level of cholesterol in the blood has been shown to be a major risk factor for developing heart disease. Dietary cholesterol is found in all animal products, but is especially high in egg yolks and organ meats. Eating foods high in dietary cholesterol and saturated fat tends to raise the level of blood cholesterol. Foods of plant origin such as fruits, vegetables, grains, and beans, peas, and lentils contain no cholesterol. Cholesterol is found in foods from the milk, meat, and fat lists.

Dietitian – A registered dietitian (RD) is recognized by the medical profession as the primary provider of nutritional care, education, and counseling. The initials RD after a dietitian's name ensure that he or she has met the standards of the American Dietetic Association. Look for these credentials when you seek advice on nutrition.

Exchange – Foods grouped together on a list according to similarities in food values. Measured amounts of foods within the group may be exchanged or traded in planning meals. A single exchange contains approximately equal amounts of carbohydrate, protein, fat, and calories.

Fat – One of the three major energy sources in food. A concentrated source of calories—about 9 calories per gram. Fat is found in foods from the fat and meat and meat substitutes lists. Some kinds of milk also have fat; some foods from the starch list also contain fat.

- **Saturated fat** – Type of fat that tends to raise blood cholesterol levels. It comes primarily from animals and is usually hard at room temperature. Examples of saturated fats are butter, lard, meat fat, solid shortening, palm oil, and coconut oil.

- **Polyunsaturated fat** – Type of fat that is usually liquid at room temperature and is found in vegetable oils. Safflower, sunflower, corn, and soybean oils contain the highest amounts of polyunsaturated fats. Polyunsaturated fats, such as corn oil, can help lower high blood cholesterol levels when they are part of a healthful diet.

- **Omega-fat** – Type of polyunsaturated fat found in fish and soybean oil known to lower triglyceride levels and protect the heart.

- **Monounsaturated fat** – Type of fat that is liquid at room temperature and is found in vegetable oils, such as canola and olive oils. Monounsaturated fats can help lower high blood cholesterol levels when they are part of a lower-fat diet.

- **Trans fatty acids** – Trans fatty acids are fatty acids made through the process of hydrogenation, which solidifies liquid oils. Hydrogenation increases the shelf life and flavor stability of the oils and the foods that contain them. These fatty acids tend to raise blood cholesterol like saturated fats do.

Fiber – An indigestible part of certain foods. Fiber is important in the diet as roughage, or bulk. Fiber is found in foods from the starch, vegetable, and fruit lists.

Gram – A unit of mass and weight in the metric system. An ounce is about 30 grams.

Insulin – A hormone made by the body that helps the body use food. Also, a commercially prepared injectable substance used by people who do not make enough of their own insulin.

Meal Plan – A guide showing the number of food exchanges to use in each meal and snack to control distribution of carbohydrates, proteins, fats, and calories throughout the day.

Mineral – Substance essential in small amounts to build and repair body tissue and/or control functions of the body. Calcium, iron, magnesium, phosphorus, potassium, sodium, and zinc are minerals.

Nutrient – Substance in food necessary for life. Carbohydrates, proteins, fats, minerals, vitamins, and water are nutrients.

Protein – One of the three major nutrients in food. Protein provides about 4 calories per gram. Protein is found in foods from the milk and meat and meat substitutes lists. Smaller amounts of protein are found in foods from the vegetable and starch lists.

Sodium – A mineral needed by the body to maintain life, found mainly as a component of salt. Some individuals need to cut down the amount of sodium (and salt) they eat to help control high blood pressure.

Starch – One of the two major types of carbohydrate. Foods consisting mainly of starch come from the starch list.

Sugars – One of the two major types of carbohydrate. Foods consisting mainly of naturally present sugars are those from the milk, vegetables, and fruit lists. Added sugars include common table sugar and the sugar alcohols (sorbitol, mannitol, etc).

Triglycerides – Fats normally present in the blood that are made from food. Gaining too much weight may increase the blood triglycerides.

Vitamins – Substances found in food, needed in small amounts to assist in body processes and functions. These include vitamins A, D, E, the B-complex, C, and K.

MEAL PLAN

Meal Plan for: _____ Date: _____

Dietitian: _____ Phone: _____

	Grams	Percent
Carbohydrate		
Protein		
Fat		
Calories		

Time	Number of Exchanges/Choices	Menu Ideas

	_____Carbohydrate Group
	        _____Starch
	        _____Fruit
	        _____Milk_____
	_____Meat and Meat Substitute Group_____
	_____Fat Group _____	

	_____ _____ _____ _____	

	_____Carbohydrate Group
	        _____Starch
	        _____Fruit
	        _____Milk_____
	        _____ Nonstarchy Vegetables
	_____Meat and Meat Substitute Group _____
	_____Fat Group _____	

	___ _____ ___ _____ ___ _____	

	_____Carbohydrate Group
	        _____Starch
	        _____Fruit
	        _____Milk_____
	        _____ Nonstarchy Vegetables
	_____Meat and Meat Substitute Group _____
	_____Fat Group _____	

	___ _____ ___ _____ ___ _____	

Last updated: 7/14/03

For more information about the best meal plan for you, call a registered dietitian (RD), the American Dietetic Association/Nutrition Information Hot Line (1-800-366-1655), or the American Diabetes Association (1-800-342-2383).

The American Diabetes Association is the nation's leading voluntary health agency working to prevent and cure diabetes and to improve the lives of all people affected by diabetes.
www.diabetes.org

The American Dietetic Association is the nation's largest organization of food and nutrition professionals, with nearly 70,000 members.
www.eatright.org

This 2003 edition was reviewed and updated by
Anne Daly, MS, RD, BC-ADM, CDE, Chair
Marion Franz, MS, RD, CDE
Lea Ann Holzmeister, RD, CDE
Karmeen Kulkarni, MS, RD, BC-ADM, CDE
Belinda O'Connell, MS, RD, LD, CDE
Madelyn Wheeler, MS, RD, FADA, CDE
Additional review by Stephanie Dunbar, MPH, RD, and Esther Myers, PhD, RD, FADA.

The Exchange Lists are the basis of a meal planning system designed by a committee of the American Diabetes Association and The American Dietetic Association. While designed primarily for people with diabetes and others who must follow special diets, the Exchange Lists are based on principles of good nutrition that apply to everyone. ©2003 American Diabetes Association and the American Dietetic Association.

For more than fifty years, nutrition experts have produced a set of nutrient and energy standards known as the Recommended Dietary Allowances (RDA). A major revision is currently underway to replace the RDA. The revised recommendations are called Dietary Reference Intakes (DRI) and reflect the collaborative efforts of both the United States and Canada. Until 1997, the RDA were the only standards available and they will continue to serve health professionals until DRI can be established for all nutrients. For this reason, both the 1989 RDA and the 1997 DRI for selected nutrients are presented here.

1989 Recommended Dietary Allowances (RDA)

AGE (YR)	(kcal) ENERGY	(g) PROTEIN	(µg RE) VITAMIN A	(mg α-TE) VITAMIN E	(µg) VITAMIN K	(mg) VITAMIN C	(mg) THIAMIN	(mg) RIBOFLAVIN	(mg NE) NIACIN	(mg) VITAMIN B_6	(µg) FOLATE	(µg) VITAMIN B_{12}	(mg) IRON	(mg) ZINC	(µg) IODINE	(µg) SELENIUM
Infants																
0.0–0.5	650	13	375	3	5	30	0.3	0.4	5	0.3	25	0.3	6	5	40	10
0.5–1.0	850	14	375	4	10	35	0.4	0.5	6	0.6	35	0.5	10	5	50	15
Children																
1–3	1300	16	400	6	15	40	0.7	0.8	9	1.0	50	0.7	10	10	70	20
4–6	1800	24	500	7	20	45	0.9	1.1	12	1.1	75	1.0	10	10	90	20
7–10	2000	28	700	7	30	45	1.0	1.2	13	1.4	100	1.4	10	10	120	30
Males																
11–14	2500	45	1000	10	45	50	1.3	1.5	17	1.7	150	2.0	12	15	150	40
15–18	3000	59	1000	10	65	60	1.5	1.8	20	2.0	200	2.0	12	15	150	50
19–24	2900	58	1000	10	70	60	1.5	1.7	19	2.0	200	2.0	10	15	150	70
25–50	2900	63	1000	10	80	60	1.5	1.7	19	2.0	200	2.0	10	15	150	70
51+	2300	63	1000	10	80	60	1.2	1.4	15	2.0	200	2.0	10	15	150	70
Females																
11–14	2200	46	800	8	45	50	1.1	1.3	15	1.4	150	2.0	15	12	150	45
15–18	2200	44	800	8	55	60	1.1	1.3	15	1.5	180	2.0	15	12	150	50
19–24	2200	46	800	8	60	60	1.1	1.3	15	1.6	180	2.0	15	12	150	55
25–50	2200	50	800	8	65	60	1.1	1.3	15	1.6	180	2.0	15	12	150	55
51+	1900	50	800	8	65	60	1.0	1.2	13	1.6	180	2.0	10	12	150	55

1997 Dietary Reference Intakes (DRI)

AGE (YR)	(µg) VITAMIN D	(mg) CALCIUM	(mg) PHOSPHORUS	(mg) MAGNESIUM	(mg) FLUORIDE
Infants					
0.0–0.5	5	210	100	30	0.01
0.5–1.0	5	270	275	75	0.5
Children					
1–3	5	500	460	80	0.7
4–8	5	800	500	130	1.1
Males					
9–13	5	1300	1250	240	2.0
14–18	5	1300	1250	410	3.2
19–30	5	1000	700	400	3.8
31–50	5	1000	700	420	3.8
51–70	10	1200	700	420	3.8
71+	10	1200	700	420	3.8
Females					
9–13	5	1300	1250	240	2.0
14–18	5	1300	1250	360	2.9
19–30	5	1000	700	310	3.1
31–50	5	1000	700	320	3.1
51–70	10	1200	700	320	3.1
71+	10	1200	700	320	3.1

Note: This National Academy Press summary table does not reflect updates for each nutrient. For further detail, please refer to the detailed DRI tables on the CD-ROM that accompanies this textbook, or visit the National Academy Press website at www.nap.edu.

Source: National Academy Press

APPENDIX D SOURCES OF NUTRITION EDUCATION MATERIALS

5 A Day Campaign: http://www.5aday.gov/

American Diabetes Association: http://www.diabetes.org

American Dietetic Association: http://www.eatright.org

American Heart Association: http://www.americanheart.org

Calorie Control Council: http://www.caloriecontrol.org

DASH Eating Plan: http://www.nhlbi.nih.gov/health/public/heart/hbp/dash/

Dietary Guidelines for Americans: http://www.nal.usda.gov/fnic/dga/

Extension Offices: Find your Extension Office (a Web directory): http://lancaster.unl.edu/office/locate.htm

FDA Food Labeling: http://www.cfsan.fda.gov/~dms/foodlab.html

Federal Citizen Information Center (click "Food"): http://www.pueblo.gsa.gov/

Food and Nutrition Information Center Consumer Corner: http://www.nal.usda.gov/fnic/consumersite/

Food and Nutrition Information Center. Foreign Language Resources: http://www.nal.usda.gov/fnic/etext/000088.html

Food Marketing Institute: http://www.fmi.org/consumer/

International Food Information Council: http://www.ific.org/

National Cholesterol Education Program: http://www.nhlbi.nih.gov/about/ncep/

National Dairy Council: http://www.nationaldairycouncil.org/

Following material ©1993, American Dietetic Association. "A Healthy Food Guide: Hemodialysis." Used with permission.

MILK CHOICES

Average per choice: 4 grams protein, 120 Calories, 80 milligrams sodium, 185 milligrams potassium, 110 milligrams phosphorus

Milk (nonfat, low-fat, whole)	1/2 cup
Lo Pro	1 cup
Buttermilk, cultured	1/2 cup
Chocolate milk	1/2 cup
Light cream or half and half	1/2 cup
Ice milk or ice cream	1/2 cup
Yogurt, plain or fruit-flavored	1/2 cup
Evaporated milk	1/4 cup
Sweetened condensed milk	1/4 cup
Cream cheese	3 T
Sour cream	4 T
Sherbet	1 cup

NONDAIRY MILK SUBSTITUTES

Average per choice: 0.5 gram protein, 140 Calories, 40 milligrams sodium, 80 milligrams potassium, 30 milligrams phosphorus

Dessert, nondairy frozen	1/2 cup
Dessert topping, nondairy frozen	1/2 cup
Liquid nondairy creamer, polyunsaturated	1/2 cup

MEAT CHOICES

Average per choice: 7 grams protein, 65 Calories, 25 milligrams sodium, 100 milligrams potassium, 65 milligrams phosphorus

Prepared without added salt

Beef	1 ounce

Round, sirloin, flank, cubed, T-bone, and porterhouse steak; tenderloin, rib, chuck, and rump roast; ground beef or ground chuck

Pork	1 ounce

Fresh ham, tenderloin, chops, loin roast, cutlets

Lamb	1 ounce

Chops, leg, roasts

Veal	1 ounce

Chops, roasts, cutlets

Poultry	1 ounce

Chicken, turkey, Cornish hen, domestic duck and goose

Fish

Fresh and frozen fish	1 ounce
Lobster, scallops, shrimp, clams	1 ounce
Crab, oysters	1 1/2 ounces
Canned tuna, canned salmon (canned without salt)	1 ounce
Sardines (canned without salt)[b]	1 ounce
Wild Game	1 ounce

Venison, rabbit, squirrel, pheasant, duck, goose

Egg

Whole	1 large
Egg white or yolk	2 large
Low-cholesterol egg product	1/4 cup
Chitterlings	2 ounces
Organ meats[b]	1 ounce

Prepared with added salt

Beef	1 ounce

Deli-style roast beef[a]

Pork	1 ounce

Boiled or deli-style ham[a]

Poultry	1 ounce

Deli-style chicken or turkey[a]

Fish

Canned tuna, canned salmon[a]	1 ounce
Sardines[ab]	1 ounce

Cheese

Cottage[a]	1/4 cup

The following are high in sodium, phosphorus, and/or saturated fat. They should be used in your diet only as advised by your dietitian.

- Bacon
- Black beans, black-eyed peas, great northern beans, lentils, lima beans, navy beans, pinto beans, red kidney beans, soybeans, split peas, turtle beans
- Frankfurters, bratwurst, Polish sausage
- Luncheon meats, including bologna, braunschweiger, liverwurst, picnic loaf, summer sausage, salami
- Nuts and nut butters
- All cheeses except cottage cheese

[a] *High sodium—each serving counts as 1 Meat choice and 1 Salt choice*
[b] *High phosphorus*

STARCH CHOICES

Average per choice: 2 grams protein, 90 Calories, 80 milligrams sodium, 35 milligrams potassium, 35 milligrams phosphorus

Breads and Rolls

Bread (French, Italian, raisin, light rye, sourdough, white) . . . . .1 slice (1 ounce)

Bagel . . . . .1/2 small

Bun, hamburger or hot dog type 1/2

Danish pastry or sweet roll, no nuts . . . . .1/2 small

Dinner roll or hard roll . . . . .1 small

Doughnut . . . . .1 small

English muffin 1/2

Muffin, no nuts, bran, or whole wheat . . . . . . .1 small (1 ounce)

Pancake[ab] . . . . .1 small (1 ounce)

Pita or "pocket" bread . . . . .1/2 6-in diameter

Tortilla, corn . . . . .2 6-in diameter

Tortilla, flour . . . . .1 6-in diameter

Waffle[ab] . . . . .1 small (1 ounce)

Cereals and Grains prepared without added salt

Cereals, ready-to-eat, most brands[a] . . . . .3/4 cup

Puffed rice . . . . .2 cups

Puffed wheat . . . . .1 cup

Cereals, cooked

Cream of Rice or Wheat. Farina, Malt-O-Meal . . . . . . .1/2 cup

Oat bran or oatmeal, Ralston . . . . .1/3 cup

Cornmeal, cooked . . . . .3/4 cup

Grits, cooked . . . . .1/2 cup

Flour, all-purpose . . . . .2 1/2 T

Pasta (noodles, macaroni, spaghetti), cooked . . . . . . .1/2 cup

Pasta made with egg (egg noodles), cooked . . . . .1/3 cup

Rice, white or brown, cooked . . . . .1/2 cup

Crackers and Snacks

Crackers: saltines, round butter . . . . .4 crackers

Graham crackers . . . . .3 squares

Melba toast . . . . .3 oblong

RyKrisp[a] . . . . .3 crackers

Popcorn, plain .1 1/2 cups popped

Tortilla chips . . . . .3/4 ounce, 9 chips

Pretzels, sticks or rings[a] . . . . .3/4 ounce, 10 sticks

Pretzels, sticks or rings, unsalted . . . . . . .3/4 ounce, 10 sticks

Desserts

Cake, angel food . . . . .1/20 cake or 1 ounce

Cake . . . . .2 x 2-in square or 1 1/2 ounce

Sandwich cookie[ab] . . . . .4 cookies

Shortbread cookie . . . . .4 cookies

Sugar cookie . . . . .4 cookies

Sugar wafer . . . . .4 cookies

Vanilla wafer . . . . .10 cookies

Fruit pie (apple, berry, cherry, peach) . . . . .1/8 pie

Sweetened gelatin . . . . .1/2 cup

The following foods are high in poor-quality protein and/or phosphorus. They should be used only when advised by your dietitian.

- Bran cereal or muffins, Grape-Nuts cereal, granola cereal or bars
- Boxed, frozen, or canned meals, entrees, or side dishes
- Black beans, black-eyed peas, great northern beans, lentils, lima beans, navy beans, pinto beans, red kidney beans, soybeans, split peas, turtle beans
- Pumpernickel, dark rye, whole wheat, or oatmeal bread
- whole wheat cereals
- whole wheat crackers

[a] *High sodium—each serving counts as 1 Starch choice and 1 Salt choice*

[b] *High phosphorus*

VEGETABLE CHOICES

Average per choice: 1 gram protein, 25 Calories, 15 milligrams sodium, 20 milligrams phosphorus

1/2 cup per choice unless otherwise indicated

Prepared or Canned without added salt unless otherwise indicated
Low potassium (0-100 milligrams)

Alfalfa sprouts (1 cup)

Bamboo shoots, canned

Beans, green or wax

Bean sprouts

Cabbage, raw

Chinese cabbage, raw

Chard, raw

Cucumber, peeled

Endive

Escarole

Lettuce, all varieties (1 cup)

Pepper, green, sweet

water chestnuts, canned

Watercress

Medium potassium (101-200 milligrams)

Artichoke

Broccoli

Cabbage, cooked

Carrots, raw (1 small)

Cauliflower

Celery, raw (1 stalk)

Collards

Corn (or 1/2 ear)[b]

Eggplant

Kale

Mushrooms, canned or fresh raw[b]

Mustard greens

Onions

Peas, green[b]

Radishes

Sauerkraut[a†]

Snow peas[b]

Spinach, raw

Squash, summer

Turnip greens

Turnips

High potassium (201-350 milligrams)

Asparagus (5 spears)[b]

Avocado (1/4 whole)

Beets

Brussels sprouts[b]

Celery, cooked

Kohlrabi

Mushrooms, fresh cooked[b]

Okra[b]

Parsnips[b]

Pepper, chili

Potato, boiled or mashed

Pumpkin

Rutabagas[b]

Tomato (1 medium)

Tomato juice, unsalted

Tomato juice, canned with salt[a]

Tomato puree (2 T)

Tomato sauce (1/4 cup)

Vegetable juice cocktail, unsalted

Vegetable juice cocktail, canned with salt[a*]

Bamboo shoots, fresh cooked[c]

Beet greens (1/4 cup)[c]

Chard, cooked[c]

Chinese cabbage, cooked[c]

Potato, baked (1/2 medium)[c]

Potato, hashed brown[c]

Potato chips (1 ounce, 14 chips)[c]

Spinach, cooked[bc]

Sweet potato[bc]

Tomato paste (2 T)[c]

Winter squash (1/4 cup)[c]

Prepared or canned with salt
Vegetables canned with salt (use serving size listed above)[a]

[a] *High sodium—each serving counts as 1 Vegetable choice and 1 Salt choice*

[a*] *High sodium—each serving counts as 1 Vegetable choice and 2 Salt choices*

[a†] *High sodium—each serving counts as 1 Vegetable choice and 3 Salt choices*

[b] *High phosphorus*

[c] *Very high potassium*

FRUIT CHOICES
Average per choice: 0.5 gram protein, 70 Calories, 15 milligrams phosphorus

1/2 cup per choice unless otherwise indicated

Low potassium (0-100 milligrams)

Applesauce

Blueberries

Cranberries (1 cup)

Cranberry juice cocktail (1 cup)

Grape juice

Lemon (1/2)

Papaya nectar

Peach nectar

Pears, canned

Pear nectar

Medium potassium (101-200 milligrams)

Apple (1 small, 2 1/2-in diameter)

Apple juice

Apricot nectar

Blackberries

Cherries, sour or sweet

Figs, canned

Fruit cocktail

Grapes (15 small)

Grapefruit (1/2 small)

Grapefruit juice

Gooseberries

Lemon juice

Mango

Papaya

Peach, canned

Peach, fresh (1 small, 2-in diameter)

Pineapple, canned or fresh

Plums, canned or fresh (1 medium)

Raisins (2 T)

Raspberries

Rhubarb

Strawberries

Tangerine (2 1/2-in diameter)

Watermelon (1 cup)

High potassium (201-350 milligrams)

Apricots, canned or fresh (2 halves)

Apricots, dried (5)

Cantaloupe (1/8 small)

Dates (1/4 cup)

Figs, dried (2 whole)

Honeydew melon (1/8 small)

Kiwifruit (1/2 medium)

Nectarine (1 small, 2-in diameter)

Orange juice

Orange (1 small, 2 1/2-in diameter)

Pear, fresh (1 medium)

Banana (1/2 medium)[c]

Prune juice[c]

Prunes, dried or canned (5)[c]

[c] *Very high potassium*

FAT CHOICES

Average per choice: trace protein, 45 Calories, 55 milligrams sodium, 10 milligrams potassium, 5 milligrams phosphorus

Unsaturated Fats

Margarine . . . . .1 tsp

Reduced-calorie margarine . . . . .1 T

Mayonnaise . . . . .1 tsp

Low-calorie mayonnaise . . . . .1 T

Oil (safflower, sunflower, corn, soybean, olive, peanut, canola) . . . . .1 tsp

Salad dressing (mayonnaise-type) . . . . .2 tsp

Salad dressing (oil-type) . . . . .1 T

Low-calorie salad dressing (mayonnaise-type) . . . . .2 T

Low-calorie salad dressing (oil-type)[a] . . . . .2 T

Tartar sauce . . . . .1 1/2 tsp

Saturated Fats

Butter . . . . .1 tsp

Coconut . . . . .2 T

Powdered coffee whitener . . . . .1 T

Solid shortening . . . . .1 tsp

[a] *High sodium—each serving counts as 1 Fat choice and 1 Salt choice*

HIGH-CALORIE CHOICES

Average per choice: trace protein, 100 Calories, 15 milligrams sodium, 20 milligrams potassium, 5 milligrams phosphorus

Beverages

Carbonated beverages (fruit flavors, root beer; colas or pepper-type)[b] . . . . .1 cup

Kool-Aid . . . . .1 cup

Limeade . . . . .1 cup

Lemonade . . . . .1 cup

Cranberry juice cocktail . . . . .1 cup
Tang . . . . .1 cup
Fruit-flavored drink . . . . .1 cup
Wine^d . . . . .1/2 cup

Remember to count these choices within your fluid allowance.

Frozen Desserts

Fruit ice . . . . .1/2 cup
Popsicle (3 ounces) . . . . .1 bar
Juice bar (3 ounces) . . . . .1 bar
Sorbet . . . . .1/2 cup

Remember to count these choices within your fluid allowance.

Candy and Sweets

Butter mints 14
Candy corn . . . . .20 or 1 ounce
Chewy fruit snacks . . . . .1 pouch
Cranberry sauce or relish . . . . .1/4 cup
Fruit chews 4
Fruit Roll Ups 2
Gumdrops . . . . .15 small
Hard candy . . . . .4 pieces
Honey . . . . .2 T
Jam or jelly . . . . .2 T
Jelly beans 10
LifeSavers or cough drops 12
Marmalade . . . . .2 T
Marshmallows . . . . .5 large
Sugar, brown or white . . . . .2 T
Sugar, powdered . . . . .3 T
Syrup . . . . .2 T

The following foods are high in poor-quality protein and/or phosphorus. They should be used only when advised by your dietitian.

- Beer^d
- Chocolate
- Nuts and nut butters

^b *High phosphorus*
^d *Check with your physician before using alcohol*

SALT CHOICES

Average per choice: 250 milligrams sodium

Salt . . . . .1/8 tsp
Seasoned salts (onion, garlic, etc.) . . . . .1/8 tsp
Accent . . . . .1/4 tsp
Barbecue sauce . . . . .2 T
Bouillon . . . . .1/2 cup
Catsup . . . . .1 1/2 T
Chili sauce . . . . .1 1/2 T
Dill pickle . . . . .1/6 large or 1/2 ounce
Mustard . . . . .4 tsp
Olives, green .2 medium or 1/3 ounce
Olives, black . . . . .3 large or 1 ounce
Soy sauce . . . . .3/4 tsp
Light soy sauce . . . . .1 tsp
Steak sauce . . . . .2 1/2 tsp
Sweet pickle relish . . . . .2 1/2 T
Taco sauce . . . . .2 T
Tamari sauce . . . . .3/4 tsp
Teriyaki sauce . . . . .1 1/4 tsp
Worcestershire sauce . . . . .1 T

BEVERAGE CHOICES

The following beverages may be used as desired within your daily fluid allowance.

- Carbonated beverages (except Moxie, colas, and pepper-type)
- Ice
- Lemonade
- Limeade
- Mineral water
- Water

The following beverages contain moderate amounts of potassium and/or phosphorus. They should be used in your diet only as advised by your dietitian.

- Beer^d
- Coffee, regular or decaffeinated
- Coffee substitute (cereal-grain beverage)
- Cola or pepper-type carbonated beverages
- Tea

- Thirst-quencher beverages
- Wine*d*

The following liquids are very high in sodium, potassium, and/or phosphorus. They should be used in your diet only as advised by your doctor or dietitian.

- Broth
- Bouillon
- Consomme
- Salt-free broth or bouillon containing potassium chloride (KCl)

Remember: anything that is liquid or melts at room temperature must also be counted in your fluid allowance (for example, ice cream, Popsicles, sherbet, gelatin).

d Check with your physician before using alcohol

INDEX